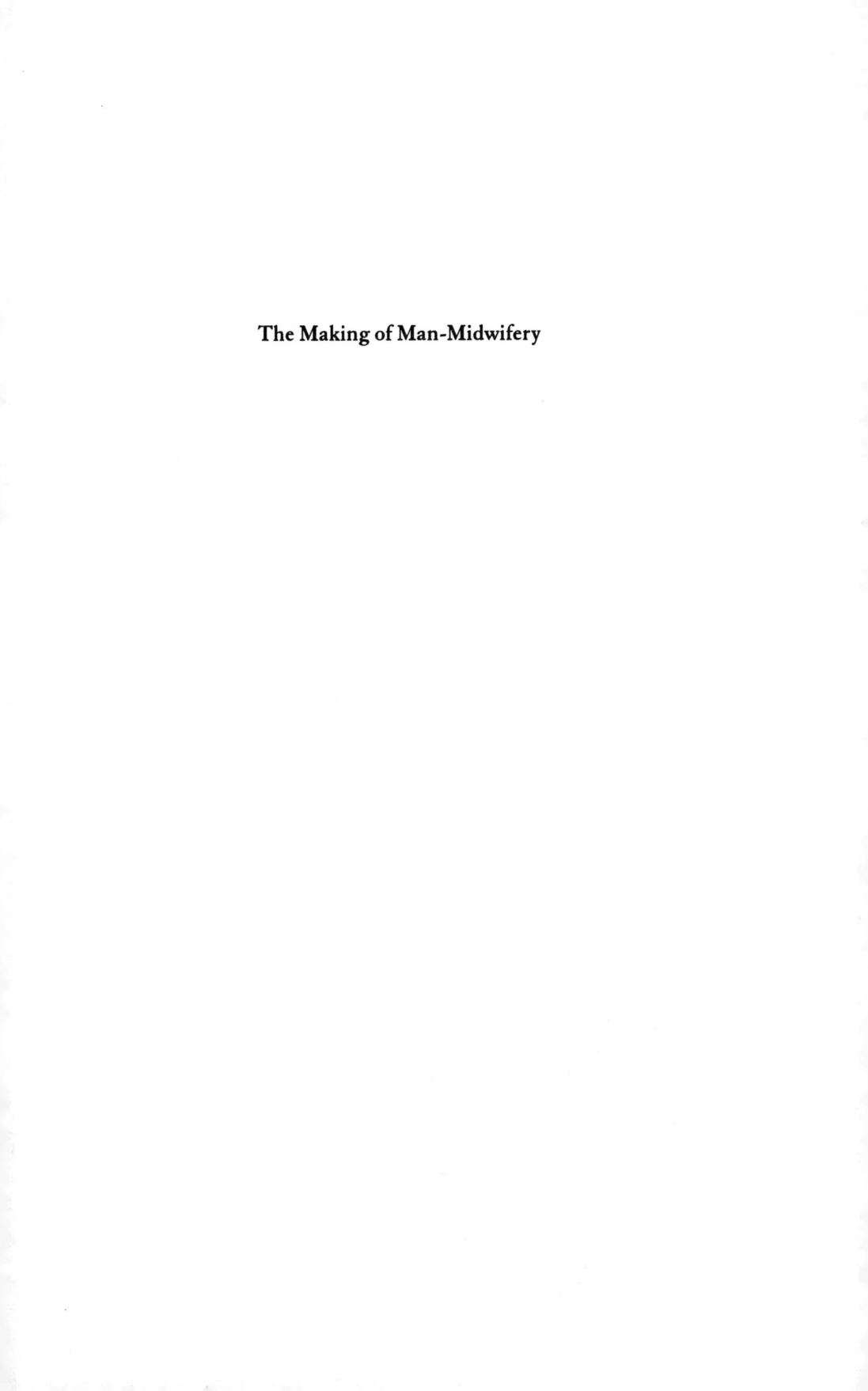

The Making of Man-Midwifery

The Making of Man-Midwifery:
Childbirth in England, 1660–1770

Adrian Wilson

Harvard University Press
Cambridge, Massachusetts
1995

Copyright © 1995 by Adrian Wilson

All rights reserved
Printed in Great Britain

Published by arrangement with UCL Press

The name of University College London(UCL) is a registered trade mark used by UCL Press with the consent of the owner.

Library of Congress Cataloging-in-Publication Data

Wilson, Adrian, 1947–
  The making of man-midwifery : childbirth in England, 1660–1770/ Adrian Wilson.
    p.   cm.
  Includes bibliographical references and index.
  ISBN 0-674-54323-8
  1. Obstetricians—England—History—18th century.
  2. Midwives—England—History—18th century.
  3. Obstetrics—England—History—18th century.
  4. Childbirth—England—History—18th century. I. Title.
RG18.G7W54 1995
618.2'00942'09033—dc20   94-38976

*In memory of my mother, Irene Gerritje Wilson
and for my father, Derek Finlay Wilson*

"The world will give me credit, surely, for having had sufficient opportunities of knowing a good deal of female characters. I have seen the private as well as the public virtues, the private as well as the more public frailties of women in all ranks of life. I have been in their secrets, their counsellor and adviser in the moments of their greatest distress in body and mind. I have been a witness to their private conduct, when they were preparing themselves to meet danger, and have heard their last and most serious reflections, when they were certain they had but a few hours to live."

William Hunter in 1783

Contents

Acknowledgements	xi
1 Introduction	1
The puzzle of man-midwifery	1
Man-midwifery's prehistory	5
Notes	7

Part I The traditional management of birth

2 The bodily processes of childbirth	11
The varieties of childbirth	11
The incidence of difficult births	15
Standard techniques for delivering difficult births	19
Notes	23
3 The practices of midwives	25
The ceremony of childbirth	25
To be a midwife	30
The problem of difficult births	33
The skills of midwives	36
Notes	39

CONTENTS

4 Traditional obstetric surgery	47
Male paths to childbirth	47
The horizon of male practice	49
The horizon transcended: the Chamberlen family	53
The female/male division transcended: Sarah Stone	57
Notes	*59*

Part II From obstetric surgery to man-midwifery

5 The Chamberlen instruments and their sale	65
The Chamberlen instruments	65
The sale of the forceps in England	67
The need for instruction	71
The Tory associations of the forceps	72
Notes	*74*

6 The forceps contested: the London Deventerians	79
Hendrik van Deventer and his obstetrics	79
The use of Deventer in London	82
Notes	*87*

7 The impact of the forceps	91
William Giffard's case-series and his practice	91
Mothers' expectations	96
Male practitioners' attitudes	98
Limits of the effects of the forceps	99
Notes	*101*

Part III Whig and Tory men-midwives

8 Conflict and initiative in London, 1720–40	107
Early skirmishes	107
The publication of the forceps, 1733–35	108
John Douglas's intervention, 1736–37	110
Manningham's Lying-in Infirmary, 1739	114
The specificity of the London pattern	116
Notes	*118*

CONTENTS

9	A new synthesis: William Smellie	123
	Life and writings	123
	The development of Smellie's methods	125
	Smellie's synthesis	130
	Notes	*131*
10	John Bamber, the vectis, and the City of London	135
	John Bamber and his associates	135
	Bamber and the vectis	137
	The vectis and the City of London	140
	Notes	*141*
11	New institutions: the London Lying-in Hospitals	145
	An overview of London's lying-in hospitals	145
	Obstetric allegiances	148
	Political orientations	151
	The significance of the lying-in hospitals	153
	Notes	*154*

Part IV The man as midwife

12	The varieties of man-midwifery	161
	Recapitulation: new practices, old forms	161
	Man-midwifery transformed	164
	Notes	*169*
13	William Hunter: the man as midwife	175
	The man as midwife	175
	Hunter, Smellie and the forceps	178
	"Their counsellor and adviser"	180
	Notes	*182*
14	Two female cultures	185
	A new female culture	185
	Ladies as mothers	191
	Notes	*192*

CONTENTS

15	Conclusion	197
	Counterattacks	197
	Prospect	199
	Notes	*206*
	Bibliography	*211*
	Index	*229*

Acknowledgements

I first became intrigued by this subject in 1974; my approach has changed a great deal since I completed a doctoral thesis on some aspects of it in 1982. A long gestation has produced many obligations, and it is a pleasure to thank those who have helped to make this book possible.

For generous financial support I am most grateful to my parents; to Clare Hall, Cambridge; to the Local Population Studies Society; and to the Wellcome Trust. Behind any history book labours an unseen army of archivists and librarians: for their unfailing courtesy and help I wish to thank the staffs of the Derbyshire County Record Office; Greater London Record Office; Leicestershire Record Office; Lichfield Joint Record Office; Lincolnshire Archives Office; Norfolk and Norwich Record Office; British Library; Cambridge University Library; Hunterian Library, University of Glasgow; Bodleian Library, Oxford; Huntingdon Library; Library of the Wellcome Institute for the History of Medicine; Royal College of Obstetricians and Gynaecologists Library; Royal College of Physicians Library; and the Royal College of Surgeons Library. The computing staff at Cambridge and Leicester have given kind and efficient help; in this connection I especially thank Richard Mobbs at Leicester. For advice and support over the years I thank my present and former colleagues at Cambridge, Leicester and Leeds: in Cambridge, at the Wellcome Unit for the History of Medicine, the History and Philosophy of Science Department, the ESRC Cambridge Group for the History of Population and Social Structure, the Centre for Family Research (formerly the Child Care and Development Group), and the History Faculty; at Leicester, the Departments of Economic and Social History, English Local History, and History; at Leeds, the History and Philosophy of Science Division of the Philosophy Department. I am also grateful for the observations and advice of my former undergraduate and postgraduate students and of the participants in seminar discussions at various universities, at the London Hospital, and at the

Halifax branch of the Royal College of Midwives.

To name here all the individual scholars who have advised me would make for a very long list; I have acknowledged much assistance in particular chapters. But here I want to thank those who have helped with the development of the book as a whole: Peter Hennock and Colin Brooks, who got me started and gave much advice and support; Roger Schofield and Willy Lamont, who helped not only as fair and critical doctoral examiners but also in other capacities; Timothy Ashplant, Andrew Cunningham, Roy Porter and Simon Schaffer, who have given invaluable historiographic guidance; Steven Gerrard, who has helped me to arrive at the shape of the book; Liz Roberts, for improving the text in many places; and Karen Adams, Rosalind Bayham, Marina Benjamin, Helen Brock, Cathy Crawford, David Cressy, Roger French, Mark Goldie, David Harley, Roger Houlbrooke, Gill Hudson, Deborah Hughes, Ludmilla Jordanova, Maria Kiely, Peter Laslett, Alan Macfarlane, Julian Martin, Elizabeth Nathaniels, Beverley Omar, Olga Parker, Linda Pollock, Martin Richards, Craig Rose, Keith Snell, Amanda Vickery, Richard Waller, Liz Whitney, Diane Wilson, Julian Wilson, Jenny Woodhouse, Mike Woodhouse, Ros Wright, Tony Wrigley and David Wykes. I am of course responsible for the errors that remain.

For permission to reproduce Figures 1.1, 2.1, 2.2, 3.1 and 6.1, I thank the Wellcome Institute Library, London, and for Figure 5.1, the Royal College of Obstetricians and Gynaecologists.

This was to have formed part of a larger work, to be entitled "A safe deliverance", spanning the seventeenth century as well as the eighteenth, but this proved to be beyond the compass of a single book. I hope to produce in due course a further study giving a more detailed treatment of the seventeenth-century themes that are summarized here in Part I. For that proposed book the title "A safe deliverance" will be appropriate – since for all its dangers and difficulties, and despite what has often been supposed, childbirth was usually a happy event for women before, as well as after, the arrival of the man-midwife.

Leeds, May 1994

Chapter One
Introduction

The puzzle of man-midwifery

In England in the seventeenth century, and doubtless for centuries before, childbirth was emphatically under the control of women. The midwife ran the birth, helped by several female "gossips"; men were excluded both from the delivery and from the subsequent month of lying-in. The enclosed female space of the "lying-in chamber" was dedicated to the mother's rest and recovery and to the collective female ritual that surrounded childbirth. Medical men were only called upon to help in difficult deliveries and as a last resort; they had no place in the management of normal childbirth. This structure defined the horizons of both male knowledge and male ambitions in midwifery. Official medicine had no concept of the mechanism of birth, and knew very little of the anatomy of the uterus or the function of the placenta. Medical men might criticize the skills of midwives, but they had no ambition to replace them; and they accepted without comment the customary procedures of women such as the darkening of the lying-in chamber and the swaddling of the newborn child.

But in the eighteenth century there came into being a new kind of practitioner: the "man-midwife", the man who acted in lieu of a midwife, the medical man who delivered normal births. These new practitioners at once created an explosion of knowledge, which has been called a "revolution in obstetrics", and a series of institutional initiatives in midwifery.[1] The works of Fielding Ould (1742), and especially of William Smellie (1752), opened the entirely new field of the accurate mechanical description of the processes of birth; and William Hunter, who in the 1760s succeeded Smellie as London's leading man-midwife, produced the definitive description of the structure and function of the placenta in his great classic *The anatomy of the gravid uterus* (1774). While Hunter was engaged upon his 20-year study, midwifery institutions were proliferating, particularly in London. These included systematic teaching (led by Smellie, who taught over 900 male pupils in the 1740s), lying-in hospitals (four between 1749 and 1767) and lying-in charities (the first in 1757). Some of these developments found echoes in provincial cities, such as Liverpool, Manchester and Newcastle; and the new male practitioners, taught by Smellie and his successors, swarmed through county and market towns from Devon to Yorkshire. Equipped with new knowledge, skills and aspirations, these men could now criticize the traditional female management of childbirth; thus the practices of women now came under attack, notably from Charles White in 1772. Correspondingly, the new man-midwifery was itself criticized — as immodest, interventionist, and a trespass on the work of midwives. Yet these polemics, which date from around 1750, had little effect. By the late eighteenth century men-midwives had achieved a permanent place in the management of childbirth, chiefly among the wealthy and urban sections of the population — that is, in the most lucrative spheres of practice. And as a result, the midwife's position of trust and respect declined to the point where she could be stereotyped, in the 1840s, as "Sairey Gamp" in Dickens's *Martin Chuzzlewit*.

How had this come about? Why did women desert the traditional midwife? How was it that a domain of female control and collective solidarity became instead a region of male medical practice? Why did a torrent of criticisms directed against "men-midwives" fall upon deaf ears? What was the relation between the new male knowledge and the new male practice? What had broken down the barrier that had formerly excluded the male practitioner from the management of birth? Was this a sudden development, or a gradual one; a matter of insidious growth, or a series of distinct steps? These are the questions that have animated this study; behind them lies a profound sense of puzzlement and surprise at the eighteenth-century transformation of midwifery from a female sphere to a central part of male medicine. The more one contemplates the achievements of the eighteenth-century men-midwives, the more one is struck by the contrasting female exclusiveness of the management of births in seventeenth-century England — and thus, the more surprising becomes the breaking down of that exclusiveness.

Such questions have particular interest today because in recent years the medical management of childbirth has come increasingly under attack. Advanced obstetrics, which has made childbirth vastly safer than ever before, finds itself in tension with modern feminism, which has given women the confidence to challenge the male control of obstetrics and to demand that childbirth be turned back from high technology to personal experience. By the 1980s the place, the personnel and the technical management of birth had all become matters of dispute, generating contests not only between different groups such as doctors, midwives and mothers, but also within a single profession as in the Wendy Savage case of 1983–84.[2] All sides in such battles necessarily develop and deploy historical arguments as weapons of struggle. Thus childbirth acquires a history: a past that had been forgotten comes to light and loses its innocence.[3] And in that history, the developments of the eighteenth century will have a central place for all protagonists – for it was between about 1720 and 1770 that childbirth became part of medicine.

There are two traditional explanations for the change: fashion and the forceps. Man-midwifery spread, it is alleged, by the process of *fashion*. At first adopted at the top of the social scale, it diffused downwards by a process of envious emulation – the "aping the quality" so much bemoaned and practised in Hanoverian England. Man-midwifery, on this argument, was rather like tea-drinking, the possession of coaches and livery servants, the taking of snuff, the wearing of wigs. But this explanation ignores the specificity of our theme; it forgets that there was a real alternative in the female midwife; above all, it begs the question as to how the process got started. What made man-midwifery fashionable in the first place? The alternative explanation is the midwifery *forceps*. Since its invention in the early seventeenth century, this instrument had been kept secret by its inventors and possessors, the successive generations of the Chamberlen family. But in the early eighteenth century, the forceps spread to other practitioners, and once its design was published in 1733–35, it was available for a few pounds from any competent instrument-maker. The release of the forceps appears to coincide with the rise of man-midwifery; the influential Smellie used and taught the instrument (and improved its design); it enabled the male practitioner to deliver a living child, where previously he could only deliver a dead one. On these grounds, the forceps has justifiably been seen as playing a crucial role in the rise of man-midwifery: as one scholar puts it, the forceps was "the key to the lying-in room".[4] Yet there are also good reasons to doubt this interpretation. As Margaret Versluysen has observed, the forceps was useful in only a tiny minority of deliveries; it was disliked by mothers; its misuse was "one of the main themes of the opponents of man-midwifery"; and it was even opposed by some of the leading men-midwives.[5] Indeed, William Hunter himself declaimed against the forceps that "where they save one, they murder twenty . . . 'tis a thousand pities that they were ever invented".[6] If this was the attitude of the acknowledged leader of the new man-midwifery, how can the forceps explain the rise of the man-midwife? The difficulties posed by these two explanations are underlined if we attempt to combine them. Fashion worked by downward social diffusion; yet forceps practice began among the poor, as indicated by the posthumously published *Cases in midwifery* (1734) of William Giffard, the first London forceps practitioner outside the Chamberlen family.[7]

Thus we have here an unexplained revolution, a massive social transformation with manifest effects but hidden causes. Moreover, both the timing and the location of this revolution were radically different from the analogous developments in medicine as a whole. Michel Foucault has taught us that it was in Revolutionary France, and specifically in the new *Ecoles de Santé* founded in 1794, that there occurred "the birth of the clinic": the genesis of that "clinical gaze" that pierces the patient's skin and literally sees the interior of the patient's body as a living, dying presence in the consultation itself. Hence the invention of the physical examination, the active deployment of the technique of percussion, the creation of the stethoscope; the routine post-mortem, using death to dissect the tissues of the body; the entire system of pathological anatomy, and anatomical pathology, founded by Bichat and continuing (with important transformations) to our own day. Hence, perhaps above all, the depersonalization of the patient, the construction of that precise form of doctor–patient relationship in which the patient's presence becomes a mere materiality.[8] Simplified though Foucault's picture may be, that picture certainly captured a real transformation in concepts, in

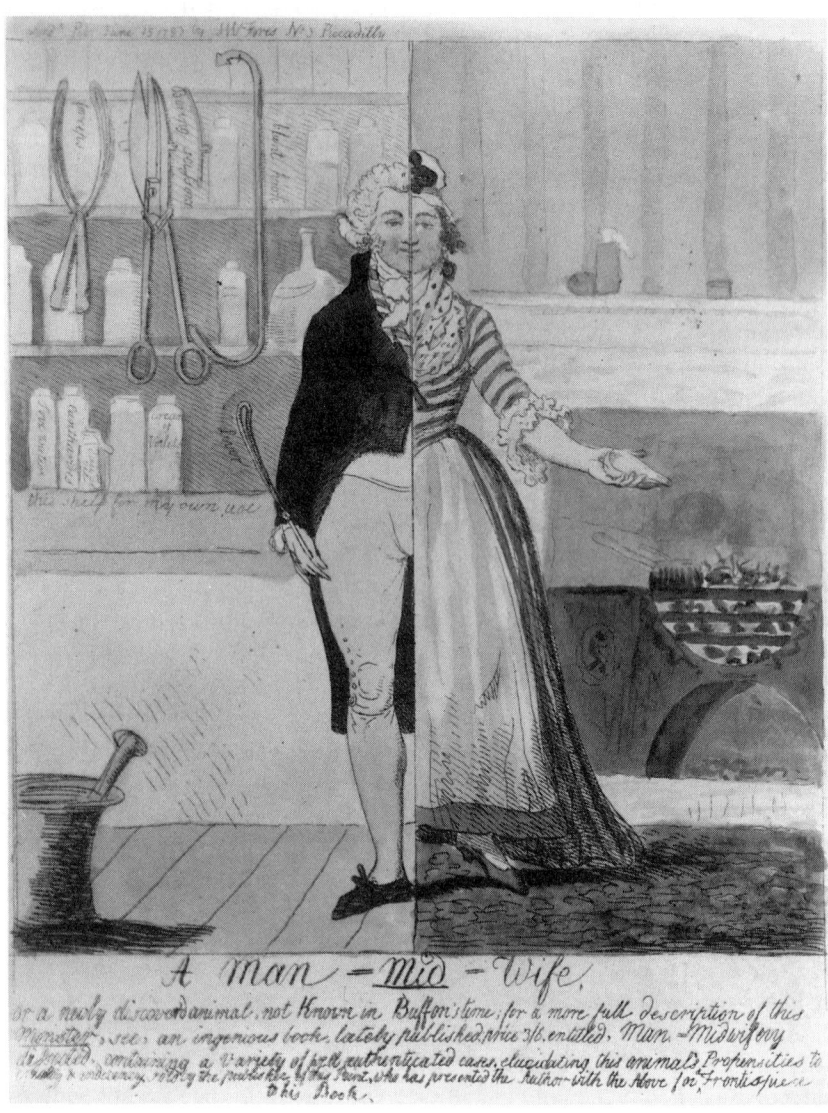

Figure 1.1 "A man-midwife" (Fores, Man-midwifery exposed, *1793*).

ways of saying and seeing, and in the nature of medical practice. And in relation to this history, the medicalization of childbirth came too early, and occurred in the wrong country. Surely it was with Hunter's practice that male medicine entered the lying-in chamber, just as it was with Hunter's *Anatomy of the gravid uterus* that male medicine entered the womb itself. Yet it was not in Revolutionary France, but in Hanoverian London, that these developments took place. Thus the transformation of childbirth from a female domain into a part of medicine cannot be assimilated to wider medical changes; it has its own, distinctive history.

Indeed, recent research suggests that the man-midwifery of eighteenth-century England was almost unique, apart from Britain's American colonies.[9] Elsewhere in Europe, although male practitioners acquired new skills, they were largely restricted to delivering difficult births until at least 1800.[10] Moreover, the intervention of Enlightened governments brought into being a new cadre of skilled female midwives in this period. Concerned to enlarge the populations they governed, State and municipal authorities set about raising the standards of midwives' practice by means of training systems, licensing schemes and sometimes the payment of salaries. The most systematic initiative of this kind took place in France, where between 1759 and 1783 the roving instructress Mme Le Boursier (later du Coudray), armed with Royal authorization, created a new kind of midwife – young, unmarried, and systematically-trained – throughout most of the kingdom: by the 1780s her pupils comprised two-thirds of the country's midwives. Less ambitious schemes worked to similar effect, although on a more limited scale and chiefly within towns, in the Dutch Republic, in the German states, in the Italian cities and in Spain. Strikingly, all these efforts focused on the midwife rather than the male practitioner – because normal births remained in the hands of midwives. True, man-midwifery did develop to some extent in France: Andre Levret in Paris paralleled Smellie in London, and Mme du Coudray began to have male rivals in the 1770s. But elsewhere the midwife's hegemony over normal births remained unchallenged. In Spain male practitioners were limited to delivering difficult births, and in the 1770s the midwife Luisa Rosado was even encroaching on this territory. In Italy, "throughout the [eighteenth] century, the presence of the man-midwife at a birth was rare". In the Dutch Republic, "obstetric doctors were generally only present to assist in . . . obstetric emergencies" and made no attempt to take over from midwives. And in Germany, "the conflict between men and women midwives never developed". The specificity of English developments shows that the rise of the man-midwife was by no means inevitable, and sharpens our explanatory puzzle.

Man-midwifery's prehistory

A simple index of the eighteenth-century change is the publication of original midwifery treatises. From 1540, when Rösslin's *Rosegarten* was translated into

English as *The birth of mankind*, the popular demand for information about midwifery and related matters was met by translating into English the advice of one or many Continental authors.[11] Before our period, almost nothing original on obstetrics had been published in English; the lead came from a distinguished French tradition – Paré, Guillemeau, Bourgeois, Mauriceau, Du Tertre, Portal, Dionis, Peu, La Motte – supplemented, after 1700, by the Dutch author Hendrik van Deventer. But all this changed dramatically from 1733, the year in which Edmund Chapman published his *Essay towards the improvement of midwifery* – the first account in print of the midwifery forceps. In the next decade (1733–42), seven authors (one a midwife, Sarah Stone, the others men) published original works on midwifery in English.[12] From this point onwards, the original English midwifery treatise was the norm; the new publications attained a high standard of technical knowledge; and a continuous tradition connects the works of Chapman and his successors with the journal-literature in obstetrics of our own day. At the level of print, the "revolution in obstetrics" was very sudden: 1733 marks a permanent watershed.

Yet at least one seventeenth-century English medical man – Percival Willughby of Derby – had written original works on midwifery. His *Observations in midwifery* and *The country midwife's opusculum or vade-mecum,* which remained unpublished in his lifetime but survived in manuscript, reveal that Willughby enjoyed a substantial practice from around 1630 to 1670 in, as he put it, "the midwife's bed".[13] Thus male practice in midwifery in seventeenth-century England may have been less of an absence than at first appears. This is underlined by the Chamberlens, the inventors and possessors of the midwifery forceps. Admittedly, the Chamberlens were of French origin: they had settled at Southampton as Huguenot refugees in the late sixteenth century, before moving to London around 1600. Yet it was in England that they made their remarkable invention, and they practised midwifery in London throughout the seventeenth century. Members of that family were involved in public initiatives over the regulation of midwives in 1617, 1634 and 1647; four of them were using the family secret in the early 1670s; they were even called "men-midwives".[14] There is no doubting the importance of their practice, although its details are obscured by the secrecy with which they guarded their instruments. It appears, then, that eighteenth-century English man-midwifery had a prehistory. What was the relation between this earlier male practice – especially revealed for us by Willughby's writings – and that which became visible from the 1730s onwards?

Approach

The story I shall be telling is based on three premises. First, childbirth was both a bodily and a social event, and these dimensions were connected, not separate as historiographic traditions have implied.[15] This means that practical obstetrics must be taken seriously in its own right, and also situated in its cultural context.

Secondly, we should seek not to evaluate but to explain the actions of our ancestors, both female and male. Thus, rather than passing judgement on the methods of eighteenth-century practitioners, we should attempt to reconstruct the actual tasks in which they were engaged. And thirdly, the women of early-modern England were not passive victims either of their bodies or of men, but active agents who made their own history.[16] On the documentary surface men appear as the more prominent agents, since most of our source-materials were written by men-midwives. Yet these practitioners owed their very existence to the choices and actions of women, and this turns out to be the key to our story.

Notes

1. Aveling, *Midwives*, p. 86.
2. Wendy Savage, a consultant at the London Hospital, tried to give her patients greater choice over practical obstetric decisions. She was dismissed for alleged malpractice, but appealed against the decision; after a prolonged enquiry, during which she was widely supported by women, she won her case and was reinstated. The case attracted considerable public interest, reaching the front pages of the British newspapers at every stage. See W. Savage, *A Savage enquiry: who controls childbirth?* (London: Virago, 1986).
3. See for instance B. Ehrenreich & D. English, *Witches, midwives and nurses: a history of women healers* (New York: Feminist Press, 1973); J. Towler & J. Bramall, *Midwives in history and society* (London, 1986); A. Rich, *Of woman born: motherhood as experience and as institution* (London: Virago, 1977); S. Kitzinger & J. Davis (eds), *The place of birth* (Oxford: Oxford University Press, 1978); S. Kitzinger, *Birth at home* (Oxford: Oxford University Press, 1979); N. Leap & B. Hunter, *The midwife's tale: an oral history of childbirth in the twentieth century* (London: Scarlet Press, 1993).
4. Radcliffe, *Milestones*, p. 30 and *passim*.
5. M. C. Versluysen, "Midwives, medical men, and 'poor women labouring with child': lying-in hospitals in eighteenth century London", in H. Roberts (ed.), *Women, health and reproduction* (London: Routledge, 1981), pp. 18–49, at p. 31. Versluysen's own suggestion, that lying-in hospitals served as exemplars for male practice (p. 39) and created an "ideological medicalization of childbirth" (p. 42; cf. p. 33), will be discussed in Ch. 11.
6. Spencer, *British midwifery*, pp. 72–3, quoting from MS notes of Hunter's lectures.
7. Giffard, *Cases*: Among Cases 1–40, of the 25 where the mother's social standing or her husband's occupation is given, two patients were described as "gentlewoman", one as "Mrs" (indicating fairly high social status), but nine were "poor" and the remaining 13 were married to men in a wide spectrum of trades: baker, chairman, waterman, hosier, cabinet-maker, servant of the Prince, apothecary, joiner, hackney-coachman, periwig-maker, printer, hatter, carpenter. This reads like a rough cross-section of London society at this time (1724–28).
8. M. Foucault, *The birth of the clinic: an archaeology of medical perception* (trans. A. M. Sheridan, London: Tavistock, 1973).
9. J. W. Leavitt, *Brought to bed: childbearing in America, 1750–1950* (New York & Oxford: Oxford University Press, 1986).
10. N. Gelbart, "Midwife to a nation: Mme du Coudray serves France", in *Art of midwifery*,

Marland, pp. 131–51; T. Ortiz, "From hegemony to subordination: midwives in early-modern Spain", in *ibid.*, pp. 95–114, at pp. 104–105; N. M. Filippini, "The church, the State and childbirth: the midwife in Italy during the eighteenth century", in *ibid.*, pp. 152–75, at p. 167; H. Marland, "The 'burgerlijke' midwife: the stadsvroedvrouw of eighteenth-century Holland", in *ibid.*, pp. 192–213, at pp. 203–204; M. Lindeman, "Professionals? Sisters? Rivals? Midwives in Braunschweig, 1750–1800", in *ibid.*, pp. 176–91, at p. 188. Cf. I. Loudon, *Death in childbirth: an international study of maternal care and maternal mortality 1800–1950* (Oxford: Clarendon Press, 1992), pp. 399–400.
11. See E. Ingerslev, "Rösslin's "Rosegarten": its relation to the past (the Muscio manuscripts and Soranos), particularly with regard to podalic version", *Journal of Obstetrics and Gynaecology of the British Empire* **15** (1909), pp. 1–25, 73–92; J. W. Ballantyne, "The 'Byrth of Mankynde'", *Journal of Obstetrics and Gynaecology of the British Empire* **10** (1906), pp. 297–325; **12** (1907), pp. 175–94, 255–74; **17** (1910), pp. 329–32.
12. Edmund Chapman, Alexander Butter, William Giffard, John Douglas, Henry Bracken, Sarah Stone, Fielding Ould; see Ch. 8.
13. Willughby, *Observations*, pp. 114, 245.
14. Aveling, *Chamberlens*; Ch. 4 below.
15. Compare the earlier medical histories by e.g. Aveling, Spencer and Radcliffe, where the history of childbirth was the history of obstetrics, with for instance Marland, *Art of midwifery*, where the body is almost absent.
16. Contrary to the argument of E. Shorter, *Women's bodies* (New Brunswick, NJ: Transaction Publications, 1990) – a unique attempt to integrate the bodily and social dimensions of childbirth, although in a very different way from what will be essayed here.

Part I

The traditional management of birth

Chapter Two
The bodily processes of childbirth

Childbirth can be easy or difficult, rapid or protracted, trouble-free or attended with complications.[1] The varieties of childbirth, their respective frequencies, and the techniques available in cases of difficulty are important for our story, since these conditioned the different experiences of childbirth of mothers, of midwives and of medical men. Although the exercise of counting the varieties of birth only began at the end of our period, we shall see that some earlier evidence can be gathered. A more difficult problem is that the very categories with which we seek to describe the bodily process of birth are themselves theory-laden in both past and present. Thus the following (simplified) account might have been accepted by some eighteenth-century observers (such as William Smellie and perhaps Sarah Stone), but would probably have been rejected by others (such as Hendrik van Deventer and Elizabeth Nihell).

The varieties of childbirth

The progress of labour depends above all on the posture of the child as it enters the mother's pelvis, which in turn determines what part of the foetus "presents" itself. Most commonly, the baby's *head* is the presenting part; less common is for the *breech* to present (effectively because the child has failed to make the usual somersault, within the womb, in the last weeks of the pregnancy); rarest of all is for the child to be lying "transversely", or "athwart the womb", which results in presentation usually of the *shoulder* or *arm*, sometimes of the back or belly, occasionally a "compound" presentation of both hand(s) and foot or feet. Between these three very broad categories, difficulty corresponds to rarity: births by the head are usually easy, births by the breech are more difficult, while births by the arm (and others arising from transverse lie) are almost invariably obstructed. At this level, there is fair agreement between the modern textbook and much earlier evidence. Thus in the Paris ordinance of 1560 regulating the practice of midwives, it was stated that midwives should get advice from physicians or surgeons if the child presents "other than head first, which is the normal delivery, or feet first, which is the next most normal delivery".[2] If we read "feet" here as breech, this implies the same broad picture shown by modern rates of presentation. Similarly, Willughby wrote a century later that arm presentation was the birth "which most amazeth and puzzleth midwives", suggesting that this was both rare (amazement) and difficult (puzzlement).[3]

Let us now consider the physical process of birth, beginning with births by the head.[4] For the child to be born by natural processes, the strength of the uterus has to be sufficient, and the foetal head and body have to pass through a bony passage that is, even at the best of times, only just wide enough for the purpose. That passage itself has a complicated shape: at its inlet its widest diameter runs from side to side, whereas at the outlet the widest diameter runs from front to back. The foetus, too, has different diameters: the head is biggest from front to back, the shoulders and hips from side to side. Consequently, the passage of the foetus through the pelvis always involves movements of *rotation*: for example, the head normally enters the mother's pelvis with the child facing more or less sideways, but must leave the pelvis with the child facing either the mother's back or (much more rarely) towards the front. But such are the dimensions of the child's head in relation to the mother's pelvis that this rotation requires some degree of *flexion*: that is, the child's head must be bent forwards, pressing its chin against its chest, to make rotation of the head possible. Finally, a further aspect of this process is the *moulding* of the child's head. The bones of the foetal head have some degree of mobility against each other, so that the head can be compressed into different shapes. This takes time, and it proceeds more effectively when the birth is relatively gradual. (The phenomenon of moulding illustrates the difficulty of giving a purely mechanical account of birth, since one of the two component parts, the foetus, is not of fixed dimensions.[5])

The baby's head can enter the mother's pelvis in any of several orientations. Thus head-presentations themselves are nowadays subdivided into a series of different types, according to two considerations: first, the way in which the child's head is bent in relation to its own body, and secondly, the orientation of its head with respect to the mother's pelvis. (The orientation is in fact achieved gradually, by the process of rotation already mentioned.) Normally, the child's head is so positioned that the top of the head, or *vertex*, presents; but if the head is tilted backwards a little, the *brow* first enters the pelvis, and further bending in the same direction ("extension" of the head, in medical terminology) makes the *face* present. Normally, too, the head is oriented more or less with the child's face to the mother's back ("face to sacrum" in eighteenth-century language, "occipito-anterior" as it is generally described today); sometimes however, this orientation is reversed, so that the child faces forwards ("face to pubis" or "occipito-

THE VARIETIES OF CHILDBIRTH

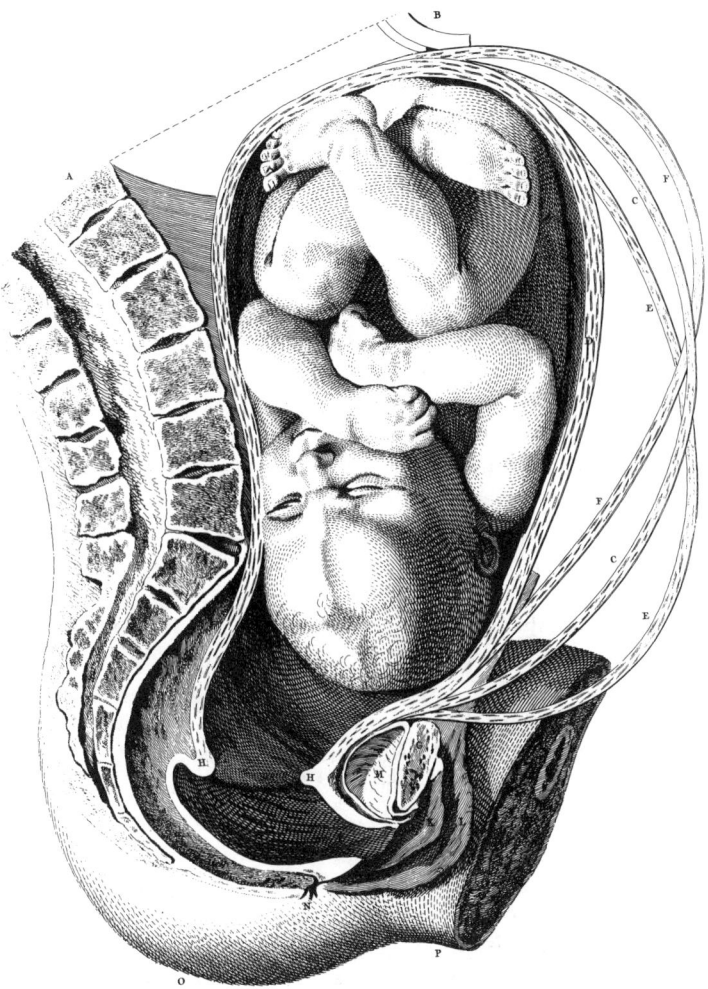

Figure 2.1   The position of the foetus (Smellie, Anatomical tables, *1754).*

posterior"). If we combine these two dimensions of variation, what we find is that the normal presentation (reached by greater or lesser degrees of rotation, depending on the starting-point) is the *occipito-anterior vertex*; in this orientation, birth is almost invariably achieved spontaneously and with relatively little difficulty. Any departure from this ideal results in some degree of difficulty: for instance, face presentations result in very protracted labour, occipito-posterior presentations tend (though not inevitably) to become obstructed.

Such in broad outline is the mechanism of birth by the head. A different mechanism, although involving similar principles, operates for birth by the *breech*. Thus breech births, too, can be regarded as natural, since such deliveries can be accomplished by the natural powers of the uterus. Nevertheless breech-presentation is much more likely to lead to difficulties, up to and including complete obstruction. Probably the commonest source of difficulty in our period was the aftercoming head, for several reasons. The breech, being smaller and softer than the head, dilates the cervix less effectively; there is not time for moulding to develop to the full; and the rotation of the head may require manual assistance. (Breech births are nowadays divided into three sub-types. The child may descend in a squatting posture, which is called a "full breech"; or with its feet to its head, known as a "frank breech"; or with one or both feet first, a "footling breech". Of these three varieties, the footling breech is the most likely to lead to obstruction.) Finally, presentation by the *arm* or shoulder, and other presentations arising from transverse lie, almost always lead to complete obstruction: only a premature foetus can be born with the arm and shoulder leading, and none can be born by the back, by the belly, or by compound presentation. We shall not err greatly if we assume that every case of transverse lie led to obstructed labour requiring manual intervention.

If difficulty is encountered, it is open to the observing attendants or practitioners to interpret that difficulty in any of a great variety of ways. Here are two examples.

1. Let us imagine that the child's head presents and is unusually large. This makes it more difficult for the head to flex; consequently, there is less chance of successful rotation; and the effect is often a face-to-pubis (occipito-posterior) orientation. The practitioner observes difficulty: what is the cause of the difficulty? Any of the stages just mentioned can be assigned causal priority – and so too can other factors.[6] Some will ascribe the difficulty to the size of the child's head; others, to impaired flexion and/or rotation; still others, to the occipito-posterior orientation. *All* of these descriptions are true; what the practitioner makes of the delivery will be a function of prior categories, past experience and present purposes. And today's impaired flexion probably corresponds to the eighteenth-century diagnoses of Sarah Stone and William Giffard that the child's head was stuck over the share-bone or pubic bone.[7]

2. Consider the case of a breech birth in which the aftercoming head is incorrectly flexed. That is one description, but another would be that the aftercoming head is in the wrong orientation; still another would be that the cervix of the uterus had closed around the child's neck; last but not least, a practitioner might with some justice assert that the fault lay simply with its being a breech birth, since breeches are always troublesome.

The potential for different interpretations is well illustrated by historical changes in the account given of obstructed births by the head. Until the mid-seventeenth century, this was ascribed simply to the *size* of the foetal head. It was François Mauriceau, writing in 1668 (and translated into English in 1673), who first pointed out that the occipito-anterior orientation led to spontaneous delivery, and the occipito-posterior to protracted or obstructed labour.[8] From this point onwards, the critical factor was usually seen as the *orientation* of the head – something that Willughby, for instance, had never even noticed. As for the movements of rotation, these were first observed by Fielding Ould in 1742 and were elaborated in great detail by Smellie in 1752.[9] Thus the categories deployed above are anachronistic, emerging as they did only gradually in the course of our period.

Childbirth is liable not only to obstruction, but also to a variety of *complications;* these can conveniently be divided into minor and major types. The minor complications included fainting, vomiting, and tearing of the perineum. Although distressing for the mother, these were not very common and seem not to have led to serious difficulty. It is also worth observing that fistulae, which are today a widespread and serious problem in parts of Africa, seem to have been uncommon in early-modern England.[10] The two major complications, attested by a variety of sources, were "flooding" (what is now called haemorrhage) and convulsions or "fits" (today known as eclampsia). Flooding was usually caused by the separation of the placenta during late pregnancy or at the onset of labour. Probably about half of these dangerous occurrences arose from the placenta being implanted near the cervix of the uterus (a condition recognized only towards the end of our period, and known today as "placenta praevia"). This was extremely serious, leading swiftly to the death of both mother and child unless a speedy delivery was enforced. Convulsions, while less often fatal, were nevertheless dangerous. A third cause of death, the most dangerous condition of all, was puerperal fever, which arose not during birth but after it. Its incidence is very difficult to assess because it was only recognized at the end of our period. Very probably it was this condition that Willughby described as "scouring" or "looseness", that is, diarrhoea – another telling instance of the historical mutability of observation categories.[11] The risk of puerperal infection was certainly increased by difficulty in the birth itself, especially by prolonged obstructed labour.

The incidence of difficult births

How frequent were cases of obstruction or difficulty? For eighteenth-century London we have three different sources of evidence. First, the cases of William Giffard offer a cross-section of *difficult* deliveries from around 1730. These can suggest the relative incidence of different types of difficulty, although for their absolute rates we shall have to look elsewhere. Secondly comes an estimate offered by William Smellie (1752), embracing both the relative and the absolute rates of births according to the presentation-type and the degree of difficulty. Smellie was the first author to put forward any such estimates; his estimates are thus of considerable intrinsic interest, although as we shall see they are less than ideal for our purpose. Thirdly, and apparently equally original in conception, in 1781 Robert Bland published an analysis of some 1897 births delivered under the auspices of the Westminster General Dispensary, classified by presentation-type and incidence of difficulty. Here we have direct observation of a large number of births, all attended by the Dispensary's midwives from the onset of labour, and thus – in contrast to Giffard's cases – not subject to any filter that might select difficult or unusual deliveries. These three sources complement each other and yield a consistent picture, once due allowance is made for their special characteristics. In addition, Felix Macdonough in 1768 provided some statistics from the General Lying-in Hospital which offer a rough corroboration.

Giffard's posthumously published *Cases in midwifery* included some 225 deliveries. From these I have selected the final 67 cases, which probably comprise a complete record of Giffard's emergency practice during the last 11 months of his life.[12] Their seasonal distribution corresponds roughly to the overall seasonality of birth; there are no gaps between successive cases of longer than 22 days, save for a five-week interval in March–April 1731 when Giffard was fully engaged "attending" a "Lady". The total number of these difficult cases, combined with the findings that will emerge below, suggests that Giffard was the chief emergency practitioner for a catchment area of roughly 4000 births per year, and this is consistent with the geographical distribution of his cases. Finally, Giffard had polemical reasons for making the case-series all-inclusive: every case was itself an argument, and both repetition (there are many forceps deliveries) and diversity were grist to his rhetorical mill. Prima facie, then, we can take these 67 cases as a full record of the difficult births Giffard attended during this period.

Table 2.1 enumerates the various sources of difficulty among these cases. There were 43 obstructed labours; 16 cases of complications (mostly flooding during labour); and 8 miscellaneous cases, not easy to classify or irrelevant to our enquiry. Of the 43 obstructed births, 24 were by the head, 5 by the breech, and 14 were transverse. There was only a single case of convulsions during labour. A noteworthy point, to which we shall return, is the contribution of rickets: 7 of the 43 cases of obstruction were attributed by Giffard to the sacrum being "very much bent inwards", or to "a narrow passage", which probably indicate a rachitic maternal pelvis.[13] (Rickets in the mother's childhood produces a characteristic pelvic deformity, involving narrowing, a change of shape, and inflexibility of the coccyx, all of which make for severe obstetric difficulty.[14])

Table 2.1   Giffard's last 67 cases.

Obstructed labour			Complicated labour				
head	breech	arm	flooding	retained placenta	fits	Other cases[a]	Total
24	5	14	11	4	1	8	67

(a) twins – 2; head not engaged — 1; funis and head – 1; inverted uterus – 1; arm and head – 1; probably not emergencies – 2.

Smellie's estimates had a specific polemical purpose, namely, "to inform young practitioners that difficult cases do not frequently occur".[15] Converted into a more accessible form, these estimates are reproduced in Table 2.2. How reliable were they? In view of his proclaimed argument, we should expect him to underestimate the incidence of difficult births, and it appears that his estimates were indeed biased in just this way. Smellie's breech-presentation rate comes to only 7 per 1000, as against usual estimates of around 30 per 1000; his transverse-presentation rate is 2 per 1000, compared with modern rates of 4–5 per 1000. But *within* the category of "laborious or praeternatural cases" Smellie's assessment of the *relative* rates of different kinds of difficulty was probably accurate; for in this respect, he could draw on almost 30 years of practice. Now among 10 imagined cases of serious difficulty, Smellie allocated six to births by the head, and two each to breech and transverse presentations – a distribution roughly compatible with what we have seen from Giffard's cases. Smellie did not offer any estimate of the rate of complications, but his actual cases included nine instances of flooding and eight of convulsions; only four of the eight cases with convulsions were inserted under this heading, which suggests that in Smellie's practice, as in Giffard's, flooding was the more frequent of the two accidents.[16] Rickets undoubtedly made a significant contribution to Smellie's overall emergency practice, although its precise influence is difficult to assess.[17]

Table 2.2 Smellie's estimates of rates of difficulty. Numbers in brackets are inferred; others were stated by Smellie.

	Head	Breech	Arm	Total
Difficult	6	2	2	(10)
Lingering	(65)[a]	(5)	(0)	(70)
Spontaneous	(920)	(0)	(0)	(920)
Total	(991)	(7)	(2)	(1000)

(a) actually 63–5.

Bland's cases are displayed in Table 2.3.[18] Here, unfortunately for our purposes, there is no indication of the incidence of breech-obstruction. A compensating advantage is that we can assess the overall rate of both breech- and arm-presentations – 28.4 per 1000 and 4.2 per 1000 respectively, levels that agree well with more recent statistics. The known obstructed births comprise 8 by the arm and 12 by the head. Bland investigated the contribution of rickets, and was able to rule it out for at least 2 of the 12 mothers who had obstructed births by the head; he inferred that "the number of women . . . who from error in their conformation were incapable of bearing live children appears to be very inconsiderable". There are nine cases of flooding, and only two of convulsions; these, too, imply rates supported by later statistics.[19]

How are we to compare and combine these three lines of evidence? The only available reference-point is births by the arm, which appear to be reasonably stable in incidence and which virtually always lead to complete obstruction. Let us suppose that their incidence was 4 per 1000 births (rounded from the 4.2 per 1000 that emerged from Bland's cases). For each of our three tabulations we can con-

Table 2.3 Bland's classification of 1897 actual deliveries. Numbers in brackets are inferred; others were stated by Bland.

	Head	Breech	Arm	Flooding	Retained placenta	Fits	Total
(a) Actual numbers							
Difficult	12	?	8	9	0	2	31 + breech
Natural	(1812)	?	(0)	(0)	(0)	(0)	(1812) + breech
						Total	1843 + 54 breech
Total	(1824)	54	8	9	0	2	1897
(b) Converted to base of 1000 births							
Difficult	6.3	?	4.2	4.7	0	1.1	16.3 + breech
Natural	(955.2)	?	(0)	(0)	(0)	(0)	(955.2) + breech
						Total	971.5 + 28.5 breech
Total	(961.5)	28.5	4.2	4.7	0	1.1	1000

vert the number of arm-presentations to 4, using the appropriate divisor or multiplier, and we can then apply this same conversion factor to each of the other categories of difficulty. The results will yield estimates of the approximate incidence of difficulty per 1000 births. Such a calculation is shown in Table 2.4. To compensate for the existence of blanks in the table, the minima and maxima are shown.

Table 2.4 Assessment of the incidence of difficult births per thousand total births, combining evidence from Giffard, Smellie and Bland (Tables 2.1–3).

	Obstruction			Complications[a]		Total
	head	breech	arm	flooding	fits	
Giffard	6.9	1.4	4.0	3.1	0.3	15.7
Smellie	12.0	4.0	4.0	?	?	20.0+
Bland	6.0	?	4.0	4.5	1.0	15.5+
minimum	6.0	1.4	4.0	3.1	0.3	14.8
maximum	12.0	4.0	4.0	4.5	1.0	25.5

(a) complicated labours: retained placenta excluded.

Let us first look at the overall result, and then break this down into its constituents. Our minimum estimate is about 15 difficult cases per 1000; our maximum, about 25. Thus, it looks as if somewhere between 1.5 and 2.5% of births involved either obstruction or major complications. If we keep in mind a figure of 2% as a working guide, we shall be reasonably close to the mark. The largest single category of difficult births, according to all three sources, was obstructed births by the head. But this was also the most variable in extent, ranging from 6 to 12 per 1000; we shall attend to this variation in a moment. The contribution of complications of labour – flooding and fits – was rather slight, amounting to less than a quarter of Giffard's difficult cases: hence, perhaps, the fact that Smellie omitted these categories. Obstructed breech births were less common than arm cases in

Giffard's series, although Smellie assessed these at the same rate; in each case, however, these were well outweighed by obstructed births by the head. So too Felix Macdonough's statistics of 1768, while indicating a higher overall rate of difficulty (4.27%), suggest that malpresentations accounted for a minority of these difficult cases.[20]

What of the marked variation in the frequency of obstructed births by the head? One possible explanation is a change in the incidence of rickets. We saw that rickets played a major role in Giffard's cases, usually leading to obstructed head-presentation, and it was undoubtedly important also in Smellie's practice. Bland was explicitly arguing that this problem was rare, and therefore he adduced evidence that some mothers had *not* had rickets; in line with his rhetorical purpose, he did not assess how many *had* suffered from the disease. Yet perhaps there was a decline in the incidence of rickets between the Giffard–Smellie period (1731, the 1740s) and Bland's time (1774–81). If such a change was real, it did not necessarily reflect a secular decline. For instance, London-born mothers may have had less exposure to sunlight in childhood, and thus a higher incidence of rickets, than mothers born elsewhere; thus if the mothers delivered by the Westminster General Dispensary between 1774 and 1781 included a relatively high proportion of immigrant women, these would have had fewer obstructed labours. An influence of this type need not have been confined to frank cases of rickety pelvis: quite minor alterations in the shape and size of the maternal pelvis could have, in the aggregate, a marked effect on the incidence of obstructed labour. This underlines the impossibility of deriving precise rates of difficulty in our period. The best we can hope for is an approximate range.

Our estimate of the incidence of serious difficulty is roughly consonant with the prevailing rates of stillbirths and of maternal mortality. If we suppose, for the sake of argument, that all obstructed births and all cases of flooding led to a stillbirth, this will contribute about 20 stillbirths per 1000 deliveries; there was ample room for such a number within the rates of 40–50 observed in the period, which will have included some stillbirths produced by other causes.[21] Maternal mortality has been estimated at around 1 or 2%, and this corresponds with the fact that the vast majority of births were normal and spontaneous.[22] Indeed, all these lines of evidence – stillbirths, maternal mortality, the probable incidence of obstruction and complications – converge towards the same conclusion: despite the very real risks of childbirth, the usual outcome was, in the words of the churching service, "a safe deliverance".

Standard techniques for delivering difficult births

Before about 1720, since no English midwives and few English male practitioners left any record of their practice, we do not know what techniques most of them deployed. But we can reconstruct the repertoire of methods described in books, that is to say, the range of *publicly known* techniques. I shall review the main techniques by their occasions – obstructed births by the head, malpresentations, complications of labour. Mention will then be made of the two Caesarean operations, whose contribution was theoretical rather than practical.

Obstructed births by the head

For obstructed births by the head the standard technique was the operation of *craniotomy*, i.e. opening the head of the child to reduce its size, and then extracting by means of traction through the skull. For this purpose a variety of instruments had been developed, some of them of great antiquity. The standard ancient authority, Soranus, had recommended the use of two hooks; Rueff proposed the use of forceps (not to be confused with the midwifery forceps), of two different kinds, smooth and toothed; Scultetus depicted two hooks with chains in place of solid handles; in the late seventeenth century Mauriceau invented a "tire-tête", while his contemporary Viardel proposed the use of the fingers alone for the purpose. But the standard device used in seventeenth-century England was a single hook, known as a "crotchet".[23] It must be stressed that while this operation appears cruel to us, its purpose was compassionate: it was designed to save the mother's life when the child had died, for a mother left undelivered in such circumstances could herself survive only for a few days. Nevertheless, craniotomy could pose serious ethical and political dilemmas. The diagnosis was often uncertain: how could it be known that the child was dead? Sometimes the diagnosis was contested: who was to decide? And if the baby was still alive but the mother's life was in danger, could the child be killed to save the mother? On rare occasions a child was indeed sacrificed to save the mother's life – two or three times in Willughby's 45 years of practice, always with the sanction of a minister of religion.[24]

There was one publicly known alternative: sometimes it was possible in such cases to turn the child from the head to the feet and to effect the delivery by traction on the feet. This manoeuvre (today known as podalic version) will be described below under malpresentations, in which it found its main application. Had it been possible to apply this in obstructed births by the head, the lives of many children could have been saved. But we shall later see that it was usually impracticable in such cases, even though a series of male practitioners tried to apply it in the hope of avoiding craniotomy.[25]

Malpresentations

For malpresentations two very different methods were available. The logical approach was to turn the child to the head, changing an unnatural presentation into a natural one. This manoeuvre, later called *cephalic version* (or more precisely,

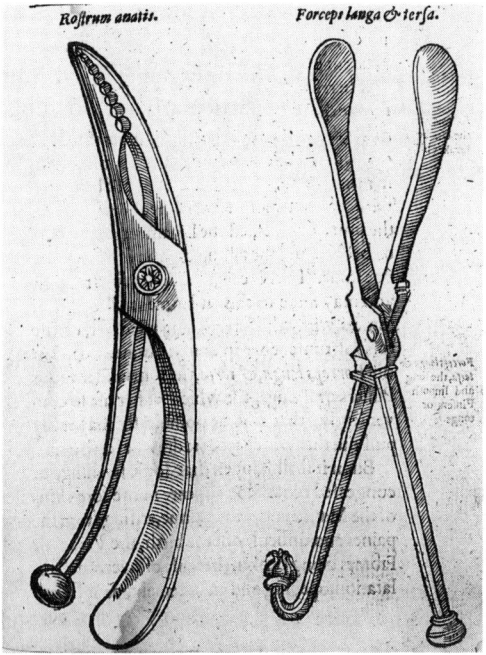

Figure 2.2   Craniotomy instruments (Rueff, The expert midwife, 1637).

internal cephalic version), was passive in intent: that is, it relied on the powers of the uterus to effect the delivery. It could therefore succeed only when performed early in the labour, and it seems that it required considerable manual skill.[26] The alternative was to turn the child to the feet, that is, to perform what was subsequently termed *podalic version*. Compared with cephalic version this was less intuitive, since birth by the feet was not a natural process. But it was more immediately effective, since by grasping the feet the operator could exert active traction; and because it did not depend on the uterus, it could be performed many hours or even days after the onset of labour.

Just as podalic version was chiefly used for malpresentations but could occasionally deliver obstructed births by the head, so, conversely, destructive instruments, although mainly applied to obstructed births by the head, were sometimes used for malpresentations. In particular, if the birth came by the arm and obstruction had been prolonged, the midwife or surgeon might cut off the arm with a knife, and then deliver by some such device as a crotchet. As with craniotomy, such an operation was usually performed only after it was agreed that the child had died.[27]

Flooding and convulsions

In cases of flooding and convulsions, the only remedy was immediate delivery. This usually meant podalic version – particularly for flooding, which was the more frequent of these two major complications; but in such cases delivery might occasionally be effected by craniotomy.

Caesarean section

One further method of delivery was theoretically available: *Caesarean section*, which could be used for any difficult birth. There were two distinct variants of this drastic operation. *Post-mortem* Caesarean section could of course only save the life of the child: canon law enjoined that this should be attempted whenever the mother had died and the child was believed to be still alive, so that the child's soul could be saved by baptism.[28] In being delayed until the mother's death and designed to save the child, this operation was symmetrically complementary to craniotomy. In contrast, Caesarean section *on the living mother* was intended by its sixteenth-century proposer, François Rousset, to save the lives of *both* mother and child. In practice, few mothers can have survived the operation in our period, since throughout Europe it was carried out only rarely, always *in extremis*, and without knowledge of aseptic precautions. Nevertheless, those who followed Rousset's lead and argued in favour of the operation always wanted to save the mother's life.[29]

Neither form of the operation was practised in seventeenth-century England – despite the requirement in canon law for the post-mortem operation (for which there must have been some occasions), and despite the fact that a few observers advocated the Rousset operation. The two different forms of the Caesarean operation served not as practical alternatives but as conceptual reference-points for ethical debate. The most advanced midwifery textbook, Mauriceau's *Diseases of women with child*, advocated the post-mortem operation and castigated the Rousset operation – a stance that probably arose from the Catholicism of its author. In contrast, James Cooke of Warwick, in the 1685 edition of his *Mellificium chirurgiae*, supported the Rousset operation. But most English practitioners probably shared Willughby's view that *both* forms of the operation were "works of cruelty".[30] In taking this view Willughby was probably reflecting the attitudes of women, who seem to have consistently favoured the life of the mother where an ethical choice was required. Nor was the Caesarean operation much promoted by English practitioners in the eighteenth century, although to this there are a few exceptions. In short, Caesarean section did not offer a practical alternative to the standard techniques already reviewed.

Notes

1. For help on technical obstetric matters I thank M. G. Elder, John & Flic Gabbay, and Jo Garcia. Remaining errors are my own responsibility.
2. T. G. Benedek, "The changing relationship between midwives and physicians during the Renaissance", *Bulletin of the History of Medicine* 51 (1977), pp. 550–64, at p. 557.
3. Willughby, *Observations*, p. 321.
4. The following account draws chiefly on McClintock, *Smellie's midwifery* and Galabin, *Manual of midwifery*.
5. It was much discussed whether the same applied to the mother's pelvis, i.e. whether the pelvic bones separated during labour. In mid-eighteenth-century Paris it was claimed on the basis of post-mortem examinations that this was indeed the case. See D. Diderot & J-R. D'Alembert (eds), *Encyclopédie ou dictionnaire raisonnée des sciences, des arts et des métiers, par une société des gens de lettres* (Paris: Briasson, David, Le Breton & Durand, 17 volumes; 1751–57, 1765), vol. I (1751), p. 85. For earlier discussions see Willughby, *Observations*, pp. 14–18; Radcliffe, *Milestones*, p. 28; McClintock, *Smellie's midwifery*, vol. I, pp. 79–81. Note also Deventer's manoeuvre (Ch. 6 below).
6. Thus McClintock wrote, of a different kind of difficult birth: "I have long held the opinion, derived from clinical experience, that pelvic capaciousness is really a predisposing cause of face presentation". Like other diagnostic opinions, this had practical consequences: McClintock was arguing that face presentation did not require forceps. See McClintock, *Smellie's midwifery*, vol. I, p. 279.
7. For Stone and Giffard, see Chs 4 & 7 below.
8. See Radcliffe, *Milestones*, pp. 24–5.
9. Radcliffe, *Milestones*, pp. 42–3; McClintock, *Smellie's midwifery, passim*.
10. Vesico-vaginal fistula: not mentioned in Cooke, *Mellificium chirurgiae*, pp. 174–8, "Of symptoms or accidents after birth". But see M. Macdonald, *Mystical bedlam: madness, anxiety and healing in seventeenth-century England* (Cambridge: Cambridge University Press, 1981), p. 273; Willughby, *Observations*, pp. 225–7; McClintock, *Smellie's midwifery*, vol. III, Cases 438–9, p. 238. Ano-vaginal fistula: "happens though seldom" according to Cooke, *Mellificium chirurgiae*, p. 176. See also Willughby, *Observations*, pp. 59, 159; McClintock, *Smellie's midwifery*, vol. III, Cases 437, 440, pp. 237–9. Cf. J. B. Lawson & D. B. Stewart (eds), *Obstetrics and gynaecology in the tropics and developing countries* (London: Edward Arnold, 1967).
11. Willughby, *Observations*, pp. 71, 89, 108, 110, 211, 217–22, 248; cf. Giffard, *Cases*, Case 72, p. 169. The source for this conception seems to have been Hippocrates: see Nathaniel Torriano, *Compendium obstetricii: or, a small tract on the formation of the foetus, and the practice of midwifery* (London, 1753; in his English translation of J. B. L. Chomel, *An historical dissertation on . . . sore throat*, French original Paris, 1749), p. 42.
12. Giffard, *Cases*. For the concept of emergency calls see Ch. 4 below; on Giffard's case series, rate of practice and catchment area, Ch. 7 below.
13. Giffard, *Cases,* Cases 182, 202.
14. Willughby, *Observations*, pp. 80–2, 109–14, 240.
15. McClintock, *Smellie's midwifery*, vol. I, p. 197.
16. *Ibid.*, vols II & III: flooding, Cases 326–34; convulsions, Cases 165–6, 234, 264, 342–5.
17. *Ibid.*, Case 3 & Cases 189–92.
18. Robert Bland, Some calculations . . . taken from the midwifery reports of the Westminster General Dispensary, *Philosophical Transactions of the Royal Society,* No. 71, Part I, 22

(1781), pp. 35–72.
19. See Galabin, *Manual of midwifery*, pp. 469, 360 (figures from Guy's Hospital Lying-In Charity, 49,145 births): flooding 4.08 per 1000 (Bland's figures imply 4.74), eclampsia 1.10 per 1000 (Bland, 1.05).
20. *An account of the rise, progress, and state of the General Lying-in Hospital, the corner of Quebec-Street, Oxford-Road* (London, 1768). Out of 8768 labours, 110 (1.25%) were "praeternatural" (probably cases of arm, compound and obstructed breech presentation) and 265 (3.02%) comprised "very difficult, tedious and lingering cases" (probably protracted as well as obstructed births by the head, and perhaps also some breech births). The higher rate of difficulty doubtless arose from the inclusion of "tedious and lingering cases". It is not clear where Macdonough classed complications of labour, nor whether his 378 "miscarriages at various periods of pregnancy" included full-term stillbirths.
21. See Wilson, *Childbirth*, n.2 to Ch. 12, drawing on T. R. Forbes, *Chronicle from Aldgate* (New Haven & London: Yale University Press, 1971), p. 65; R. Finlay, *Population and metropolis* (Cambridge, 1981), p. 37; R. S. Schofield, Perinatal mortality in Hawkshead, Lancashire, 1581–1710, *Local Population Studies*, No. 4 (1970), pp. 11–16, at p. 13; and K. Wrightson, "Infanticide in earlier seventeenth-century England", *Local Population Studies*, No. 15 (1975), pp. 10–22, at p. 18.
22. R. Schofield, "Did the mothers really die? Three centuries of maternal mortality in 'the world we have lost'", in L. Bonfield et al. (eds), *The world we have gained* (London, 1986), pp. 230–60.
23. Willughby, *Observations, passim*; Cooke, *Mellificium chirurgiae*, 1685 edn, pp. 167–8; J. Rueff, *De conceptu et generatione hominis* (Zurich, 1554), illustration facing p. 31; J. Scultetus, *The chyrurgeon's store-house* (trans. J. Ruding, London, 1674) Table XVII, p. 43; Radcliffe, *Milestones*, p. 26; C. Viardel, *Observations sur la pratique des accouchemens* (Paris, 1671, reprinted 1673, 1674), *passim*., e.g. pp. 186, 223–5; S. A. Brody, "The life and times of Sir Fielding Ould: man-midwife and master physician", *Bulletin of the History of Medicine* 52 (1978), pp. 228–50, at p. 245; Glaister, *Smellie*, p. 143.
24. Willughby, *Observations*, pp. 103–4 (Mrs Dutton or Dubton), 109–11 (Mrs Charles), 112–14 (Mrs Allestree).
25. See Chs 4 & 9 (Willughby, Smellie). The other notable practitioner who tried to use podalic version to obviate craniotomy was La Motte, *Midwifery*.
26. Galabin, *Manual of midwifery*, pp. 694–5.
27. Willughby, *Observations*, p. 99 (contrast pp. 55–6, 249, 250, 322–5); Cooke, *Mellificium chirurgiae*, 1685 edn, p. 170.
28. Edmund Gibson, *Codex Juris Ecclesiae Anglicani* (2nd edn, 2 volumes; Oxford, 1761), vol. II, p. 372.
29. See Young, *Caesarean section*, and E. Turner, "Bibliographie de François Rousset", *Annales de gynécologie* 14 (1881), pp. 1–25.
30. Young, *Caesarean section*, pp. 28, 31–2, 34, 224–5; Cooke, *Mellificium chirurgiae*, 1685 edn, pp. 172–3; Willughby, *Observations*, p. 340.

Chapter Three
The practices of midwives

The ceremony of childbirth

In England around 1700, as for centuries before, childbirth was a social occasion for women.[1] In the later months of her pregnancy, the mother-to-be would issue invitations to her female friends, relatives and neighbours. Her midwife would probably know when the birth was due, for as we shall see, the midwife usually lived nearby, and she might well have been giving advice on the management of the pregnancy.[2] When the mother's labour-pains began, there fell upon her husband (perhaps assisted by a servant or neighbour) the duty of what in East Anglia was known as "nidgeting": that is, going about from house to house to summon the midwife and the other women to the birth.[3] Within an hour or so, the group of women – probably five or more of them as a rule – would be assembled in the mother's bedroom. Meanwhile, the father-to-be would have to make his own arrangements for passing the ensuing hours – for he was excluded from the all-female childbirth ritual.[4] In fact these rapid preparations were moving the mother away from the world of men (centrally, her husband) and into the collective culture of women, where birth belonged.

The invited women were known as "gossips", and the history of this word attests to the importance of childbirth both in women's individual lives and in their collective culture.[5] Originally, "gossip" was a corruption of "god-sib" or "god-sibling", that is, someone invited to witness the birth for the subsequent purpose of the child's baptism. By the seventeenth century, "gossiping" was used for women's getting together both at childbirth and elsewhere. (Men of the period used the word with a certain hostility, producing the modern, derogatory usage.[6]) Correspondingly, a woman's "gossips" were her close female friends.[7] It was those friends, and often also her own mother, whom the mother-to-be invited to attend her delivery.

As essential as the gossips was the midwife, or, as she was known in some areas, the "grace-wife".[8] Occasionally a birth might take place without a midwife – for instance, because the labour was so swift that the mother had been delivered before the midwife could arrive. But deliveries without a midwife were rare, and the presence of the midwife was a universal norm. "Midwife" meant "with-woman", suggesting that the midwife was the woman who would *be with* the mother during the delivery.[9] In practice, her role was more specific than this. The midwife took charge as soon as she arrived, and expected to remain in charge thereafter. It was even possible for a young and inexperienced midwife, probably of no higher than yeoman status, to defy a mother who was a lady, that is, the wife of a gentleman, a member of the ruling class.[10] Power, then, was a defining feature of the midwife's office. Correspondingly, she was paid for her services – although not by any fixed amount, and often in the form of a gift or "grace", whence her alternative name of "grace-wife".[11] She might receive two shillings from the parish officers for delivering a pauper woman; six or ten shillings for a birth in a town; several guineas from a gentlewoman or an aristocratic lady; a hundred pounds for delivering the Queen.[12] The midwife's remuneration did not end here, for a few days later she would receive tips from the godparents at the child's baptism. Beyond power and payment, the midwife probably had a further defining characteristic: it seems likely that she alone was entrusted with the right to touch the mother's "privities" – her labiae, vagina and cervix.

The birth was not only contained within a distinct social space, but also physically and symbolically enclosed. Air was excluded by blocking up the keyholes; daylight was shut out by curtains; and the darkness within was illuminated by means of candles, which were therefore standard requirements for a delivery.[13] Thus reconstituted, the room became the *lying-in chamber,* the physical counterpart of the female social space to which the mother now belonged. Somewhere in this room, if it had a fireplace, or perhaps elsewhere in the house, some of the gossips were preparing the mother's *caudle* – the special drink associated with childbirth, consisting of ale or wine, warmed with sugar and spices.[14] As the gossips and midwife arrived, as the room and the caudle were being prepared, the birth itself was gradually advancing. Delivery, too, was a matter of culture, not simply of Nature: as we shall see, different midwives had their own chosen methods, and this practical discretion reflected their authority over the birth. But once the child had been delivered, the "navel-string" tied and cut (perhaps by one of the gossips), and the child washed, such variability gave way to constancy with the *swaddling* of the child – either performed or supervised by the midwife. Once swaddled, the child was shown to the mother.[15]

Although swaddling completed the birth, the childbirth ritual was only beginning – for this comprised the ensuing month of *lying-in*. It was for this, as much as for the birth itself, that the room had been prepared; hence its description as the lying-in chamber. The mother had been "brought to bed", she had completed her "crying out"; but she was still "in the straw", and she would remain in that state for what was called "the month" or "her month".[16] Throughout this time she was treated as an invalid, recovering in a series of steps. At first she was confined to bed, for anything from three days to a fortnight, and during this time the room remained darkened. Then came her "upsitting", when the bed-linen was changed; after this she remained in her room for a further week or 10 days, not confined to bed but still resting. In the third and final stage of lying-in, she moved about the house, but did not venture out of doors; this stage, too, seems to have lasted for about 10 days.[17] The timing of these changes depended on the mother's perception of her strength, for as she recovered she resumed her usual household tasks. In the first two stages of lying-in, the housework was performed either by a hired nurse or by a relative or friend, who would also look after the mother.[18] In the third stage the mother would become, as Ralph Josselin wrote on one such occasion, "busy through mercy in the family".[19] Yet she could not work out of doors, and thus her husband had to carry out some of her traditional tasks, "fetching meal from the mill and such other like".[20] Corresponding to these shifts in physical space were a series of movements in social space. At first, only women could visit the mother: the "upsitting" appears to have been an important social occasion, and there is some evidence to suggest that a women's feast was held a little later, during the second stage of lying-in.[21] In addition to such group occasions, there were individual visits, during which the female guest would drink the mother's caudle. Thus the celebratory, collective female character of the birth continued through the lying-in. Correspondingly, male access to the mother was restricted: initially, only men who were the mother's own relatives could visit her, although by the final stage of lying-in this restriction was apparently relaxed, and it may have been easier for a man to pay a visit if he was accompanied by his wife.[22]

Lying-in also involved a further difference from normal married life: the suspension of sexual activity. Thus the diarist Nicholas Blundell wrote in 1704 that "my wife's month being now out we lay together"; and indirect evidence suggests that Ralph and Jane Josselin, half a century earlier, usually followed the same practice.[23] Other fragments attest to the husband's distinct and solitary condition during the lying-in month, or as it was called, his "gander-month". In 1655 John Stewkly of Preshaw, Hampshire, wrote during his wife's pregnancy to Sir Ralph Verney that he "desired a man's society during his gander-month". And Henry Newcome, in 1649, took separate lodgings – apparently in an inn – for "that month in which my wife lay in".[24]

The end of the lying-in month was marked by the ecclesiastical rite of *churching*; originally "purification", this had since 1552 been "the thanksgiving of women after childbirth" in the Reformed Church of England.[25] In theory, the mother could not go outdoors until she was churched – so for the journey to the church she was symbolically and socially enclosed, wearing a veil and accompanied by her midwife and gossips.[26] Once inside the church she would kneel, according to the 1662 rubric, "in some convenient place, as hath been accustomed, or as the Ordinary shall direct"; in fact there was often a specific "uprising seat" or "churching pew" for the mother, midwife and gossips.[27] The priest then exhorted her to "give hearty thanks unto God" for her "safe deliverance . . . in the great danger of childbirth", and recited Psalm 116 or 127. There followed a *Kyrie eleison,* the Lord's Prayer, three specific versicles and responses, and a concluding short prayer of thanks and supplication. Finally, the woman made her "accustomed offerings" of a few pence each to the priest and to the parish clerk. The churching service probably took about 10 minutes; it could be held at any time, but it seems that women usually came to be churched during divine service. The baby's *baptism* was supposed to take place before the mother's churching, for the *Book of Common Prayer* required that the child was baptized on the first or second Sunday after delivery.[28] In theory baptism did not involve the parents, only the three godparents or "sponsors", but sometimes baptisms were delayed until the day of churching, so that mothers could attend. This was probably why the typical interval between birth and baptism drifted in the eighteenth century from a few days to three weeks or so, in contravention of the Prayer Book.[29] In fact there were many links between baptism, churching, birth and lying-in.[30] The midwife customarily attended the baptism; she and the gossips sat in the "churching pew" – whence its alternative designations as the "midwives' seat" or "chrisning seat"; the sponsors would tip the midwife, as we have seen, and also the lying-in nurse.[31]

Unlike baptism, churching was neither compulsory nor systematically recorded; but it was very popular with mothers. Wherever we have numerical evidence – that is, in parts of London at scattered dates – we find that at least 90% of mothers were churched: in the early seventeenth century, in the late nineteenth century, and in the 1950s.[32] For the eighteenth century we lack such statistics, but all the indications are that churching was routinely observed. Thus in 1722 Charles Wheatly declaimed against the custom of being churched at home but did not mention non-observance as a problem.[33] So too the wider childbirth ritual, although its details are more visible among mothers of high wealth and social status, was followed by women of all social classes. Although poor mothers living in one- or two-roomed cottages did not have the luxury of a separate room, and may have been unable to afford the curtains, the candles, and the paid nurse, they adapted and improvised – by shortening the "month", by using the bed itself as the lying-in space, or by lying in at the house of a more wealthy relative or friend.[34] The parish overseers of the poor paid for the traditional customs, supplying the unmarried Grace Pearson with a nurse for three weeks, and "a pint of liquor for Anne Barne's lying-in".[35] And late eighteenth-century evidence strongly suggests that the lying-in ritual was universally observed.[36] Hence the fact that wealthy mothers made an expensive display of their lying-in chamber: mere lying-in did not demonstrate their social status, which had to be shown by other means.[37]

To move from describing to explaining the ceremony of childbirth is to pass from fragmentary evidence to documentary silence; yet this has not deterred historians. The prevailing view sees lying-in as required by the churching of women, and churching as arising from "the primitive view of woman as shameful and unclean", itself associated with a supposed "universal belief" in her "inferior capacity". According to this account, childbirth had defiled the mother and churching was needed to purify her.[38] This interpretation, derived from Puritan polemics, precisely inverts the meaning of these rituals. Churching was popular because lying-in was popular; it was women who made it so; and if they believed that childbirth was defiling, they behaved very strangely indeed, thronging around the mother as they did from the birth itself through her lying-in to the moment of her churching. In fact the ceremony of childbirth was created by women, and its customs are intelligible in the context of women's lives. One case in point is the swaddling of the child. Swaddling was an excellent child-care practice: by sending the baby to sleep it elegantly satisfied the needs of both mother and child, and by implementing it from the moment of birth the women of early-modern England were practising it in the ideal way.[39] Another aspect of the ritual with a sound practical foundation was the darkened room: in the late nineteenth century medical men discovered that this prevented eclampsia.[40] Both in darkening the room and in swaddling the child, women had worked out what was best for them.

But the meaning of the ritual was also political, because marriage was a contract of inequality. At her wedding the bride vowed to "obey and serve" her husband; wifely obedience was a central normative value, and correspondingly the power of the husband was a major ideological resource.[41] Under the common law the husband owned the wife's worldly goods, her physical labour and its fruits, and her sexuality.[42] And the effect of the lying-in month was to withdraw from the husband his wife's physical labour and her sexual services. Her physical labour was replaced by that of the nurse; the payment to the nurse was a subsidy from husband to wife. So too were the festivities, as Thomas Turner noted in 1756: "While we were at Mr French's, Mr Piper came to call Mrs French to his wife, who, it seems, had sent for the midwife and many more good women – now, the poor old creature's purse!".[43] Thus the ceremony of childbirth inverted the normal pattern of conjugal relations; the wife's bodily energies and sexuality now, for the space of "the month", belonged to her; what marriage had taken from her, the childbirth ritual temporarily restored. Hence the collective female character of the ritual. The presence of other women may have served to police the lying-in – to ensure that the husband respected the norms; the mother's immersion in a female collectivity inverted the conjugal relation of individual male property. In short, the ritual was constructed and maintained by women *because it was in the interests of women*.

What, then, did men make of the childbirth ritual? Their usual response was passive acceptance, shown both by diarists such as Josselin and by medical writers such as Willughby. Yet we also find a few signs of male hostility. The Puritans of the early seventeenth century criticized churching along with other ecclesiastical ceremonies, and some male Puritan attacks on churching extended to the whole process of lying-in.[44] After the Restoration, William Sermon constructed the fantasy that lying-in was not observed by American wives, and suggested that English women should similarly return to their wifely duties immediately after birth.[45] *The woman's advocate* of 1683 attributed to a husband some aversion to women's sociability during lying-in, and then defended the women in the following terms:

> for gossips to meet... at a lying-in, and not to talk, you may as well dam up the arches of London Bridge, as stop their mouths at such a time. 'Tis a time of freedom, when women ... have a privilege to talk petty treason.[46]

Notice the obliqueness of this criticism: this anonymous male author gave voice to men's resentment only through the mouth of an invented husband, taking care to distance himself from such a critical attitude. The ceremony of childbirth was almost beyond the reach of explicit criticism in print; such muffled resentment, like the more usual passive acceptance, eloquently attests to the hegemony of the ritual. Through the ceremony of childbirth women secured a period of rest and recovery, and they kept childbirth under their own collective control.

To be a midwife

Who were the midwives? Most were probably married women or widows, of middling social status and of mature years, who had already had children. Yet this was a pattern, not a rigid framework, for we find much variation in midwives' marital status, age and wealth.[47] Examples are known of unmarried midwives,[48] of teenage midwives and of midwives in their eighties,[49] of rich midwives and of poor.[50] However, the *literacy* of midwives may present a more consistent pattern. It is true that there are known instances of midwives who could sign their name and of others who could only make a mark, suggesting variation in this respect as well.[51] Yet it is possible that all or most midwives in our period could read, for as Margaret Spufford has argued, this capacity was much more widespread than the ability to write or to sign.[52] And there are indications that literacy of both kinds was higher among midwives than among their clientele as a whole. As early as 1634 it was asserted that most London midwives could read; by the 1660s it seems that country midwives could do so too, in an age when female literacy was still very low.[53] Midwives' signing-literacy was remarkably high (of the order of 80%) both in London around 1700 and in Bury, Lancashire in the first half of the eighteenth century; even the signing rate of 20% among the midwives of rural Cheshire in this period was probably relatively high for their sex in the villages they served.[54]

It is also tempting to speculate that one common characteristic of midwives was a certain boldness, self-confidence, or strength of character. Medical men saw this as stubbornness, defiance, and refusal to accept help or instruction; thus in the 1660s Willughby sighed that "midwives will follow their own ways, and will have their own wills", and Giffard complained around 1730 of midwives' "self-sufficiency".[55] Nor is it only from the frustrated medical man that we get such indications of midwives' boldness. Sarah Marlton of Wickhambrooke, a midwife who began practice around 1710, asserted in 1723 that her parish priest was "unfit to administer the sacrament" (and got away with it).[56] Four years later the Oxford midwife Mrs Kite was described as "very forward" – which probably meant both self-assertive and flirtatious – by the antiquary Thomas Hearne.[57] It is at least a hypothesis worth exploring that it was, on the whole, women of strong character who became midwives – whether on their own initiative or (more interestingly) at the behest of their prospective clientele.[58] This would fit with the midwife's authority over the birth, which as we have seen could run against the normal distinctions of rank and status.

If it is difficult to generalize about who midwives were, there is one important respect in which we can now say who they were *not*. Historiographic tradition has long suggested that in sixteenth- and seventeenth-century England there was some association between midwives and witches – an association that historians have located either in the minds of the witch-persecutors or in reality. Such a connection had certainly existed in the fantasies of the two fifteenth-century Dominican authors of the *Malleus maleficarum*, who produced elaborate theories linking the activities of supposed witches with those of allegedly infanticidal midwives. But in early-modern England, as David Harley has recently shown, there is no evidence for any such connection, even in the minds of those who conducted persecutions for witchcraft.[59] Instead, the supposed link between "the midwife and the witch" has been the product of historians' imaginations.

What particularly eludes recovery is the process by which midwives were *recruited*. This surely involved an element of collective choice among the midwife's prospective clientele; yet such transactions among women left few documentary traces. Recruitment was seldom mentioned in the testimonials which, as we shall see below, were required for licences from the Church. Typically, a testimonial like that for Elizabeth Cornwallis of Norwich (1702) would "certify" that she "hath for some time past exercised the art of a midwife with good success"; these signatories went on that they "do further esteem her to be a woman of good judgment in the said art, and well qualified to practise the same".[60] Such bland commendations reveal nothing of how Elizabeth Cornwallis had become a midwife in the first place. Nor did Willughby discuss this question, beyond asserting that some women embarked on the practice of midwifery "for the getting of a shilling or two, to sustain their necessities".[61] Even for the restricted group of poor midwives this was barely an explanation: there were many poor women, only some of whom became midwives. Indeed, we are entitled to suspect that Willughby wrote nothing about the recruitment of midwives because he knew nothing about it. Like our other informants – medical writers, diarists, ecclesiastical officers – he encountered midwives only *after* they had entered practice.

In mid-seventeenth-century London the recognized way to start practice was to serve as a *deputy* to an established midwife, perhaps for as long as seven years –

but this remarkable system, apparently created by the midwives themselves many decades earlier, was fast declining by 1700.[62] Elsewhere no such system is known, although Mary Griffin of Deal in Kent paid £5 in the 1690s for three years' instruction from Mrs Anne Slap.[63] Occasionally, however, we encounter a process of *mother–daughter instruction*. Ellen Fletcher of Liverpool had been trained by her mother before 1691. In the West Country soon after this, "the famous Mrs Holmes" of Bridgwater trained her daughter Sarah; subsequently Sarah, now Mrs Stone, became the first English midwife to write an original midwifery treatise, and her *Complete practice of midwifery* (1737) announced that she was training her own daughter in turn. Ruth Rogerson of Northwich stated in 1724 that she had been "instructed both by her grandmother and mother".[64] The same procedure was followed around this time in the family of George Ballard: his mother was a midwife at Campden, Gloucestershire, and (as Thomas Hearne observed in 1730) his "ingenious sister, who is now 26 years of age, is . . . designing to be a midwife by the assistance of her mother, who hath followed that employment many years." George's sister had wider interests as well, for she was "very curious in coins and physic", and "reads very much in physic and history, and procures many of the best books that way"; surely it was her example that inspired George to produce 20 years later his celebration of female accomplishments, the *Memoirs of several ladies of Great Britain*.[65] Such mother–daughter instruction was probably unusual, although its incidence is very difficult to assess.[66] (How had Mrs Holmes herself acquired her skill? What became of Sarah Stone's daughter?) It was surely no accident that, as we shall later see, Mrs Stone acquired outstanding skills.[67] For such training made it possible to pass on the otherwise fragile gains of technical prowess acquired through practical experience.

Just as London midwives had constructed the deputy system, so also there were several seventeenth-century attempts to create in the capital a corporation of midwives analogous to those of the physicians, surgeons and apothecaries. Peter Chamberlen II promoted such an initiative in 1617; his son, Dr Peter Chamberlen, repeated the attempt in 1634; and in 1687 the Catholic midwife Mrs Elizabeth Cellier put to James II a scheme for a "college of midwives". But these attempts came to nothing: the Chamberlens were frustrated by the College of Physicians, and Mrs Cellier by the abdication of her Royal patron.[68] The failure of these attempts left the power to regulate midwives, in London as elsewhere, in the hands of the bishops of the Church of England. For midwives were subject to licensing by the bishops, under a *de facto* extension of their power to license physicians and surgeons conferred by Parliament in 1512.[69] To be awarded an episcopal licence a midwife had to bring a testimonial, as we have seen; swear an oath, which sometimes had many clauses, sometimes just one or two; and pay a huge fee, of the order of a pound or more, equivalent to hundreds of pounds at today's prices. Had it been systematically enforced, episcopal licensing would have restricted the practice of midwifery to women of at least the yeoman or artisan class, who alone could afford the fee. But licensing was only implemented patchily and with limited success. The methods of its enforcement varied greatly both between different dioceses and over time: it was imposed more systematically when the incomes of ecclesiastical officers were under pressure, typically in the early eighteenth century. Subsequently it declined, disappearing at different dates in different dioceses (from 1720 in London to 1818 at Peterborough).[70] At no stage did church licensing regulate the entry of women into midwifery; even when enforced, it merely ratified the previous choice made by the midwife's clientele (examples are known of midwives licensed after 20 or 30 years' practice).[71] Nor did it serve as an effective test of the midwife's skill; on the contrary, as some contemporaries observed, it made it easier for an unskilled midwife to embark on practice, since a midwife could prepare an impressive testimonial after handling only a few deliveries.[72] Indeed, in London after the Restoration it was perhaps ecclesiastical licensing, with its stress on client testimonials, that led to the decline of the deputy system.[73]

The problem of difficult births

Qualified observers of both sexes routinely claimed that few midwives could deliver difficult births. The most graphic testimony of this kind is that of Willughby, whose *Observations in midwifery* included dozens of case-histories attesting to the limited skills of seventeenth-century Derbyshire midwives. A few decades later Sarah Stone's *Complete practice of midwifery* gave a similar account of her colleagues in the West Country, and her critical account was matched at this time by William Giffard in London, Edmund Chapman in Essex and Henry Bracken in Lancashire.[74] Moreover, the very existence of these practitioners points in the same direction, for their work mainly consisted of delivering difficult births that midwives had been unable to manage. Yet we are also confronted by a very different testimony, that is, the actions of mothers, who went on summoning to their deliveries those same "ignorant midwives" castigated by observers like Willughby and Stone. No statute required a midwife to be present at the birth; the very existence of midwives was sustained solely by popular demand. Thus mothers evidently had confidence in their midwives.[75] How are we to reconcile this with the indications that midwives were unskilled?

The paradox is resolved if we attend to the material framework of midwives' practice, that is, to the types of births they encountered and the experience they acquired. As we have seen, the vast majority of births – of the order of 98% – were normal. Thus most mothers were never confronted with the limitations of midwives.[76] Further, a midwife could only accumulate experience of difficult births by attending a large number of deliveries, but few midwives ever acquired such experience. For in the rare instances when we can assess the numbers of midwives in a substantial rural area, we find about two midwives to every three settlements; and their average case-load seems to have been 20 deliveries per year or less. Two examples – from West Suffolk in the mid-1720s and from part of Lincolnshire some 80 years later – are set out in Table 3.1; these conform with other, more patchy evidence.[77] It seems that the smallest parishes had no midwife of their own, while a larger parish might have two or three midwives. But the typical settlement was a village of a few hundred people, among whom perhaps 10–20 births took place each year, and such a village usually had its own midwife. This suggests that there were six or seven thousand midwives practising in early eighteenth-century England.[78] Although low case-loads meant that most midwives gained little experience of difficult births, the large number of midwives had several advantages. It doubtless enabled mothers and midwives to know each other personally. It meant that the midwife was usually close at hand when the summons came – thus at Earles Colne in the mid-seventeenth century, only once in Jane Josselin's eight recorded births did the midwife arrive late.[79] And it kept to a minimum those occasions, which occurred more frequently than we might expect, when a midwife found two of her clients falling into labour at the same time.[80]

Opportunities for more intensive practice arose in the larger settlements – ranging from "great towns" (roughly, market towns), with populations of 1500 or so, through county towns (4000–10,000) and regional capitals like Bristol, Exeter, Newcastle, Norwich and York (10,000–30,000), to London (about 575,000 in 1700).[81] If a market town with a population of 1500 had just one midwife, she would practice at an 'urban' rate of about 50 deliveries per year. The opportunities were still greater in larger towns, and in such places we do indeed find midwives who practised at a substantially higher rate. At Kendal in the early 1670s, the local midwife attended around 70 births per year.[82] At Taunton about half a century later Sarah Stone was delivering, so she claimed a while afterwards, "at least three hundred children a year".[83] Mrs Mary Hopkins of Wilton, Wiltshire, sustained a case-load of over 200 births a year for over 40 years, between the 1720s and the 1760s; so did Mrs Phoebe Crewe of Norwich, practising between 1777 and 1817.[84] Such midwives must have accumulated repeated experience of difficult births and thus probably became capable of delivering them.

Yet some towns had several midwives, with much lower case-loads than were theoretically possible. At Bridgwater, where Mrs Stone had practised before moving to Taunton, there were three or four midwives in 1736, sharing between them about 100 births a year.[85] At both Ipswich and Bury St Edmunds in the early eighteenth century there were about 220–260 births per year; these could have been shared between two or three midwives, practising at a high rate, yet in each of these towns we find at least seven midwives at this time.[86] Thus the practice of midwives in towns was subject to two mutually contradictory influences, one leading to an "urban" pattern of low numbers and high case-loads, the other pushing them towards the complementary, "rural" pattern. Both tendencies are attested at Bungay, Suffolk in the early eighteenth century, where there were probably about 50 or 60 deliveries each year: here the number of midwives fluctuated between one and three, implying that case-loads varied between 20 and over 50 births per year.[87] Indeed, around 1700 there is evidence of low case-loads even

Table 3.1 Two examples of the distribution of midwives in rural areas.

Region, date	Number of parishes	Estimated births p.a.	Number of midwives	Case-load (births p.a.)
Three hundreds in West Suffolk, 1723–25	83	1089	55	20
Part of Lincolnshire, 1805	103	930	63	15

West Suffolk, 1723–25: Numbers of midwives from two episcopal visitations combined; midwives were identified by name in apparitors' citation lists (NNRO, VIS/13 and/14). The region concerned, in which citation of midwives was unusually complete, comprises the deaneries of Clare, Thedwastre, and part of Sudbury (the part administered visitationally at Bury St. Edmunds), corresponding respectively to the hundreds of Resbridge, Thedwestry and Babergh. Numbers of births estimated using 1801 Census, *Parish register abstracts* and Wrigley & Schofield, *Population history*.

Lincolnshire, 1805: Number of midwives from a count made by the Lincolnshire Medical Benevolent Society: see Edward Harrison, *Remarks on the ineffective state of the practice of physic in Great Britain: with proposals . . . and the resolutions of the members of the Medical Benevolent Society in Lincolnshire* (London, 1806). Numbers of medical practitioners, including midwives, were given for just two of the ten "divisions" into which the society partitioned Lincolnshire; precise administrative boundaries were not specified and have to be inferred. Numbers of midwives given here are for the "Horncastle division"; this "comprehends the market towns of Horncastle, Spilsby, Alford and Tattersall" (p. 38), which belonged respectively to the Soke of Horncastle, the East Soke of Bolingbroke, the Wold Division of the Hundred of Calceworth, and the South Division of the Wapentake of Gartree (*1801 Census*). Comparison with a map suggests that the region also included the West Soke of Bolingbroke, the Wold Division of the Wapentake of Candleshoe, and the entire Hundred of Hill. The figure of 930 births per year is the sum of separate estimates for these various administrative areas. For most of these areas, baptisms were taken from the *Parish Register Abstracts* and inflated to compensate for the missing registers (identified by collation with the *1801 Census*); and births were then estimated by a further inflation of 1.406 to compensate for under-registration and nonconformity. But two variations were required. (1) For the Soke of Horncastle the number of baptisms in 1800 was implausibly low (38, surely a misprint, since the population of the Soke was 4983 in 1801); here the national birthrate of 36.6 per thousand was applied, yielding an estimate of 182 births per year. (2) For the Hundred of Calceworth baptisms in 1800 were given only for the whole hundred; baptisms for the Wold division were estimated as a proportion, using 1801 population figures for the two divisions. The national birthrate and inflation factors for under-registration and nonconformity were taken from Wrigley & Schofield, *Population history*.

in London, the largest concentration of births in the kingdom. Mrs Cellier assumed an average case-load of between 8 and 16 births per year (or even less) – for her plan would have divided London's 16,000 annual births among 2000 midwives, of whom the "first thousand" were apparently to have the lion's share of practice (and she envisaged some deputies as well).[88] This probably reflected her perception of existing reality: she would not have wanted to raise the number, since she intended to regulate the recruitment of midwives. Subsequently, we find that a London midwife who practised throughout the entire metropolitan area between 1694 and 1723 delivered only about 23 births per year.[89] In fact, late seventeenth-century London midwives probably comprised two layers: many hundreds who had low case-loads and correspondingly limited skills, and a small, skilled élite (doubtless including Mrs Cellier) who practised at a high rate.

The skills of midwives

Probably, therefore, most midwives in both town and country were indeed unable to deliver difficult births: their low case-loads fit with the comments of such authors as Willughby, Giffard and Stone. Yet this picture, although true in its own terms, is one-sided, for the criticisms of Willughby et al. were produced from a particular point of view. As specialists in the management of difficult births, they not only tended to see midwives' failures rather than their successes; they also had a particular conception of what counted as skill. In the eyes of any given practitioner, skill was what she or he was good at; other activities, even quite closely related ones, were invisible. Hence the fact that the swaddling of the newborn child – an essential task for the midwife, and vitally important for both mother and child – was ignored by Willughby, Stone, Chapman and Giffard, and actively disdained by Bracken.[90]

More generally, the management even of normal birth was a domain of skill. Take the case of one common practice of midwives repeatedly denounced by Willughby: "to stretch the labiae vulvae with their hands and fingers, when the throes approached".[91] If we join Willughby in his critical stance, we can castigate such practices as "meddlesome midwifery".[92] But we learn from William Smellie, who routinely used this technique, that it was effective in stimulating the labour-pains.[93] Presumably, then, some midwives had learnt from experience that stretching the mother's labiae enhanced the pains and thus speeded the labour. Of course, there would have been occasions when this did not work, and it was precisely those births to which a practitioner like Willughby might be called. Experiences such as this convinced Willughby that "hauling, with pulling, and stretching their bodies" did "never any good". Or rather, these experiences were part of what convinced him of this; the other source of this learning was the contrasting custom of other midwives, of "keeping the labouring woman warm and quiet", and "desisting from using violence".[94] Thus different midwives used different methods towards the same end: a swift and safe delivery. This was the purpose of the various *birth-postures*, which seem to have varied by region. In the Midlands, it appears that kneeling was the usual posture; in London, midwives used a stool in the mid-seventeenth century (though this subsequently went out of use); in early eighteenth-century Taunton, midwives often delivered women standing up; and in Manchester, the mother would sit in another woman's lap.[95] We also find that midwives had a variety of techniques to *revive* both child and mother if they were in a weak condition after the delivery.[96] (It is notable that these emerged fortuitously in Willughby's case-descriptions; he did not elevate this task into his normative accounts of the midwife's role.) The purpose of all these methods was the comfortable and speedy management of normal birth. And it was this that mattered to mothers – for most births were normal.

Furthermore, the activities of midwives were not restricted to childbirth but extended outwards into a wide and unbounded sphere. To begin with, midwives practised what we now call antenatal care.[97] Sometimes this was occasioned by a

C A P V T II.

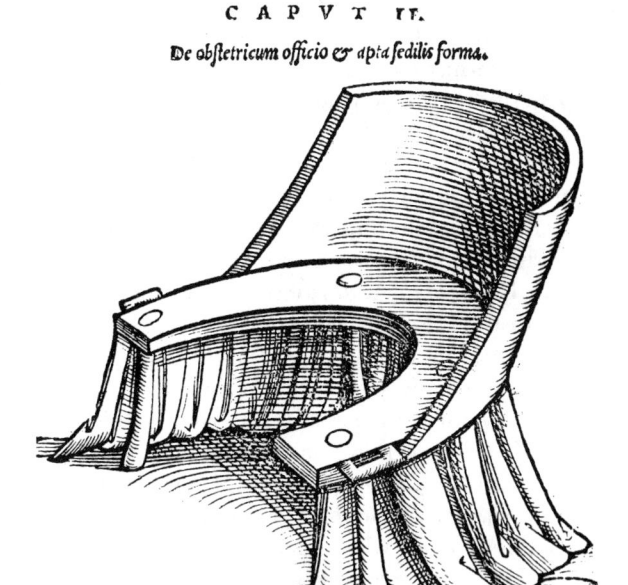

De obstetricum officio & apta sedilis forma.

Figure 3.1 Birth stool (Rueff, De conceptu et generatione hominis, 1554).

problem experienced during pregnancy.[98] In other cases a midwife might be paid by a wealthy mother simply to take care of her during her pregnancy: thus in 1725 Lady Fitzwalter paid a country midwife two guineas for this service, even though the actual delivery was to take place in London.[99] Similarly, gentlewomen and even some mothers of the yeoman class engaged their midwives to reside in the house for some time before the birth itself.[100] Just as the midwife's attendance might begin before birth, so it may also have continued after delivery. Here we lack direct evidence – probably because our usual, male informants were themselves not much engaged in this task, as is true of swaddling. But it is suggestive that Sarah Stone's case-descriptions often include mention of "a good lying-in"; in this respect Mrs Stone may have been intermediate between the typical midwife and the male practitioner.[101] And since the midwife was routinely present at the mother's churching, it seems likely that she would have been visiting the mother, and perhaps supervising the lying-in nurse, during the intervening four weeks.

Beyond this, midwives are known to have practised medicine, surgery and bloodletting. For example, Sarah Seeley of Dalham and Alice Webb of Stradishall (Suffolk), both described in 1716 as practising "bleeding and surgery", in 1723 turned out to be midwives.[102] Other indications suggest that the picture revealed by these fluctuating descriptions was not untypical.[103] Thus in 1668 Dr Whistler referred Bulstrode Whitelocke's wife, still unwell some three months after a suspected miscarriage, to the help of "Mrs Kent the famous midwife".[104] An early eighteenth-century case-history of Daniel Turner's reveals what was probably a very common pattern: his female patient consulted first other women, then a midwife, and finally Turner himself.[105] Hence the fact that in 1709, when Claver Morris "visited Mrs Goold at Sharpham, who was ill of a tertian ague", he found that "Mrs Erney the Shaftesbury midwife was there".[106] This range of healing activities suggests a certain continuity between the humble village midwife and exceptional individuals such as Mary Houlden of Sudbury, Suffolk, who published almanacs for 1688–89 and is described as "midwife, astrologer, and physician for women's diseases", or Elizabeth Blackwell of London, author of the very beautiful *A curious herbal* published in 1737.[107]

Nor were midwives' activities confined to healing, for it seems that in times of great personal distress women reposed a special trust in their midwives. Thus in 1732 Miss Wright of Oxford, driven to distraction both by the death of her six-month-old illegitimate baby and by allegations that she had poisoned the child, ran away to Cowley with the intention of committing suicide. But before she ran off, she "put ten shillings (being what money she had) into the hands of one Mrs Holdship, a midwife".[108] Hence the various indications – from episcopal accusations to the tales in Defoe's *Moll Flanders* – that midwives assisted unmarried mothers to cover up their lapses.[109] Most of the newborn babies left at the London Foundling Hospital, when its doors were opened in the late 1750s, were probably brought not by their mothers but by other people, and it is tempting to speculate that midwives performed this role. Midwives may well have been drawn into helping unmarried mothers, given their general role as supporters of women and the essential continuity between illegitimate and legitimate births.[110] Conversely, midwives were recruited by male institutions for various juridical functions pertaining to women.[111]

The midwife was so important because childbirth itself and the associated ritual were central in women's lives. The popular ceremony of childbirth both reflected and helped to maintain a *collective culture of women*. That culture conferred on the midwife her authority over the birth; conversely, in exercising her office she confirmed and maintained women's collective control over this, the pivotal event in their lives. Moreover, the wide range of midwives' activities puts their low case-loads in a very different light. If the midwife participated in the management of pregnancy and lying-in, then even a midwife with a case-load of, say, 15 births per year would nevertheless have had a more or less continuous burden of responsibilities. In addition, her other healing activities would have augmented both her duties and her income. Adding to this her attendance at baptisms, churchings and the associated festivities, such a midwife was probably busy in one way or another every week of the year. The management of childbirth stood at the centre of her activities, but represented a starting-point rather than a boundary of practice. The midwife was the women's doctor, and perhaps the women's confidante, of early-modern England.

Notes

1. See my "The ceremony of childbirth and its interpretation", in V. Fildes (ed.), *Women as mothers in pre-industrial England: essays in memory of Dorothy McLaren* (London: Routledge, 1990), pp. 68–107, where further documentation is given.
2. See below, at *n*.79 and *n*.98.
3. *OED*, "nidget", verb (2); Josselin, *Diary*, pp. 50, 415, 118; Hearne, *Remarks*, vol. viii, pp. 323–4 (23 January 1724/5, recorded by Hearne on 25 January); D. Vaisey (ed.), *The diary of Thomas Turner 1754–1765* (Oxford: Oxford University Press, 1985), p. 70.
4. See below, at *n*.24. But at Royal births male witnesses were always present, because of the dynastic importance of such deliveries.
5. *OED*, "gossip".
6. See the 1603 woodcut *Tittle-tattle: or, the several branches of gossipping*, cited in V. Pearl, "Change and stability in seventeenth-century London", *The London Journal* 5 (1979), pp. 1–34, plate facing p. 25 (I thank Vivien Brodsky for this reference).
7. N. Culpeper, *A directory for midwives* (1st edn, 1651; London, 1675), p. 119.
8. *OED*, "grace", noun, (21b).
9. *OED*, "midwife".
10. Willughby, *Observations*, pp. 142–5, 226.
11. *OED*, "grace", noun, (21b).
12. J. Lane, "The administration of an eighteenth century Warwickshire parish: Butlers Marston", *Dugdale Society Occasional Papers*, 21 (1973), p. 20; Donnison, *Midwives*, pp. 9–10, 208 (*n*. 66); J. R. Magrath (ed.), *The Flemings in Oxford* (3 vols., Oxford, 1904–24), I, p. 451 and *passim*; R. Trumbach, *The rise of the egalitarian family: aristocratic kinship and domestic relations in eighteenth-century England* (New York: Academic Press, 1980), p. 181; Aveling, *Midwives*, p. 31.
13. C. White, *A treatise on the management of pregnant and lying-in women* (London, 1772), pp. 4–5, 248–9; Willughby, *Observations*, p. 65; Cooke, *Mellificium chirurgiae* (1648 edn), p. 257; M. Thale (ed.), *The autobiography of Francis Place* (Cambridge: Cambridge University Press, 1972), p. 184.
14. *OED*, "caudle" (noun, verb); Giffard, *Cases*, Case 72, p. 169.
15. J. Sharp, *The midwives book* (London, 1671), pp. 372–4; J. Maubray, *The female physician* (London, 1724), p. 327; H. Bracken, *The midwife's companion, or, a treatise of midwifery; wherein the whole art is explained* (London, 1737), pp. 207–8.
16. *OED*, "bed" (noun, 2b, 6c); "bring" (8c); "cry" (verb, 21c); "crying" (noun, 2); "straw" (noun, 2b); "month" (3f, 6).
17. Willughby, *Observations*, p. 212; Giffard, *Cases*, Case 52, p. 117; E. Hobhouse (ed.), *The diary of a West Country physician AD 1684–1726* (London: Simpkin Marshall, 1934), p. 57.
18. Aveling, *Chamberlens*, p. 141; R. Barret, *A companion for midwives, childbearing women, and nurses* (London, 1699); R. Gough, *The history of Myddle*, David Hey (ed.) (Harmondsworth: Penguin, 1981), p. 207; L. Pollock (ed.), *A lasting relationship: parents and children over three centuries* (London, 1987), p. 28.
19. Josselin, *Diary*, p. 503 (the 29th day); and cf. pp. 415–19, 465–6.
20. M. Spufford, *Contrasting communities: English villagers in the sixteenth and seventeenth centuries* (Cambridge: Cambridge University Press, 1974), pp. 254–5.
21. *OED*, "upsitting" (1); Trumbach, *Rise of the egalitarian family*, p. 184; J. J. Cartwright (ed.), *Wentworth Papers 1705–39* (London, 1883), p. 325; Josselin, *Diary*, p. 167; *The good nurse* (London, 1825), pp. 153–5.

22. Hobhouse (ed.), *Diary of a West Country physician*, p. 90 (19 January 1722); Trumbach, *Rise of the egalitarian family*, pp. 184–5; R. C. Matthews & W. Latham (eds), *The diary of Samuel Pepys* (11 volumes; London, 1970–83), viii, pp. 177, 200 (courtesy of Linda Pollock).
23. Blundell quoted in Trumbach, *Rise of the egalitarian family*, p. 178; Josselin, *Diary*, p. 118.
24. *OED*, "gander", 4, and references; M. M. Verney (ed.), *Memoirs of the Verney family* (4 volumes; London: Longmans, 1892–9), vol. III, p. 229 (editor's paraphrase); R. Parkinson (ed.), *The autobiography of Henry Newcome, MA, vol. I* (Chetham Society, *Remains Historical and Literary* 26, 1852), pp. 13, 153.
25. F. Proctor & W. Frere, *A new history of the Book of Common Prayer, with a rationale of its offices* (London, 1905), pp. 638–9.
26. W. P. M. Kennedy, *Elizabethan episcopal administration* (3 volumes; London, 1924), vol. III, pp. 149–50; P. Cunnington & C. Lucas, *Costume for births, marriages and deaths* (London, 1972), p. 18; Hobhouse (ed.), *Diary of a West Country physician*, p. 57.
27. W. M. Campion & W. J. Beaumont (eds), *The Prayer Book interleaved with historical illustrations* (10th edn, London, 1880), p. 219; *OED*, "uprising" (noun, 2c); *Notes and Queries*, 9th series, 2 (1898), pp. 5, 255; 3 (1899), p. 212.
28. Campion & Beaumont, *The Prayer Book interleaved*, p. 188.
29. C. D. Linnell (ed.), "The diary of Benjamin Rogers, Rector of Carlton, 1720–71", *Publications of the Bedfordshire Historical Records Society*, 30 (1950), at p. 32; B. Midi Berry & R. S. Schofield, "Age at baptism in pre-industrial England", *Population Studies* 25 (1971), pp. 453–63.
30. Another indication of this was the word "chrisom". See *OED*, "chrisom"; Campion & Beaumont, *The Prayer Book interleaved*, p. 219; W. E. Tate, *The parish chest: a study of the records of parochial administration in England* (Cambridge: Cambridge University Press, 1969), pp. 59–60; *Local Population Studies*, No. 32 (1984), pp. 62–3, & No. 33, p. 71.
31. R. Paulson, *The art of Hogarth* (London: Phaidon, 1975), plate 14 and discussion; Tate, *The parish chest*, p. 104; W. J. Pressey, "Some seating experiences in Essex churches", *Essex Review* 35 (1926), pp. 1–11, at pp. 8–9; H. M. Moody, "The Monnington letters 1720–25", *Worcestershire Recusant* 3, No. 21 (1973), pp. 8–19, at p. 11; John Beresford (ed.), *The diary of a country parson: the Reverend James Woodforde. Vol. I, 1758–1781* (Oxford: Clarendon, 1924), p. 168.
32. J. Boulton, *Neighbourhood and society: a London suburb in the seventeenth century* (Cambridge, 1987), pp. 276–9; figures from Booth's survey, kindly communicated by Hugh McLeod; J. Cox, *The English churches in a secular society: Lambeth, 1870–1930* (Oxford: Oxford University Press, 1982), pp. 88–9; M. Young & P. Willmott, *Family and kinship in East London*, 3rd edn (Harmondsworth: Penguin, 1986), p. 57.
33. C. Wheatley, *A rational illustration of the Book of Common Prayer of The Church of England* (1st edn, 1710; 4th edn, London, 1722), pp. 519–29.
34. Boulton, *Neighbourhood and society*, pp. 276–9; White, *Management of pregnant and lying-in women* (2nd edn, 1777), Appendix, p. 58; Willughby, *Observations*, p. 120; A. Clark (ed.), *The life and times of Anthony Wood, antiquary, of Oxford, 1632–1695, described by himself* (5 volumes; Oxford, 1891–1900), vol. I, pp. 440, 447, 489–90; Hearne, *Remarks*, vol. IX, p. 146.
35. D. Marshall, *The English poor in the eighteenth century: a study in social and administrative history* (London: Routledge, 1926), p. 210; A. Warne, *Church and society in eighteenth-century Devon* (Newton Abbot, 1969), p. 156.
36. See Ch. 15 below.

NOTES

37. Cartwright (ed.), *Wentworth papers*, p. 325; Hearne, *Remarks*, vol. VI. p. 261.
38. K. Thomas, *Religion and the decline of magic: studies in popular beliefs in seventeenth-century England* (first publ. 1971; Harmondsworth: Penguin, 1978), pp. 42–3; idem, "Women and the Civil War sects", *Past & Present*, No. 13 (1958), p. 43; W. Coster, "Purity, profanity and Puritanism: the churching of women, 1500–1700", in W. J. Sheils & D. Wood (eds), *Women in the church* (Oxford: Blackwell, for the Ecclesiastical History Society, 1990), pp. 377–87. For a more balanced view, see D. Cressy, "Purification, thanksgiving, and the churching of women in post-Reformation England", *Past & Present*, No. 141 (1993), pp. 106–46.
39. Wilson, "The ceremony of childbirth"; E. L. Lipton et al., "Swaddling, a child care practice: historical, cultural and experimental observations", *Paediatrics*, Supplement, 35 (1965), pp. 519–67.
40. See Garrison, *History of medicine*, p. 739.
41. Campion & Beaumont, *The Prayer Book interleaved*, pp. 203–7; P. Higgins, "The reactions of women, with special reference to the women petitioners", in *Politics, religion and the English Civil War*, B. Manning (ed.)(London, 1973), pp. 179–222, esp. 179–82. 203, 211–13; S. M. Okin, "Women and the making of the sentimental family", *Philosophy and public affairs* 11 (1982), pp. 65–88; S. D. Amussen, "Gender, family and the social order, 1560–1725", in *Order and disorder in early-modern England*, J. Stevenson & A. Fletcher (eds) (Cambridge: Cambridge University Press, 1985), pp. 196–217, esp. pp. 197–205.
42. J. H. Baker, *An introduction to English legal history* (2nd edn, London, 1979), pp. 391–407; P. Crawford, "From the woman's view: pre-industrial England, 1500–1750", in *Exploring women's past*, Crawford (ed.) (2nd edn, Sydney, 1984), pp. 49–85; K. Thomas, "The double standard", *Journal of Historical Ideas* 20 (1959), pp. 195–216, esp. pp. 210–16.
43. D. Vaisey (ed.), *The diary of Thomas Turner 1754–1765* (Oxford: Oxford University Press, 1985), p. 70.
44. Thomas, *Religion and the decline of magic*, pp. 68–9.
45. A. Fraser, *The weaker vessel: woman's lot in seventeenth century England* (2nd edn, London, 1985), pp. 511–12.
46. Quoted in M. Roberts, "'Words they are women, and deeds they are men': images of work and gender in early-modern England", in *Women and work in pre-industrial England*, L. Charles & L. Duffin (eds) (London: Croom Helm, 1985), pp. 154–5.
47. See D. N. Harley, "Ignorant midwives – a persistent stereotype", *Bulletin of the Society for the Social History of Medicine*, No. 28 (1981), pp. 6–9, and the following valuable essays in Marland, *Art of midwifery*: D. Evenden, "Mothers and their midwives in seventeenth-century London" (pp. 9–26); D. Harley, "Provincial midwives in England: Lancashire and Cheshire, 1660–1760" (pp. 27–48); A. G. Hess, "Midwifery practice amongst the Quakers in southern rural England in the late seventeenth century" (pp. 49–76); H. King, "The politick midwife: models of midwifery in the work of Elizabeth Cellier" (pp. 115–30).
48. For example, Eleanor Willughby (fl. 1654–62), Hannah Brancker (fl. 1679–99), George Ballard's sister (1730), Mary West of Blackburn (1747), Margaret Strettell, Hannah Sutton of Knutsford (1760). See Willughby, *Observations*, pp. 119, 130, 134–7 and Wilson, *Childbirth*, Appendix E; Harley, "Provincial midwives", pp. 32–4; Hearne, *Remarks*, vol. X, p. 320, 21 August 1730.
49. Eleanor Willughby practised between the ages of 17 and 22; one midwife at Norwich applied for a licence at the age of 73; two midwives in their eighties applied for licences in Restoration London. NNRO, TES/8, file I, item 60; T. R. Forbes, *The midwife and the witch*

(New Haven, Conn.: Yale University Press, 1966), p. 153. Cf. Willughby, *Observations*, pp. 8, 30, 72, 73 (young midwives), 24, 134, 135, 172 (old midwives). For an indication that "an elderly woman" was sometimes preferred see Stone, *Complete practice*, Observation II.

50. For some wealthy midwives (1662) see Harley, Provincial midwives, pp. 31–2. Two examples of poor midwives from Norwich testimonials: Elizabeth Barber of Acle, widow, 1693, "so poor that she was never able to purchase a licence"; Jane Crome of Northelmham, 1703, who has "ver[y little] or nothing else to maintain herself and her poor children withal" (NNRO, TES/8, file I, items 60, 229).
51. Harley, Ignorant midwives, p. 8; T. R. Forbes, "The regulation of English midwives in the sixteenth and seventeenth centuries", *Medical History* 8 (1964), pp. 235–44, at p. 242.
52. M. Spufford, *Small books and pleasant histories: popular fiction and its readership in seventeenth-century England* (Cambridge: Cambridge University Press, 1981), pp. 19–44.
53. Donnison, *Midwives*, p. 14; Willughby, *Observations*, p. 2.
54. P. Earle, "The female labour market in London in the late seventeenth and early eighteenth centuries", *Economic History Review*, 2nd series, 42 (1989), pp. 328–53, at p. 343; Harley, Provincial midwives, p. 34.
55. Willughby, *Observations*, p. 126 (cf. pp. 44, 151, 156); Giffard, *Cases*, pp. 305–6.
56. NNRO, VSB/3, comperta process for Clare, 1723. Mrs Marlton had been licensed on May 3 1710 (VSC/6, 1723 book, p. 303).
57. Hearne, *Remarks*, vol. IX, pp. 375–6 (28 & 30 November 1727). Hearne also knew of two other Oxford midwives: Mrs Holdship (*ibid.*, vol. XI, pp. 90–1, cf. below) and Mrs Tredwell (vol. VIII, p. 377).
58. For a much later individual instance (Nanny Holland, c.1830s) see M. E. Fissell, *Patients, power and the poor in eighteenth-century Bristol* (Cambridge: Cambridge University Press, 1991), p. 40. I thank Mary Fissell for drawing my attention to this story.
59. See David Harley, "Historians as demonologists: the myth of the midwife-witch", *Social History of Medicine* 3 (1990), pp. 1–26.
60. NNRO, TES/8, file I, item 203, 20 October 1702, endorsed "Fiat Licentia" on the same day.
61. Willughby, *Observations*, p. 72.
62. J. Hitchcock, A sixteenth-century midwife's license, *Bulletin of the History of Medicine* 41 (1967), pp. 75–6; Aveling, *Chamberlens*, p. 37; Willughby, *Observations*, p. 73; Donnison, *Midwives*, pp. 229–31; Aveling, *Midwives*, pp. 76–82. The deputy system seems to have disappeared by 1736, since it was not mentioned by John Douglas (see Ch. 8).
63. Donnison, *Midwives*, p. 8.
64. Harley, Provincial midwives, pp. 28–9; Stone, *Complete practice*, pp. xxi, 148.
65. Hearne, *Remarks*, vol. X, p. 320, 21 August 1730; G. Ballard, *Memoirs of several ladies of Great Britain* (Oxford, 1752); see *DNB* and Todd, *Women writers*, pp. xvii, xxi.
66. Systematic assessment of its frequency would require large-scale identification of midwives across two generations (which we are unlikely to find), together with nominal record-linkage complicated by the problem that female surnames changed on marriage.
67. Ch. 4 below.
68. Aveling, *Chamberlens*, pp. 20–6 (and see pp. 36, 44, 45), 34–60; Clark, *College of Physicians*, i, pp. 236–8, 253–4; Aveling, *Midwives*, pp. 76–82; King, The politick midwife.
69. Wilson, *Childbirth*, Chs 3 & 4.
70. Evenden, Mothers and their midwives; Donnison, *Midwives*, p. 22; WIHM, Haggis MSS. For some other examples see CUL, EDR, G1/11 (Ely, 1733); Harley, Provincial midwives, pp. 32, 36 (Chester, 1776); Wilson, *Childbirth*, Ch. 4 (Norwich, 1791).
71. Harley, Provincial midwives, p. 31.

NOTES

72. See Aveling, *Chamberlens*, pp. 49–59 (Dr Peter Chamberlen's *A voice in Rhama*, 1647); Aveling, *Midwives*, pp. 76–82 (Mrs Cellier).
73. See Evenden, Mothers and their midwives, pp. 13, 21 and *passim* (who interprets this differently).
74. Willughby, *Observations*; Chapman, *Essay* (1733); Giffard, *Cases*; Stone, *Complete practice*; H. Bracken, *The midwife's companion, or, a treatise of midwifery; wherein the whole art is explained* (London 1737)
75. Cf. Evenden, Mothers and their midwives, pp. 22–3.
76. Ch. 2 above. If 2.5% of births were difficult, then a mother who had seven deliveries had a chance of better than 83% that all of these were normal.
77. Wilson, *Childbirth*, Ch. 5.
78. Assuming 10,000 settlements and two midwives to every three settlements, we reach 6667 midwives. Starting from 160,000 births per year in 1700, allowing one-third of these to take place in towns, and assuming case-loads of 20 (rural) and 50 (urban) births per midwife per year, we arrive at 6400 midwives.
79. Josselin, *Diary*, p. 415.
80. If births were evenly spaced throughout the year, a midwife who attended just 23 births per year would each year have a 50% chance that two mothers fell into labour on the same day: see M. R. Spiegel, *Theory and problems of probability and statistics* (New York: McGraw-Hill, 1975), p. 31. The rate of practice associated with a 50% annual chance of "overlap" will have been even less than 23 per year, since births were more frequent in the midwife's busy period around March than in the slack season around August (see E. A. Wrigley & R. S. Schofield, *The population history of England: a reconstruction* (1981), pp. 286–93).
81. C. G. Clay, *Economic expansion and social change: England, 1500–1700* (2 volumes; Cambridge, 1984), vol. I, pp. 20, 169.
82. In the six years 1669–74, this midwife attended 52, 53, 67, 82, 89 and 73 births (median 70, mean 69.3): Cumbria Record Office, Kendal midwife's account-book, 1665–75, *passim*. I thank the archivist for a photocopy and Ann Hess for a transcript of this document.
83. Stone, *Complete practice*, p. 139.
84. When she died in 1767, it was recorded that Mrs Hopkins had "during the space of forty-five years past, delivered upwards of 10,000 women, with the greatest success, and is therefore greatly lamented by all who knew her": *Adams's Weekly Courant*, 9 June 1767, cited by C. Morsley, *News from the English countryside 1750–1850* (London: Harrap. 1979), p. 60. Mrs Crewe died in 1817, and her tombstone recorded that in 40 years she had delivered 9730 children: Donnison, *Midwives*, p. 60 & p. 212 n. 82.
85. Letter from Dr Allen of Bridgwater to Mr Stone, in Stone, *Complete practice*, p. xxi. According to the *1801 Census* Bridgwater had 86 baptisms in 1730 and 89 in 1740, suggesting perhaps 90–105 births per year depending on the degree of Nonconformity.
86. Wilson, *Childbirth*, Table 5.1.5.
87. *Ibid.*, p. 107; NNRO, VIS/11–19.
88. London births in the 1680s can be estimated at 16,237 per year, using evidence from Wrigley & Schofield, *Population history*, Tables 3.7 & 5.25; see Wilson, *Childbirth*, n.54 to Ch. 5. For Mrs Cellier's scheme see Aveling, *Midwives*, pp. 76–82 (deputies, p. 80).
89. The midwife attended 676 deliveries in these 30 years: Evenden, "Mothers and their midwives", pp. 11–12, 14.
90. Willughby, *Observations*, p. 143; Bracken, *The midwife's companion*, pp. 207–8.
91. Willughby, *Observations*, p. 6.

92. E. Shorter, The management of normal deliveries and the generation of William Hunter, in *William Hunter*, Bynum & Porter (eds), pp. 371–83, at pp. 372, 374–6.
93. McClintock, *Smellie's midwifery*, Cases 230, 231, 235, 236, 246, 257, 264, 266, 269, 270, 271, 273. By 1750 Smellie began to be critical of this practice, but he was still using it occasionally (Cases 226, 265).
94. Willughby, *Observations*, p. 6.
95. Kneeling: Willughby, *Observations*, pp. 133, 160. London birth-stools and their decline: *ibid.*, pp. 8, 10, 71, 73–4; Cooke, *Mellificium chirurgiae* (1685 edn), pp. 166, 255; McClintock, *Smellie's midwifery*, vol. I, p. 200; Hunter, lectures, p. 90. Standing: Stone, *Complete practice*, p. 55. Sitting in a woman's lap: White, *Management of pregnant and lying-in women*, pp. 285–306, Cases 8, 9, 11–14 (cf. Willughby, *Observations*, pp. 71, 133, 224).
96. Revival of the child: Willughby, *Observations*, pp. 40, 66, 82 (but contrast p. 186); Cooke, *Mellificium chirurgiae*, 1685 edn, p. 167; N. Culpeper, *A directory for midwives* (London, 1651), p. 176; Donnison, *Midwives*, p. 50 (Mrs Ann Newby); Bracken, *The midwife's companion*, p. 207. Revival of the mother: Willughby, *Observations*, pp. 49, 234, 256.
97. L. Pollock suggests that this was unusual: "Embarking on a rough passage: the experience of pregnancy in early-modern society", in *Women as mothers in pre-industrial England: essays in memory of Dorothy McLaren*, Valerie Fildes (ed.) (London: Routledge, 1990), pp. 39–67, at p. 52. But many antenatal consultations with the midwife surely went undocumented.
98. Willughby, *Observations*, pp. 184 (two examples), 197; Giffard, *Cases*, Cases 184–6; and for indirect evidence see Stone, *Complete practice*, p. xviii; Sir Richard Manningham, *An abstract of midwifery for use in the lying-in infirmary* (London, 1744), p. 32 (cf. Ch. 9 below).
99. R. Trumbach, *The aristocratic family in England, 1690–1780. Studies in childhood and kinship* (PhD thesis, Johns Hopkins, 1972), p. 31.
100. Willughby, *Observations*, pp. 162, 266.
101. Stone, *Complete practice*, e.g. pp. 29, 32, 43; and see Ch. 5 below.
102. NNRO, VSB/2, 1716 process for Clare (bound up in the book as an example), VIS/13 (1723 process for Clare).
103. Cf. Harley, Provincial midwives, p. 29; C. Goodall, *The College of Physicians . . . established by law* (London, 1684), pp. 421–2; Willughby, *Observations*, pp. 55–6, 153–6, 203, 224; Gough, *History of Myddle*, pp. 172–3.
104. R. Spalding (ed.), *The diary of Bulstrode Whitelocke 1605–1675* (British Academy: Records of Social and Economic History, New Series, XIII; Oxford University Press, 1990), p. 733 (September 1668). This was doubtless Frances Kent of Reading, for whom see Hess, Midwifery practice amongst the Quakers, pp. 64–7.
105. D. Turner, *The art of surgery* (2nd edn; London, 1725), vol. II, p. 419.
106. Hobhouse (ed.), *Diary of a West Country physician*, p. 56.
107. B. Capp, *Astrology and the popular press* (London: Faber, 1979), p. 313. See also *ibid.*, p. 323 for Dorothy Partridge, perhaps pseudonymous, midwife and almanac-writer of 1694. Mrs Blackwell, who called Smellie on at least one occasion, was one of the subscribers to Ballard, *Memoirs of several ladies of Great Britain*. She is in *DNB* (as are her husband Alexander, his brother Thomas and his father Thomas), and is discussed by Donnison, *Midwives*, p. 209 *n*.68; Aveling, *Midwives*, pp. 113–14; and A. Calder-Marshall, *The grand century of the lady* (London: Gordon and Cremonesi, 1976), p. 100.
108. Hearne, *Remarks*, vol. XI, pp. 90–1 (1 August 1732); cf. A.C. Underwood, *A history of the English Baptists* (London: Baptist Union/Kingsgate Press, 1947), pp. 99–100.

NOTES

109. *Second report of the commissioners appointed to inquire into the rubrics, orders, and directions for regulating the course and conduct of public worship, &c.* (London: HMSO, 1868), Appendix E, p. 517; Donnison, *Midwives*, p. 34; Harley, Provincial midwives, p. 41.
110. A. Wilson, "Illegitimacy and its implications in mid-eighteenth-century London: the evidence of the Foundling Hospital", *Continuity & Change* 4:1 (1989), pp. 103–64.
111. Harley, "Provincial midwives", pp. 40–1; H. C. Johnson & N. J. Williams (eds), *Warwick County Records Volume IX: Quarter Sessions records Easter, 1690, to Michaelmas, 1696* (Warwick, 1964), pp. 42, 43; G. R. Quaife, *Wanton wenches and wayward wives: peasants and illicit sex in early seventeenth century England* (London: Croom Helm, 1979), pp. 89–90; G. Keynes, *The life of William Harvey* (Oxford: Clarendon, 1966), pp. 209–10.

Chapter Four
Traditional obstetric surgery

We know that some seventeenth-century medical men practised, as Willughby put it, "in the midwife's bed". Such men were usually called "surgeons", rather than "men-midwives", and this tends to conceal their obstetric practice. Indeed, we usually become aware of it only through some public initiative, such as an original midwifery treatise – and such initiatives were few and far between before the 1730s. As a result, male practice of midwifery appears at first sight to have been exceptional in the seventeenth century. Yet this appearance is deceptive, for we shall see that midwifery was a routine part of seventeenth-century surgery – along with such other staples as bloodletting, curing wounds, drawing teeth, bonesetting, and healing venereal disease. But what then was the nature of this obstetric practice? Given the exclusively female childbirth ritual, how did male practitioners come to attend deliveries at all? How often did this take place? What were its occasions? What did these men do, and what were they expected to do, once summoned? Our most detailed evidence is supplied by the cases Willughby recorded, arising from his practice in Derby between about 1630 and 1670, with short stays in Stafford (1654–56) and London (1656–60). Other, more patchy indications, such as the handful of cases in James Cooke's *Mellificium chirurgiae*, confirm that Willughby's practice was characteristic of his day, and early eighteenth-century writings suggest that this style of practice remained typical until around 1720.[1]

Male paths to childbirth

With very rare exceptions, seventeenth-century male practitioners only attended childbirth *as an adjunct to the midwife*. Willughby acted in lieu of a midwife for only three mothers, all exceptional individuals;[2] and all other accounts of birth, for instance from diaries, took it for granted that the mother would be delivered by a midwife, not by a male practitioner.[3] This applies at every social level, all the way up to Royal births: for instance, on 10 June 1688 it was Judith Wilkes who delivered Mary of Modena of the boy James Francis Edward Stuart, whom some were later to call James III of England.[4] Thus we shall not err very far if we assume that whenever a male practitioner attended a birth, a midwife was there as well.

Nevertheless, male practice took a variety of forms, for medical men were called to childbirth by some five different "paths", distinguished by the timing of the call and by whether it had been anticipated.[5] In the dimension of timing we can distinguish three types of call. In an *advance* call, the practitioner was summoned by the mother to reside in her house at some stage of her pregnancy, to advise her on her diet and course of life, to remain until the birth itself, to be in attendance during the birth, and to continue for some time afterwards to supervise her recovery. An *onset* call summoned the practitioner to the delivery as soon as labour commenced; this was only practicable if he lived reasonably near. In each of these cases, the male practitioner was initially at one remove from the birth itself; a further, subsidiary "call" was required to bring him into the lying-in chamber. Thirdly, an *emergency* call sent for him only after some serious difficulty had arisen.

The dimension of anticipation involved a distinction between *booked* and *unbooked* calls. The male practitioner could be "engaged" or "bespoke" for attendance, and this comprised a booked call; if there had been no such prior arrangement, the call was unbooked.[6] All advance calls were by definition booked; onset and emergency calls, by contrast, could be either booked or unbooked. The booking amounted to an engagement to attend on the due summons, and that summons could itself be of the onset or emergency type. The effect of such an engagement was probably that the practitioner had to refuse all other calls, except emergencies close to hand. Some of these paths mirrored the different ways in which midwives were called. Wealthy mothers often had their midwives staying in the house before the birth (advance calls); most mothers probably booked the midwife and sent for her when the labour-pains began (booked onset calls); if difficulty arose a second midwife could be summoned, and indeed a third and even a fourth midwife (unbooked emergency calls).[7]

Just as important as the type of call was *who made* the call, and *why* they did so. It seems that advance and onset calls came from mothers, although the process of booking also involved their husbands; while the subsidiary call into the lying-in chamber, if this came at all, might be made by the midwife. Emergency calls could come from a wide variety of agents: the mother herself; her husband; the midwife; the attending gossips; and combinations of these, such as the mother and her husband, or "all the women". As to the reasons for calling the male practitioner, we shall see below that this was occasioned by difficulty, or expected difficulty, in the birth.

The various calls came to different extents from different social classes, and commanded different payments. Advance calls could only be made by mothers of the gentry or merchant classes, who had the large houses required for entertaining the male practitioner as a living-in guest. Again, advance calls must have earned very large payments, since they tied the practitioner down; in theory, he was not permitted to accept any other engagement, although leave might be granted to answer an emergency call or to attend from its onset the delivery of a regular patient. Onset calls came from a slightly wider circle of patients – the "semi-gentry" or wives of clergymen and professionals as well as the gentry – while emergency calls took the male practitioner to mothers of all social classes. Prior booking, which was usually made by wealthy mothers or by their husbands, probably enhanced the payment.[8] In addition, payments were probably conditioned by the wealth of the patient, and by the practitioner's reputation. Advance calls probably commanded tens of pounds, onset calls one or a few pounds or guineas, and emergency calls perhaps a pound or less. On some occasions, particularly emergency calls, a practitioner might give his services free of charge.

Most seventeenth-century male practice in midwifery consisted of emergency calls. For example, over 70% of the cases Willughby included in his "Observations" were of this type, and in this respect those cases were probably representative of his practice.[9] Since emergency calls were occasioned by difficulty in the delivery, this means that most of Willughby's experience concerned difficult births. Moreover, even advance and onset- calls were also associated with difficulty. To begin with, such calls were only made by mothers who had previously experienced troubles in childbirth, or who anticipated difficulty with the birth ahead. For example one "Lady", a "kinswoman" of Willughby's, had previously had serious troubles with the afterbirth; Mrs Clark had had epilepsy since childhood; Mrs Hoden of Aston "being in a consumption, and short-winded, through weakness, had her neck and body distorted"; Judith Ward had "a narrow passage". Correspondingly, no male practitioner was involved in any of the 42 deliveries collectively recorded by the four diarists Thornton, Josselin, Fleming and Whitelocke.[10] Further, when it came to the delivery, Willughby was only called to help if difficulty arose: he would usually wait in a nearby room, and if the birth went smoothly both he and the mother left the delivery entirely to the midwife. As a result, his practice was overwhelmingly concentrated upon difficult births.

The horizon of male practice

Emergency calls – the dominant form of male practice – were constrained by the profile of difficult births and by the suite of available techniques. We saw in Chapter 2, from eighteenth-century evidence, that by far the commonest source of difficulty was an obstructed birth by the head, and the same was true for Willughby in the 1660s.[11] The established technique for delivering such a birth was craniotomy, usually with the sharp hook or crotchet. Thus all that the male practitioner could usually do was to deliver a dead child. Hence the fact that in Willughby's experience, most emergency calls came only after the child had died – typically not until three to four days after the onset of labour, and sometimes after even longer delays. *The surgeon was called to save the mother – not the child.* While these long delays were centrally occasioned by obstructed births by the head and by the associated technique of craniotomy, emergencies of other kinds produced similar delays and were again only made after the child had died, or was thought to have died – or, in the case of bleeding, when the mother was at death's door. And the less detailed evidence emanating from other practitioners confirms that in these respects Willughby's practice was typical. For instance, Cooke, who practised in and around Warwick at about the same period as Willughby was working in Derby, routinely performed obstetric surgery as part of a wider surgical practice. The chief part of his obstetric work was the delivery of a dead child in obstructed births by the head, and he, like Willughby, was sometimes called several days after the child had died.[12]

The reason for these long delays was something Willughby rarely mentioned, yet which was probably at work in all the difficult births to which he was called: fear of the male practitioner, and dread of the operation of craniotomy.[13] For that operation must have been truly horrendous to a mother. It invaded her body; it destroyed her child; and since it was only used when the child was already dead or as a last resort to save her own life, she must have already been close to death and must have known this. Thus women were terrified of craniotomy, and they expressed that fear by delaying for as long as possible before sending for the surgeon. As Cooke observed,

> I shall conclude this dreadful operation with that saying of Sennertus
> ... which amounts to this, that women will seldom or never admit of
> these operations, but rather submit the business to God, and Nature.

Cooke's gloss on Daniel Sennert is not to be taken literally, for this would mean that surgeons like Willughby and himself never had to use their craniotomy instruments. In fact his own cases make it clear that such operations were routine for him just as for Willughby; indeed, after describing one such delivery, Cooke added 'Were it not to swell the book, I could multiply observations'. Rather, his remark confirms that although surgeons were called to use the crotchet, this was with extreme reluctance and dread on the part of mothers.[14] But this means that mothers' fears effectively conspired with the material circumstances – the bodily processes of birth, the prevailing arrangements for its management, and the available technology – to produce a *self-perpetuating system*. Long delays ensured that the child was usually dead before the surgeon was called, which reinforced the practical dominance of craniotomy.

Thus, contrary to what many historians have supposed, mothers were not afraid of childbirth in general: rather, they were afraid of *calling the male practi-*

tioner. As I have shown in detail elsewhere, the best-documented series of births suggest that maternal fear was in fact unusual and arose specifically when the birth became difficult. Alice Thornton's autobiography mentioned fear in only two of her seven pregnancies; Jane Josselin's attitude, in the eight pregnancies reported by her husband Ralph, was usually "cheerful"; Daniel Fleming recorded 12 of his wife's deliveries, never suggesting that she was afraid.[15] And just once in 15 recorded pregnancies (of three wives) did Bulstrode Whitelocke write that his wife was "full of pain and fears" – illustrating the fact that in pregnancy just as in delivery, fear was occasioned by troublesome symptoms, not by childbearing itself.[16]

After some three days of difficult labour, the mother, midwife and gossips gave up hope for the child. A few midwives would thereupon deliver the child with makeshift instruments; but the usual course of action in such cases was to summon a male practitioner to remove the child.[17] Nevertheless, contrary to the women's belief, the child might still be alive, as Willughby and Cooke sometimes found on such occasions – but this did not mean that they could save the child. If the difficulty arose from a malpresentation they could deliver the child alive by turning it to the feet. But this was seldom possible in obstructed births by the head, for the child's head was usually so far advanced in the bony passage that turning to the feet was impracticable. Indeed, even Willughby – who extolled delivery by the feet in "all difficult and cross births" – in fact saved only a few children presenting by the head by this method.[18] Precisely because the call had come so late, craniotomy was generally the only way to deliver, even when the child was still alive. In such a case everyone concerned – mother, husband, midwife, gossips, surgeon – was faced with a severe ethical dilemma; and this could occasion conflict between the different parties. Such conflict might be resolved by waiting still further until all were agreed that the child had died. Or the surgeon might consult a local minister of religion as to whether the child could be sacrificed to save the mother's life. Only with this sanction, and with the further agreement of all present, did Willughby use the crotchet on a living child.[19] Cooke may have been more sanguine, since he twice managed to deliver a living child with the crotchet – fixing the instrument "slightly into the skull" in a case near Warwick, "in the lesser corner of the eye" in a delivery at Church Wotton. But this was a rare and exceptional achievement, which he attained only twice in some 40 years' practice.[20] Thus whenever the child was alive – or possibly alive – and the mother's life was in danger, a difficult ethical decision was required, for which it seems that there was no guidance in law. Such decisions were always made collectively, generally by the women who ran the birth.

In advance and onset calls, the male practitioner had much earlier access to the delivery. But although difficulty had usually been expected, which is why he was present, such births usually turned out to be normal, and were therefore delivered by the midwife. Thus these calls reinforced the pattern that normal births were the midwife's business, not the man's; and Willughby shared this attitude with his patients. For example, in the delivery of Lady Broughton in 1648, his contribution ("rewarded with gold") was simply to advise the mother to resist for as long as possible the midwife's endeavours to deliver her. As soon as "labour came upon her", Willughby "went forth of the room, putting her under the midwife's hands": the labour-pains were the signal for him to relinquish control to the midwife.[21] Correspondingly, he was only asked to intervene when difficulty occurred, and he himself deferred acting until the last possible minute. Thus in a case of around 1666 he delivered Judith Ward by turning the child, but only after "she had suffered above twenty-four hours in extremity, and ... all hopes of delivery by a natural and usual way were extinct".[22]

In this light we can begin to understand Willughby's seemingly paradoxical attitudes towards midwives. For while he held a low opinion of most midwives' technical capacities, he also had a fundamental respect for the midwife's office.[23] If the existing midwife was all too often deficient, this was a contingent problem, to be redressed by instruction. It was for precisely this reason that Willughby's wrote his "Observations" in the 1660s and his "Opusculum" in 1671; that he voiced a "hearty wish that some public good order might be made for the better educating of all, especially the younger midwives"; and that a few years later he begged the Countess of Huntingdon to translate into English the *Observations Diverses* of Louise Bourgeois.[24] Knowing as he did that *some* midwives were skilled and judicious – he acknowledged that he had learnt a lot from them – he wanted *all* midwives to be brought to this condition, by "persuasion", "entreaty", education. The corollary was that the role of the male practitioner was strictly limited. "Let her not be too hasty to send for a young chirurgion", he enjoined the midwife: the male practitioner was to be kept at arm's length, and his own master-method, turning to the feet, should become the possession of midwives.[25] The only specifically male preserves were to write prescriptions and to perform craniotomy – and even these boundaries Willughby broke, incorporating many prescriptions in his treatise and inserting (though with great reluctance) detailed instructions on the use of the crotchet.[26] These views were underlined by Willughby's scornful and critical attitude to "men-midwives". His use of the term was always hostile, and referred specifically to those rare occasions when men transgressed what he regarded as the legitimate bounds of their practice – by being called when there was no real emergency; by using instruments covertly; by practising obstetric surgery without the necessary training.[27] The role of the male practitioner was to deliver a dead child, usually with the crotchet, which required a surgical training, whereas the technique of turning the child belonged to midwives, precisely because this permitted a live birth.

Willughby's experiences were characteristic of traditional obstetric surgery. Confirmation that obstetric surgery was routine, and that this consisted chiefly of the delivery of a dead child with instruments, comes from surgical textbooks – most notably Cooke's *Mellificium chirurgiae*, the standard text of the late seventeenth century, which went through six editions between 1648 and 1717.[28] In this respect English authors were in line with their Continental predecessors, such as Ambroise Paré, Pierre Franco, Daniel Sennert, Wilhelm Fabry von Hilden and

Johannes Scultetus – all of whom treated the delivery of a dead child simply as one of the many tasks of the surgeon. The routine presence of obstetric surgery in textbooks reflected practical reality; Willughby in Derby and Cooke in Warwick were merely the most visible of some dozens of such men. Within a 10-mile radius of Derby there took place about 1000 births per year, and it was the 20 or so difficult births among these that created the demand for Willughby's emergency practice. Much the same situation prevailed throughout the kingdom. Thus most county towns probably had at least one resident practitioner who practised along similar lines to Cooke and Willughby, combining obstetric surgery with other forms of medical and surgical practice, and some market towns had them as well. For example, around 1700 we can identify such men not only at Canterbury, Kent (Dr Peters, "very famous for his skill" in managing difficult births) and Norwich (Charles Hacon), but also at Braintree, Essex (the prominent apothecary Samuel Dale) and Woodbridge, Suffolk (Benjamin Freeman, whose testimonial for a licence included a tribute from a midwife to his skill in delivering "an extraordinary difficult case as can be found").[29] All these men were described by the conventional labels – as physicians, apothecaries, or especially surgeons; it is only a chance item of information that tells us that midwifery was part of their practice. And whenever we have any information about such men's practice, we find that it was bounded by the same horizon as prevailed for Willughby and Cooke. The normal birth of a living child, comprising the vast majority of deliveries, was the province of the midwife; the surgeon's task was the delivery of a dead child in the tiny minority of difficult births.

The horizon transcended: the Chamberlen family

Nevertheless, this horizon was transcended, in seventeenth-century London, by a small group of male practitioners – the Chamberlen family. And the usual boundary between female and male forms of practice was crossed by one early eighteenth-century midwife – Sarah Stone. We must now consider these important exceptions to the prevailing rule.

From before 1620 until around 1730 members of the Chamberlen family were known in London as practitioners of midwifery.[30] They spanned four generations: the brothers Peter I and Peter II, who were surgeons; Peter II's son, Dr Peter, who was a physician; three of his sons, of whom the best known was Hugh (we shall call him Hugh I); and Hugh I's son, Hugh II, together with his two cousins the Walker brothers – Middleton Walker, who practised in London, and (probably) Chamberlen Walker, who practised in Dublin.[31] This continuity was no accident, for the Chamberlens passed their methods on from one generation to the next.[32] They were by no means the only male midwifery practitioners in the capital: others included John Nowell around 1600, James Blackbourne in 1612, a Mr Doughton around the same time, Nicholas Downing in 1635, a Mr Boudin around 1658, Sir John Hinton from 1633 until his death in 1682, Robert Barret in the 1690s, and a Dr Johnson in 1702.[33] But the Chamberlens were consistently the most prominent of such practitioners, and from an early stage they claimed a special expertise. Thus, as we have seen, Peter II attempted to create an incorporation of London midwives in 1617, and his son, Dr Peter, repeated this initiative in 1634; and from time to time the Chamberlens were referred to as "men-midwives" – in the seventeenth century a very unusual description.[34]

In 1673, about halfway through the family's long practising life, their special skill was asserted more explicitly. For in that year Hugh I announced that in the case of "a child that comes right, and yet because of some difficulty or disproportion cannot pass" (i.e. an obstructed birth by the head) his family had "long practised a way to deliver women . . . without any prejudice to them or their infants; tho all others . . . do, and must endanger, if not destroy one or both with hooks". That is, Hugh was claiming that he and his family – alone in Europe – could deliver a *living* child in such cases. The use of "hooks", he explained,

> has much caused the report, that where a man comes, one or both must necessarily die; and is the reason of forbearing to send, till the child is dead, or the mother dying. But I can neither approve of that practice, nor those delays

– since his family's method enabled the child's life to be saved. He went on

> to offer an apology for not publishing the secret I mention we have to extract children without hooks, where other artists use them, viz. there being my father and two brothers living, that practise this art, I cannot esteem it my own to dispose of, nor publish it without injury to them.

This claim, which Chamberlen made in the preface to his English translation of François Mauriceau's *Traité des maladies des femmes grosses*, was the first suggestion that the horizon of traditional obstetric surgery could be transcended.[35] A few years later, probably in 1678, either Hugh or his father, Dr Peter Chamberlen (1601–83), put forward to the Crown a proposal

> to prevent the loss of 2,100 or more children yearly, who are calculated to be destroyed at birth by want of medical aid, by confiding his particular secret to two or more discreet persons in each county of England and Wales: the King being supposed to lose £10 by the loss of each subject and the public 100 times as much.[36]

But nothing came of this, nor of a subsequent petition by Hugh in 1687 to the College of Physicians for "a patent relating to midwifery". Although his translation of Mauriceau achieved some success (it was reprinted in 1683), the claim he made in his preface seems to have attracted little or no interest at this time.[37] Nor was it clear whether the Chamberlen family's alleged secret method was manual or instrumental.

Moreover, in 1694 there emerged, in Mauriceau's own *Observations*, a story which cast grave doubt upon Hugh's claim. Mauriceau now revealed that Hugh had visited Paris in 1670 – that is, three years before translating Mauriceau's *Traité* and proclaiming his family's secret. And while in Paris, "boasting that he could deliver the most desperate and abandoned cases in less than half a quarter-hour, he had ... proposed to the King's premier physician that if he were given ten thousand crowns in reward, he would communicate his pretended secret". After Hugh had spent six months in the French capital, Mauriceau (whom the king's physician had doubtless consulted over Hugh's approach) had found a suitable test for his claims. He offered him the opportunity to deliver

> a tiny woman aged 38 years, who had been in labour of her first child for eight days ... [The child] came head first, but the face upwards, [and] stayed always in the same place, without advancing in the passage. [The mother] ... had such a narrow passage ... and the sacral bone [was] so curved on the inside, that it was quite impossible for me to introduce my hand to deliver her, although my hand is small enough.[38]

Mauriceau himself had already "declared the impossibility of delivering this woman", who evidently had a severely rachitic pelvis. Hugh Chamberlen boasted that he could effect the delivery; but he failed in the attempt, and this put paid to his claims in Paris. (In using his translation of Mauriceau as the vehicle for announcing his family secret three years later, Hugh was perhaps wreaking a subtle revenge on Mauriceau for aborting his approach to the French court. Mauriceau's account of the case 20 years later was a delayed riposte.)

Had this anecdote been available in English it could have served as a perfect counter to Hugh's earlier claim. But in fact no such counter was needed, for in all probability few people believed him. His readers doubtless saw it as self-advertisement, of a familiar kind: the alleged possession of secret remedies was a standard method of medical self-promotion. Moreover, in the 1690s Hugh I became a notorious figure for quite other reasons, and this may have damaged his credibility. Having been brought up as a Baptist, he had naturally been among the Whigs when the Exclusion Crisis split the political nation in 1679; indeed, in 1685 he joined Monmouth's ill-fated rebellion.[39] But he was not among those Whigs who prospered politically under William and Mary; for his solution to the growing problem of public credit was to promote a Land Bank, and he did not accept the victory in 1695 of the alternative scheme, the Bank of England.[40] This drove him first into clandestine opposition, and then into political exile – first to Scotland in 1700, then in 1705 to the Dutch Republic (where he died, at an advanced age, around 1720).[41] Perhaps Hugh I's political notoriety helps to explain the fact that his obstetric claim had still attracted no comment as late as 1730, even though five further editions of his translation of Mauriceau appeared, complete with his preface, between 1697 and 1727.

Meanwhile the family practice of midwifery had passed to Hugh I's son, Hugh II (c.1664–1728), and to his cousin Middleton Walker. Hugh II never went into print on the subject of midwifery; he was perhaps content to let some readers think that he, rather than his father, had produced the commercially successful translation of Mauriceau's treatise. A quieter figure than his father, Hugh II developed very different religious and political allegiances. He had apparently joined the Church of England early in life; by Anne's reign, his associations were Tory, and they remained so until his death in 1728, even acquiring a Jacobite tinge. (Queen Anne herself did not use him as her man-midwife, preferring the Whig Sir David Hamilton – probably for his capacity as a political mediator.[42]) Hugh II was one of Swift's drinking companions after the change of ministry, and the associated transfer of Swift's allegiance, in 1710.[43] He was chosen as a man-midwife by the strongly Tory Strafford family (1713); he subscribed to books by the Tory authors Thomas Hearne, Matthew Prior and John Gay (1717–1720); and he received no known favours from the court of George I (in contrast to Richard Manningham, a rival man-midwife who was knighted in 1721). In the 1720s he was associated with the Buckingham family; after his death in 1728, his epitaph was written by the exiled Jacobite Francis Atterbury, deprived Bishop of Rochester. As a fitting symbol of his membership of the Church of England, Hugh II was given a monument in Westminster Abbey in 1729. Appropriately, too, he received an obituary notice in the opposition journal *The Craftsman*, which added that "he was the last of the ancient family who practised the art of midwifery in the kingdom, except Dr Walker in Great Suffolk Street" – that is, Middleton Walker.[44]

The deaths of Hugh II and his cousin Middleton Walker in 1728 and 1732 brought the Chamberlen dynasty to an end. Around this time there began to come into the public domain, in Britain, France and the Dutch Republic, three instruments that answered the very purpose of the alleged Chamberlen secret: the midwifery forceps, the vectis, and the fillet. Although some of these newly published instruments were described as the Chamberlen secret, no evidence was produced to link them to the Chamberlens.[45] Indeed in England, where the midwifery forceps was published in 1733 and held to be the Chamberlen secret, some male practitioners now conjectured that while there had been a Chamberlen secret, this was not the forceps but some manual technique.[46] But from about 1750 the standard view in England was that the forceps, by now a well-known instrument, was the former Chamberlen secret.

In fact the Chamberlens had indeed possessed a valuable secret, and this was instrumental, not manual – but it comprised three different devices: the forceps *and* the vectis *and* the fillet. We know this thanks to the remarkable discovery, in 1813, of a box of Dr Peter Chamberlen's midwifery instruments under the attic floorboards of the house where he had died 130 years earlier – Woodham Mortimer Hall, Essex. For the box contained each of these instruments, together with the traditional sharp hook or crotchet.[47] Thus *all the three early-modern instruments for delivering a living child by the head originated with the Chamberlens.* The instruments had been invented long before their publication in the eighteenth century – indeed, probably before 1620. This makes intelligible the fact that the Chamberlens were called "men-midwives" – a term that reflected their ability to deliver a living child. It shows that the claims of Hugh Chamberlen I were genuine. And it helps to explain the earlier ambitions of Peter Chamberlen II in 1617 and Dr Peter Chamberlen in 1634 to regulate the midwives of London: their ability to transcend the practical limitations of traditional obstetric surgery made them more critical of midwives than were any of their contemporaries. Thus the instruments had significant effects from the outset, even though their secrecy doubtless limited their social impact throughout the four generations of the Chamberlens' own practice.

The uniqueness of the Chamberlens' achievement reveals that the invention of their instruments was a very special moment or process. With the single and important exception of Hendrik van Deventer, whom we shall meet in due course, the imagination of all other male practitioners of midwifery in Europe was confined within the horizon of traditional obstetric surgery, both before and after Hugh Chamberlen I's announcement of 1673.[48] The most striking example is Mauriceau, an obstetric surgeon of great experience, skill and knowledge, whose practical achievement was nevertheless limited to perfecting the methods of delivering a *dead* child. But the same is true of Willughby, a compassionate man who was deeply troubled by the grim business of traditional obstetric surgery, and of Cooke, who held strong religious convictions and was capable of surgical innovation.[49] Willughby's ingenuity was confined to extending the use of podalic version; Cooke's, to adapting the application of the crotchet so as to save the child. Only with the publication in the eighteenth century of the Chamberlen instruments and of Deventer's methods did the imaginative horizon of male obstetric practice shift beyond the delivery of a dead child.

The female/male division transcended: Sarah Stone

We have seen that at the turn of the seventeenth century, most county towns probably had their own obstetric surgeons, who had the task of delivering those difficult and obstructed births that proved beyond the capacities of the local midwives. Yet in one locality, at least, a different system prevailed. In Taunton, Somerset around 1705–20, according to the retrospective testimony of Sarah Stone, there was "no man-midwife" – which meant no obstetric surgeon – and so all the emergency obstetric work of the town and its hinterland fell to her.[50] Earlier we saw that Mrs Stone practised at an unusually high case-load, and that she had the advantage of training from her mother, Mrs Holmes of Bridgwater (a training apparently completed by 1702).[51] Here we must observe that during her stay in Taunton she transcended the usual dichotomy between male and female practice. How did Mrs Stone respond to the practical tasks that confronted her? Although she sometimes had to deliver a dead child, she almost never used instruments for this purpose: when it was absolutely necessary, she performed craniotomy with a knife, but she had only been forced to do this four times in 35 years of practice.[52] Instead, she had her own manoeuvre, which could also be used while the child was still alive. The following is a case-history that explained this manoeuvre. In this instance the child was still alive, although the mother had been in labour for 48 hours before Mrs Stone was called.[53]

> ... her pains were short, by reason the child's head fixed on the *Os Pubis* (or share-bone). I have observed, in all such labours, the pains are very short, and extreme sharp. The reason is, the pains force the child's head on the *Os Pubis*, which proves injurious both to mother and child. The practice of midwives, in general, in this case, is to press hard on the back part of the body;[54] when, indeed, they have not the least occasion to press anywhere; but to pass by, or through the *Vagina*, and gently feel for the entrance or mouth of the womb; and if it be in a wrong situation, to place it right, or dilate it, as there is occasion: which I shall show as my Observations give me leave. In this case, I examined the *Matrix*, and found the inner orifice lay very high to her back, and open enough to admit of my fore-finger, which I soon dilated to the admittance of my next finger, and with them both gently drew the matrix (or womb) towards the *Os Pubis* (or share-bone); and as I dilated with my two fingers, at the same time, I relieved and kept back the child's head from the *Os Pubis*. Which practice I have always found successful: for by such proceeding the child is retarded (or kept back), the pains strengthened, and the labour happily finished in a little time; as it hath happened to me innumerable times, in such labours. I delivered this woman in two hours, as I assured her she would be, when I first came to her; she seemed not to credit me, but found it truth. I have attended the same woman divers times; all her labours are near the same, yet she and the child do well, and hath tolerable lyings-in.

This method enabled the labour-pains to effect the delivery; Mrs Stone's treatise suggests that it almost invariably worked. Probably the precondition of such astonishing success was a much *earlier* emergency call than most male practitioners experienced. And what presumably propelled Mrs Stone (and perhaps her mother before her) to develop this manual technique was the midwife's customary aversion to the use of instruments.

Yet Mrs Stone also had an affinity with male practitioners, for her diagnosis of this case – that "the child's head fixed on the *Os Pubis* (or share-bone)" – was identical to a description used by her male contemporary William Giffard.[55] This double affiliation can also be seen in her practical method, for this apparently combined the use of the hand in the manner of a vectis (which we may see as a male technique) and the manipulation of the cervix (later described by Mrs Nihell as a female method).[56] And, indeed, Mrs Stone's views at large were *intermediate in character between those of typical female and male practitioners*. She differed from most men in opposing instruments, and from all of them in observing that the hand is painful to the mother, in commenting upon the course of lying-in, and in criticizing male pretensions to knowledge derived from training in anatomy.[57] But in several other respects she wrote more like a male practitioner than like a midwife. For instance, she argued that "the disorders of teeming women do not belong to midwives; but they ought to commit themselves to the care of a physician"; she never mentioned the swaddling of the child; she disapproved of standing and kneeling postures for deliveries; and she repeatedly criticized her fellow midwives.[58] In short, Sarah Stone's proclaimed attitudes and her practical methods harmonized with the social form of her obstetric practice: in each of these respects she was poised between the traditional midwife and the traditional obstetric surgeon.

So far as I am aware, Mrs Stone's manoeuvre was never subsequently discussed by any obstetric author, nor has it been considered in the technical histories. We might imagine that midwives would have taken up Mrs Stone's method; but the subsequent burgeoning of male practice strongly suggests that neither in London nor in the provinces was any significant use made of this resource. Perhaps there were other midwives who, like Mrs Stone, enjoyed a large-scale emergency practice and who could also deliver obstructed births by the head without instruments; if so, they have left few documentary traces. All the evidence – including later developments – suggests that most county towns, with their surrounding villages, were served by emergency male practitioners like Willughby, Cooke and Peters, whose central practical resource was the sharp hook or crotchet. Such was the traditional obstetric surgery that prevailed until around 1720.

Notes

1. Cooke, *Mellificium chirurgiae*; see J. H. Aveling, Biographical sketches of British obstetricians: James Cooke, *Obstetrical Journal of Great Britain and Ireland* 1 (1873–74), pp. 449–52; H. E. Clark, *A rare medical book and its author* (Glasgow: Macdougall, 1899); R. A. Cohen, "Documents concerning James Cooke, surgeon, of Warwick", *Medical History* 1 (1957), pp. 168–73; H. C. Johnson & J. H. Hodson (eds), *Warwick County Records Volume VIII: Quarter Sessions records Trinity, 1682, to Epiphany, 1690* (Warwick, 1953), pp. lxxx, xcviii.
2. Lady Byron, Jane Molyneux (later Wildbore), and an unnamed "gentlewoman" who may well have been his own daughter Eleanor. See Willughby, *Observations*, pp. 40–42; 22, 140, 149, 170; 38, 86, 179, 254–5, 281; Wilson, *Childbirth*, Appendix E.
3. J. R. Magrath (ed.), *The Flemings in Oxford* (3 volumes; Oxford Historical Society, 1904–1924) vol. I, pp. 396, 398, 402, 416, 426, 432, 439, 451, 457, 463, 467, 473; C. Jackson

(ed.), *The autobiography of Mrs Alice Thornton, of East Newton, Co. York* (Surtees Society Publications, vol. LXII), 1873, pp. 84–98, 123–7, 139–51, 164–7; Josselin, *Diary*, pp. 37–50, 101–111, 145–65, 231–57, 313–25, 399–415, 453–65, 496–502; R. Spalding (ed.), *The diary of Bulstrode Whitelocke 1605–1675* (British Academy: Records of Social and Economic History New Series, XIII; Oxford University Press, 1990), *passim*.

4. For this episode see J. P. Kenyon, "The birth of the Old Pretender", *History Today* 13 (1965), pp. 418–26; Aveling, *Chamberlens*, pp. 148–51. Hugh Chamberlen I was also summoned but arrived too late; after his downfall James II tried to recruit him as a witness. See *CSPD*, 1692, pp. 263–4 (April 1692).
5. This discussion is adapted from my "William Hunter and the varieties of man-midwifery", in *William Hunter*, Bynum & Porter (eds), pp. 343–69.
6. "Engaged" was Willughby's word; the term "bespoke" was later used by Smellie. Cf. Giffard, *Cases*, Case 100, p. 245: a woman "whom I had promised to attend whenever she fell into labour".
7. For two or more midwives see Willughby, *Observations*, e.g. pp. 84, 89, 109, 120, 125, 131, 134–5, 162.
8. Willughby, *Observations*, p. 205.
9. See my William Hunter and the varieties of man-midwifery, p. 356.
10. Willughby, *Observations*, pp. 64–7, 211–12, 217, 45–6, 40–2, and London version, p. 11 (Judith Ward); *n*.3 above.
11. Wilson, *Childbirth*, pp. 258–9.
12. Cooke, *Mellificium chirurgiae* (1685 edn), pp. 167–70.
13. Willughby, *Observations*, pp. 43, 164.
14. Cooke, *Mellificium chirurgiae*, 1685 edition, pp. 170–1. Mother's fears of craniotomy were also attested by forceps practitioners, whose testimony, though far from disinterested, was probably accurate on this point. See below, at *n*.35 (Hugh Chamberlen I); Chapman, *Treatise* (1735), p. xviii; Giffard, *Cases*, Cases 55 and 101, pp. 123, 252.
15. See my "The perils of early-modern procreation: childbirth with or without fear?" *British Journal for Eighteenth-Century Studies* 16:1 (1993), pp. 1–19, and Magrath (ed.), *The Flemings in Oxford*.
16. Spalding (ed.), *Diary of Whitelocke*, p. 399 (9 January 1654/5).
17. Willughby, *Observations*, pp. 55–6, 153–6, 224; R. Gough, *The history of Myddle*. D. Hey (ed.) (Harmondsworth: Penguin, 1981), pp. 172–3.
18. Willughby, *Observations,* pp. 101, 164, 207, 209, 240; Wilson, *Childbirth*, pp. 282–8.
19. Willughby, *Observations*, pp. 103–4, 112–13, 191–2.
20. Cooke, *Mellificium chirurgiae*, pp. 167–8; cf. E. Baynard, Appendix to Sir John Floyer, *The history of cold bathing both ancient and modern* (4th edn, London, 1715), p. 340.
21. Willughby, *Observations,* pp. 37–8; London version, p. 3; Wilson, William Hunter and the varieties of man-midwifery, Appendix.
22. Willughby, *Observations,* p. 46; London version, p. 11.
23. Willughby, *Observations*, pp. 11–12.
24. Willughby, *Observations*, London version, p. 20; Henry E. Huntingdon Library, San Marino, California: letter from Percival Willughby to the Countess of Huntingdon, 26 April 1678.
25. Willughby, *Observations*, pp. 6, 45, 49, 57.
26. *Ibid.*, pp. 151–3, 175–9, 188–90, 199–202, 216–21, 231–2.
27. *Ibid.*, pp. 22–3, 88, 248–9.
28. Cooke, *Mellificium chirurgiae* (edns 1648, 1662, 1676, 1685, 1693, 1717). See also H.

NOTES

Crooke, *Microscosmographica* (2nd edn, 1631), pp. 332–5; T. Brugis, *The marrow of physic. Or a learned discourse of the several parts of mans body* . . . (London, 1648), pp. 34–5, 41–2, 38, 123; A. Read, *Chirurgorum comes, or the whole practice of chirurgery* (1687), sig. A4v, pp. 537–94; W. Cowper, *The anatomy of humane bodies* (1698); J. Drake, *Anthropologia nova* (1707).

29. Dr Peters of Canterbury: Northampton Record Office, Finch-Hatton papers, Elizabeth Thanet to her sister-in-law, n.d., (*c.*1690s), kindly supplied by Linda Pollock. Samuel Dale (d. 1739; see *DNB* and Wallis, *Medics*): Cowper, *Anatomy of humane bodies*, Table 56. Hacon & Freeman: NNRO, TES/8, file I, items 96 (1695), 188 (1701).

30. For early practice of midwifery by Peter I and Peter II see Aveling, *Chamberlens*, pp. 9, 35 and T. R. Forbes, "A jury of matrons", *Medical History* 32 (1988), pp. 23–33, at p, 27.

31. For the Walkers, see Radcliffe, *The secret instrument*, p. 72; Radcliffe, *Milestones,* p. 32. In Dublin the forceps may have descended to the Walkers' son-in-law, Fielding Ould.

32. See Aveling, *Chamberlens*, pp. 49–59, and below.

33. D. S. Pady, "A London medical satire of 1607", *Journal of the History of Medicine and Allied Sciences* 33 (1978), pp. 409–16, at p. 415 (Nowell); S. Young, *The annals of the Barber-Surgeons' Company, compiled from their records and other sources* (London: Blades, East & Blades, 1890), pp. 330–1, 335–6 (Blackbourne, Downing); Charles Goodall, *The College of Physicians . . . Established by Law* (London, 1684), p. 368 (Doughton); Willughby, *Observations*, p. 23 and London version, p. 6 (Boudin; cf. pp. 17, 88, 111); Munk, *Roll* (Hinton); Robert Barret, *A companion for midwives, childbearing women, and nurses* (London, 1699); H. Brock, "James Douglas of the pouch", *Medical History* 18 (1974), pp. 162–72, at pp. 163–4 (Johnson; cf. Ch. 5 below).

34. Ch. 3 above.

35. Hugh Chamberlen (trans.), *The accomplisht midwife* (1673), "The Translator to the Reader"; later editions entitled *The diseases of women with child*.

36. *CSPD*, 1678, p. 610; dated "after 1676"; since it is in the State Papers of the reign of Charles II, it was probably before 1685.

37. Clark, *College of Physicians*, vol. I, p. 362. However, it seems that in 1679 Groeneveldt became aware of the use of some speculum-like instrument by "Dr Chamberlen". See R. Bland, *Some account of the invention and use of the lever of Roonhuysen* (London, 1790), p. 15, citing Groeneveldt's *Tutus cantharidum in medicina usus internus*, p. 129. For John (Johannes) Groeneveldt or Greenfield (?1647–?1710) see *DNB*, Munk, *Roll*, and H. J. Cook, *The decline of the old medical regime in Stuart London* (London: Cornell University Press, 1986), pp. 240–51.

38. See Aveling, Chamberlens, pp. 130–32; Radcliffe, *Milestones*, pp. 41–2.

39. See *CSPD*, 1686–7, p. 163; Aveling, *Chamberlens*, pp. 136–8, 150; W. McD. Wigfield, *The Monmouth Rebels, 1685* (Gloucester: Alan Sutton, 1985), p. 30.

40. J. K. Horsfield, *British monetary experiments 1650–1710* (London: Bell, 1960), pp. 156–79, 268–9; Aveling, *Chamberlens*, pp. 154–71; Dennis Rubini, "Politics and the battle for the Banks", 1688–1697, *English Historical Review* 85 (1970), pp. 693–714.

41. By 1699 he was an agent of the leading disaffected Whig Charles Mordaunt (Earl of Peterborough, former Earl of Monmouth). G. P. R. James (ed.), *Letters illustrative of the reign of King William III* . . . (3 volumes; London: Colburn, 1841), vol. II, pp. 371, 438; vol. III, p. 93; I thank Paul Hopkins for these references. For his exile see Aveling, *Chamberlens*, pp. 171, 179. He was still alive in 1720: see *DNB*.

42. See P. Roberts (ed.), *The diary of Sir David Hamilton 1709–1714* (Oxford: Clarendon, 1975), pp. xxxi–xlv.

43. Aveling, *Chamberlens*, p. 190; J. Swift, *Journal to Stella,* Harold Williams (ed.) (2 volumes; Oxford, 1948), pp. 82–3 (5 November 1710, Letter viii).
44. See Aveling, *Chamberlens*, pp. 191, 193, 196–203; Randolph Trumbach, The aristocratic family in England 1690–1780: studies in childhood and kinship (PhD thesis, John Hopkins University, 1972), p. 31. For details of his subscriptions see Wallis, *Medics* and Phibb, *Subscriptions;* for allegiances of their authors, *DNB*.
45. See Radcliffe, *The secret instrument*.
46. H. Bracken, *The midwife's companion, or, a treatise of midwifery; wherein the whole art is explained* (London, 1737); B. Exton, *A new and general system of midwifery* (London, 1751), 1766 edn, p. 5. The latter was noticed in Bland, *Some account of the lever of Roonhuysen*, p. 19.
47. There were three each of the vectis, fillet and crotchet, and four pairs of forceps. See H. H. Carwardine, Brief notice presented to the medico-chirurgical society with the original obstetric instruments of the Chamberlens, *Medico-Chirurgical Transactions* 9 (1818), pp. 181–4. (The author's name was here mis-spelt "Cansardine", but this was corrected in the errata, p. 500, and in the volume's index, p. 496. The name has sometimes been spelt "Cawardine".) For Henry Holgate Carwardine (1779–1867), and his family, see W. Berry, *County pedigrees: Essex* (London: Sherwood, Gilbert & Piper, 1840), and *Essex Review*, 52 (1943), pp. 57–65. For more on Woodham Mortimer Hall, see P. Morant, *The history and antiquities of Essex* (2 volumes; London, 1768), vol. I, p. 342. Later accounts of the find include Aveling, *Chamberlens*, pp. 218–20; Radcliffe, *Milestones,* p. 32; Radcliffe, *The secret instrument*, pp. 1–2.
48. For Deventer see Ch. 6 below.
49. Willughby, *Observations*, pp. 206–7; Cohen, Documents concerning James Cooke, p. 169.
50. Stone, *Complete practice*, pp. xiii, 40, 137. Her move to Bristol took place in 1721, and she had by that date practised in Taunton "for many years" (p. 138). On Mrs Stone see also I. Grundy, "Sarah Stone: Enlightenment midwife", in *Medicine and the Englightenment*, R. Porter (ed.) (Amsterdam: Rodopi, 1994).
51. Ch. 3 above.
52. Stone, *Complete practice*, pp. xiv, xviii, 18–19, 36–7.
53. *Ibid.*, pp. 8–10.
54. This seems to refer to Deventer's manoeuvre (see Ch. 6).
55. Giffard, *Cases*, e.g. Cases 83, 86, 87, 217; cf. Cooke, *Mellificium chirurgiae*, 1685 edition, p. 602.
56. On the vectis see Ch. 5 below; for Mrs Nihell's approach see Ch. 15 below.
57. Stone, *Complete practice*, pp. 36–7 (opposition to craniotomy); 42–3 (the hand painful); 10 (quoted above), 29, 32, 43 (lying-in); xi–xii (men criticized).
58. *Ibid.*, pp. 55, 65, 85, 127 (criticism of midwives); xviii ("disorders of teeming women"); 55, 69 (postures). In addition, Mrs Stone thought that the second twin should be fetched immediately (p. 65), and supported turning to the feet rather than to the head for malpresentations (pp. 34–5); these were characteristically male attitudes (see Ch. 12).

Part II
From obstetric surgery to man-midwifery

Chapter Five
The Chamberlen instruments and their sale

The Chamberlen instruments

The Chamberlens' three instruments worked in different ways to achieve the same effect – the delivery of a living child in obstructed births by the head. The *vectis* (which simply means lever) consisted of a single blade, one end curved so as to fit around some part of the foetal head (probably the occiput, the back of the head), the other end serving as a handle. Its main use was to rectify the presentation: the head could be variously flexed or rotated, according to the specific requirements and possibilities of the particular delivery. But the vectis also permitted some traction on the head, under the right conditions. (One might think of the vectis as modelled upon the crotchet.) The *midwifery forceps* comprised two blades, each somewhat similar to the vectis. By inserting the blades separately the operator could grasp the foetal head, reduce its size in imitation of the natural moulding process, and exert traction. (One possible model was the various surgical forceps, whose blades were however joined by a permanent hinge; another was the speculum, an instrument designed to dilate the mouth of the uterus for the purpose of inspection.[1]) Both vectis and forceps had several different designs: for instance, the blade or blades could be fenestrated (window-like) or unfenestrated (a continuous sheet of metal), the handles of the forceps crossed or uncrossed. The *fillet* had two detachable parts: a strip of some pliable material such as silk or leather, perhaps two inches broad (the fillet proper), and a rigid handle of metal, wood or whalebone. The strip was passed in a loop over the child's head, and secured at each end on the handle, making a noose through which traction was exerted on the head by pulling the handle.[2] Some of the Chamberlen designs are shown in Fig. 5.1.

British histories of the subject have focused on the forceps, largely forgetting the vectis and fillet. This reflects the fact that from the late nineteenth century, the

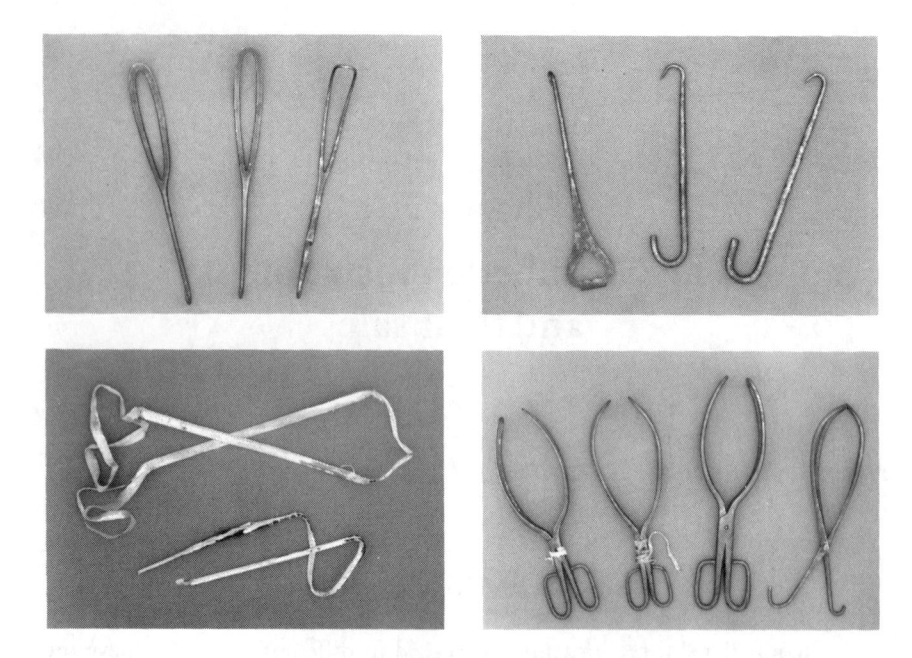

Figure 5.1   The Chamberlen instruments.

forceps came to triumph in British obstetric practice – whence a teleological history, in which only the forceps ever counted since only the forceps eventually mattered.[3] The vectis can be rescued from this neglect, since it enjoyed a well-publicized support in the intervening period. But the fillet presents a different and confusing picture as to both its origin and its value. In origin, it appears to have been a Chamberlen device, yet it was also used by Deventer, and apparently by Mauriceau.[4] As to its value, we find in the early eighteenth century – when the fillet had its heyday – a conflicting pattern of testimony: widespread use, suggesting considerable practical value, yet disparagement even by men who used it, suggesting limited utility.[5] Perhaps this paradox can be resolved by the fact that the fillet was, by all accounts, very difficult to use. Probably its application required very special skills, and conceivably it could be used for only some cases of obstruction. But much remains to be learnt about the fillet, as we shall see again in Chapter 6. (After about 1750, it appears to have gone out of use, except for a brief revival in the 1860s and '70s.[6])

Until the 1690s, there is no indication that anyone outside the Chamberlen family possessed the forceps or vectis.[7] Yet by the early 1730s, various forms of these instruments were being used by other practitioners in the Dutch Republic, in France (whence they passed to at least one Scottish practitioner, Alexander Butter), and in England. The provenance of all these instruments is highly obscure: only one individual (Jean Palfyn) claimed independent invention, and all the others concealed the means whereby they had acquired the instruments.

Thus the very passage of the vectis and forceps into public knowledge was shrouded in secrecy, just as their earlier use had been. The most plausible reconstruction is that all these instruments were sold by the Chamberlens at around this time. In the Dutch Republic it is known that Hugh Chamberlen I sold both instruments around 1694 to a party of surgeons led by Rogier van Roonhuysen, and that Roonhuysen and his successors maintained a tradition of secret sale until about 1750.[8] In France the story is less clear, but circumstantial evidence suggests that either Hugh I or his son, Hugh II, sold the forceps – but probably not the vectis – to several French surgeons around 1710–20.[9] To reconstruct those episodes is beyond my scope here. The key point for us to observe is that the instruments that emerged in these two contexts were different, both from each other and from those of Dr Peter Chamberlen. Dr Peter's instruments (as later found in the attic of Woodham Mortimer Hall) were fenestrated, rigid, and broad-bladed; and his forceps was hinged in the middle. The Dutch instruments were unfenestrated, elastic (they were apparently used not only to move the foetal head but also to dilate the maternal soft passages), and with narrower blades; and the Dutch forceps was hinged at the end of the handle.[10] The French forceps were different again: they resembled Dr Peter's instruments in their rigidity and broad blades, but the Dutch instruments in being unfenestrated.

It is also notable that the French forceps only imperfectly realized the instrument's life-saving potential. The German surgeon Heister, who had obtained a forceps from Palfyn, commented:

> I have indeed used this instrument of my friend Palfinus, but without success; for if you compress the head with it but gently, the foetus is held too firm to give way to it, and if you press too strongly, there is danger of wounding its tender head. I therefore endeavoured to amend the instrument, by joining its two parts together with a hinge, but even then it did not answer expectation: so that in this deplorable situation of the foetus we have no remedy left but the Caesarean section, or to extract the foetus either dead or alive with hooks . . . or other instruments, to preserve the life of the mother.[11]

Conversely, La Motte, although extolling the advantages of the forceps, did not suggest that they could save the child's life: he simply assimilated them to the existing suite of craniotomy instruments.[12]

The sale of the forceps in England

In England it was a variant of the forceps that came to light in the early eighteenth century. We know of several men outside the Chamberlen family who were using it before the extinction of the Chamberlen dynasty in 1732; and the instrument was published in the following year. By contrast the vectis, if it was sold in England at all, was probably restricted to a much narrower audience, since it was many decades before it came to light in this country.[13] Ironically, the first known use of the forceps outside the Chamberlen family was by someone who in all probability then abandoned that instrument. This was James Douglas, who recorded the following description of an obstetric emergency in London, dated 20 September 1702.

> I was sent for by Mrs Agnew the midwife to lay a poor woman. I went to work *a modo nostro* but could never fasten the things so as to be able to pull by reason they were not made right; and after ¾ of a hour's endeavour to bring away the child one of them locked so as to become straight whereby it was rendered useless and I forced to leave the woman unlayed. I tried to put a fillet round its neck but could not effect it. I went for young Dr Hugh Chamberlen but he excused himself from coming saying that he did not doubt but that nature would do it provided I gave her a poached egg, a glass of wine or some nourishing broth and a grain of opium. Dr Johnson was sent for; he lessened the head and so brought it away (which I could not do by reason I had not a hook).[14]

Clearly this botched attempt involved an instrument that was secret (*"a modo nostro"*, in our way), had two parts ("the things", etc.), and was designed for traction ("to pull") on obstructed births by the head. The instrument was not a fillet, since that was tried subsequently (again without success). In short, this must have been the forceps.

How had Douglas obtained the forceps? Since he had studied in Utrecht in 1696, he might have travelled to Amsterdam and bought the instrument from the Roonhuysen group. But he only embarked on midwifery in 1699 – whence his failure with the instrument in 1702, doubtless due to inexperience.[15] The fact that he expected help from "young Dr Hugh Chamberlen" (Hugh II, then aged 38, doubtless called "young" to distinguish him from Hugh I) indicates that the provider was some member of the Chamberlen family; the fact that Hugh II "excused himself" suggests that he was not that provider. It thus appears that Douglas had acquired the instrument from Hugh Chamberlen I. Amid the recent triangular movements of both Hugh I and Douglas himself between Scotland, London and the Dutch Republic, they may have had some opportunity for contact. By the same token, it appears that at the time of this delivery, Douglas was cut off from his source of instruction, and at this date Hugh I was in Scotland. The circumstantial evidence, then, points to Hugh I as the source of Douglas's forceps, which fits with the equally circumstantial point that both Hugh I and Douglas were Whigs, unlike Hugh II.[16] How long Douglas continued to use the forceps after this early disappointment we do not know, but as we shall see in due course, all later evidence (from 1719 onwards) suggests that he turned to other methods.[17]

The forceps is next known in England in the hands of three identifiable practitioners, at dates of 1720, 1726, and pre-1728.
1. Edmund Chapman practised at Halstead, Essex, where he was using the forceps by 1720. In 1732 he moved to London, probably to exploit the opportunity presented by the recent deaths of three London forceps practitioners – Chamberlen, Giffard and Walker.[18] To advertise his practice in the capital he wrote his *Essay towards the improvement of midwifery*, published in the following year. This first announced in English the existence and use of the midwifery forceps – and gave the instrument the name it retains today.
2. William Giffard had preceded Chapman by a few years in moving from Essex to London; he hailed from Brentwood, about 26 miles from Halstead, and probably arrived in the capital in late 1724.[19] In January 1725 he began writing down some of his midwifery cases, apparently with a view to publishing these along the lines of the *Observations* of Mauriceau, Portal, or La Motte.[20] From 8 April 1726 he began to record the use of an instrument he called "my Extractor" or "Eductor"; his descriptions make it clear that this was a midwifery forceps. By the time he died in late 1731, Giffard had written down 225 cases. His manuscript passed to Edward Hody, MD, who published it as *Cases in midwifery* (1734), with a frontispiece engraving of Giffard's forceps and also of the forceps as "improved by Mr Freke" – John Freke, surgeon of St Bartholomew's Hospital.[21]
3. John Drinkwater was a surgeon at Brentford, Middlesex, who began practice in 1688, received a bishop's licence in surgery in 1694, and died in 1728. Thanks to the later testimony of Robert Wallace Johnson, we know that Drinkwater had a forceps. Its pattern, wrote Johnson in 1769, "exactly agrees with those of Giffard and Chapman, save only that that the hooks of the handles are turned outwards".[22] All these three instruments had crossed handles and fenestrated blades.[23]

To these three known early English users of the forceps we may perhaps add four or five more.
4. As we have seen, John Freke "improved" the forceps – specifically by adding a sharp hook, folded for safety and concealment, at the end of one of the handles. Freke, who practised in the City, was a general surgeon of some ingenuity; his "improving" the forceps perhaps suggests that he was using the instrument himself.[24]
5, 6. Chapman mentioned a "brother practitioner in the country" who had used a forceps "for some years, but seldom with success or advantage"; and another man, "a very ingenious practitioner, now living in the country", who seems to have helped him with the use of the forceps at a time when he was having difficulties. These remarks add two unnamed early users of the forceps – unless the former individual was Drinkwater or Giffard, in which case only one man has to be added to the list.[25]
7. In Oxford, the surgeon Nally Wood (or Woods) may have been using the

forceps at this time. On 22 December 1723 Thomas Hearne wrote: "In Oxford lives now Mr Woods ... a very eminent chirurgeon. ...This Mr Woods hath a most admirable skill in midwifery. ... Two instances of this happened last week". He added of one such case that Woods could have saved the child's life "had he been sent for sooner". Similar anecdotes recur in Hearne's diary in 1725 and 1727.[26]

8. Finally, there was John Bamber, a City practitioner who used the forceps at some stage in his very long working life (from before 1700 to around 1750). It is not known when he acquired his forceps, but this could well have been in the 1720s, when he apparently began to practise midwifery.[27]

Of these men only Chapman and Giffard left written descriptions of the forceps and its use – and neither stated how they had acquired it. Although Giffard described it as "my Extractor" or "my Eductor", this did not mean that he had invented it; when extolling its benefits, he referred to it as "this Instrument", not as something of his own contriving. He commended "Dr Chamberlen" for his opposition to "forcing medicines" in childbirth, but did not link Dr Chamberlen with the instrument; he was probably referring to the translation of Mauriceau made by Hugh I, who had left England in 1699, long before Giffard acquired his instrument.[28] Chapman, too, deliberately left his acquisition of the forceps shrouded in obscurity. He asserted that this was the Chamberlen secret, but did not back this up with any account of how he had obtained it.[29] He praised various men who had earlier taught or helped him, but did not link any of them with the forceps.[30] And he claimed that the forceps was "now well known to all the principal men of the profession, both in town and country" (that is, in London and elsewhere), thus suggesting that it was in widespread use – but this claim was too self-serving for us to trust it.[31]

The shared design of these instruments and the similar timing of their acquisition suggest a common origin. That origin was surely in England, since none of these men is known to have travelled abroad; and it was probably in or near London, since they all lived and worked either in the capital (Giffard from 1725, Freke, Bamber) or at least within reasonable reach (Giffard in Brentwood, Essex until 1724; Drinkwater in Brentford, Middlesex; Chapman in Halstead, Essex; Wood at the relatively distant site of Oxford). Thus they had probably obtained the forceps either from Hugh Chamberlen II or from his brother-in-law Middleton Walker. But Walker's forceps had a special feature – an asymmetry that was perhaps in the lock, perhaps between the blades – not shown by the instruments of Chapman, Giffard, Freke or Drinkwater.[32] Probably, therefore, all the English forceps had come from Hugh Chamberlen II, the last surviving member of the Chamberlen dynasty. Having no male heir, Hugh II had no family interest to protect; aged 56 by 1720, he may have wanted to retire (his health was declining in 1722–24); and being able to command a fee of 100 guineas for an advance call (1713), he would not have needed or wanted the emergency work for which the forceps was chiefly used.[33] A hint that he passed on at least one of the family's midwifery instruments comes from his epitaph, in which Atterbury suggested – before the forceps was published – that Hugh II had "too freely imparted the resources of his skill" to others, "even to those whose opinions were not his".[34]

Despite the common focus of London, notice the geographical dispersal of the known or possible recipients, who were strung along an east–west line – Halstead, possibly Brentwood, London, Brentford, Oxford. Those in London were also largely spaced apart: Giffard in Westminster, Middleton Walker in Southwark, Bamber and Freke in the City. Thus only Bamber and Freke could have shared a common catchment area, and we shall later see that Bamber may have been distinct in also receiving the vectis. It is as if Hugh II chose his recipients in such a way as to avoid competition between them.

The need for instruction

To us the advantages of the forceps seem obvious. So familiar is the instrument, and so ingrained its objective – the delivery of a living child in obstructed births by the head – that we implicitly regard its very existence as inscribed in the natural order. Yet the forceps appeared in a very different light in the early eighteenth century. In the first place, many English practitioners opposed the instrument, as we shall see in later chapters. Secondly, as the responses of Heister and La Motte show, it was by no means obvious that the forceps could deliver a living child. But the third and most striking corrective to our assumptions comes from the early English forceps users themselves. Just as Heister "used this instrument of my friend Palfinus, but without success", so we have seen that James Douglas failed in 1702, with the ignominious result that the child had to be delivered with "a hook". Giffard's first use of his "Extractor", on 8 April 1726, resulted in a similar experience: he "was not able to fix it, the parts giving way and slipping back when I made any pressure upon them", and after a day and a half he resorted to craniotomy.[35] Presumably Giffard then went off to Hugh Chamberlen II for further instruction in the use of the forceps. As we shall see in Chapter 7, his case-series contains a gap of some 20 months soon after this unsuccessful attempt. Not until 28 June 1728 – over two years after this case – did Giffard next record using his "Extractor"; this time the operation was successful, and indeed most of his subsequent essays with the instrument proceeded more or less smoothly.[36] During the gap in his case-series he was probably using the forceps, sometimes successfully, sometimes not; by the time he resumed writing down his cases, he had evidently mastered the instrument.[37] What it is vital for us to grasp is that such routine use of the forceps – as of any technique – had to be *achieved*.

Edmund Chapman, the other early English forceps practitioner who left some record of his experiences, doubly confirms this picture. Not only did he mention a "brother practitioner in the country" who had used a forceps "for some years, but seldom with success or advantage"; he also stated that he had himself abandoned the forceps for some years, because of the difficulty of using them. Although his testimony is not quite explicit, it appears that it was the help of another colleague, "a very ingenious practitioner, now living in the country", which enabled him to take up the instrument again, this time with success.[38] In short, the experience of the early forceps users outside the Chamberlen family was consistent: they all failed in their first attempts to use the instrument. Douglas probably then abandoned the forceps for good. Chapman certainly gave it up for some years and probably only resumed using it thanks to the help of a colleague. Giffard's course of action is unclear, but both the gap in his case-series and his subsequent success with the "extractor" suggest an intervening period of instruction.

Thus it is with the use of the forceps as with other practical manoeuvres, in this and later periods, which have been investigated by historians of science: technical skill has to be *taught* directly, by a prior adept who is physically present and can explain by ostensive definition.[39] A picture of an instrument on a page, even detailed written instructions on its use, are meaningless on their own, detached from the site of their application and removed from their practical context. Ironically, the veil of secrecy with which the Chamberlens shrouded the forceps was probably superfluous: mere publication would not have persuaded anyone of the value of the instrument, and still less would it have enabled anyone to achieve successful imitation. This means that when the Chamberlens sold their instruments – whether forceps or vectis – they would also have had to deliver, as part of the deal, a period of sustained *instruction* in their use. After a certain point, the pupil could work on his own and could even improvise with success, but to get him to that point required careful and delicate nurturing, without which he would fail. In the 1720s Chapman and Giffard were in a position to receive such help; in 1702 James Douglas was not.

The Tory associations of the forceps

All Hugh Chamberlen II's associations suggest that he was a Tory, perhaps even leaning to Jacobitism: as we have seen, his very epitaph was written by the exiled Atterbury.[40] We might therefore expect that it was to men of his own party that he sold the instrument; yet Atterbury suggested that Hugh had passed on "the resources of his skill" to men "whose opinions were not his". Who were the recipients? Although the evidence on this point is fragmentary, it consistently suggests that they were Tories. To begin with the simplest case, *John Freke's* Tory credentials were impeccable; unlike some men of the period, he retained his convictions throughout his life.[41] For *William Giffard* we have two strands of indirect evidence. He was excluded, in December 1726, from the Court spectacle of Mary Toft.[42] And the one named physician who called him to a case – Dr George Wharton, in 1730 – was at this time aligned with the Nonjurors.[43] With *Edmund Chapman* we are on less clear ground: his patron, Edward Milward, was at this time a very obscure physician whose own allegiance is not easy to establish.[44] But when Chapman became engaged in heated argument with John Douglas in 1736–37, we find as one of the byways of this exchange that Douglas, as a good Whig, sneered at physicians who took their degrees in "Popish" universities – and Chapman's counter-shot was directed against those practitioners who had been "complimented" with a degree from Leyden, from a Scottish university, or by Royal Mandate at Cambridge or Oxford.[45] Since the physicians who secured the latter qualifications at this time were chiefly Dissenters and Whigs, this gibe suggests that Chapman was a Tory.[46] So too does Chapman's concern, stressed in both text and title-page of his *Reply* (1737), to vindicate "the character of the late Dr Chamberlen . . . from [Douglas's] indecent and unjust aspersions".[47]

The other known or possible early forceps practitioners were probably also Tories, although for each of these men either their political or obstetric allegiance is somewhat obscure. We know that *John Drinkwater* had a forceps, but cannot specify his politics – although the local minister's signing a 1694 testimonial for his episcopal licence in surgery suggests a Tory allegiance, since most of the clergy were of that party.[48] *Nally Wood* of Oxford was a complementary case: it is only a conjecture that he was using the forceps, but his politics must have been Tory, given the commendation of the Jacobite and Nonjuror Thomas Hearne. If *John Bamber* acquired his forceps around 1720, he would fit the Tory pattern, for his early associations were Tory, including his appointment in 1721 as lithotomist to St Bartholomew's Hospital.[49] But around 1724 he apparently aligned himself with the Court, securing first a Cambridge MD by Royal mandate (1725) and then a Fellowship in Hans Sloane's College of Physicians (1726).[50] Yet some of his later book-subscriptions suggest lingering Tory loyalties in the 1730s.[51]

Thus it seems that contrary to Atterbury's claim, Hugh Chamberlen II sold the forceps specifically to Tories. Certainly this is what we would expect in the polarized political world of the time, not least because of the secrecy shrouding the instruments even after their sale.[52] We may presume that those who bought the instruments were bound in oath not to publish what they had acquired; hence the fact that it was only after the deaths of Hugh Chamberlen II and Middleton Walker that the forceps came to light. Such secrecy had monetary value: as long as the instruments remained private property, they could probably command a high price. This would remain true even if men like Chapman and Giffard had acquired their forceps not from Hugh Chamberlen II directly but instead through some intermediary. The secrecy of these transactions, while frustrating for the historian, commands attention as a phenomenon in its own right. The forceps was doubtless exchanged not only for a sum of money but also for a pledge of silence, and shared political allegiance helped to guarantee that pledge. Moreover, in early Hanoverian England the forceps was perhaps specifically attractive to Tory practitioners. We know of three London medical practitioners of (presumptive) Whig allegiance who had some connection with the forceps before 1740 – and all three subsequently abandoned the instrument. James Douglas has already been mentioned (we shall meet him again in Chapter 6). Edward Hody, although he published Giffard's *Cases* and thus surely supported the forceps in

1734, was later (1748) said not to use the instrument.[53] And Brudenell Exton was a pupil of Chapman's in the 1730s, but then went on to learn from the anti-forceps Sir Richard Manningham, whose doctrines he subsequently espoused.[54] Whether through the accidents of patronage or through elective affinity, the forceps was specifically a Tory instrument in London until about 1740.

Notes

1. For the speculum see Radcliffe, *Milestones*, p. 46.
2. *Ibid.*, p. 47.
3. As for instance in the very title of Aveling's *The Chamberlens and the midwifery forceps*; cf. also Radcliffe, *The secret instrument*, subtitle and pp. 67–8, and K. Das, *Obstetric forceps: its history and evolution* (Calcutta: The Art Press, 1929, Reprinted by Medical Museum Publishing, Leeds, 1993).
4. Deventer, *Midwifery improv'd*, p. 326; McClintock, *Smellie's midwifery*, vol. I, pp. 250–51; vol. II, p. 290, Case 220. The Arab writer Avicenna had recommended the use of a fillet and a forceps: see *ibid.*, vol. I, p. 50, and R. Bland, *Some account of the invention and use of the lever of Roonhuysen* (London, 1790), note on pp. 16f. It is unclear whether this was for the delivery of a living or a dead child. If Avicenna's fillet and forceps had been designed to deliver a living child, it does not seem that this exerted any subsequent influence, since it was only after the Chamberlen forceps had been released in the eighteenth century that Avicenna's use of a forceps was interpreted in this way.
5. Chapman suggested that most fillets were used for drawing the child's feet, not head (*Treatise*, 1735, p. 17; this in order to claim priority for himself for the use of the fillet on the head). This interpretation was criticized by John Douglas, in *A short account of the state of midwifery in London, Westminster, &c.* (London, 1736) p. 60 (for discussion of this work see Ch. 8 below).
6. See note in McClintock, *Smellie's midwifery*, vol. I, pp. 254–5, and cf. Radcliffe, *Milestones*, p. 47.
7. See Radcliffe, *The secret instrument*, and Radcliffe, *Milestones*. Late eighteenth-century histories include M. G. Herbinieaux, "Histoire raisonnée du levier de Roonhuysen, et de ses usages", in his *Traité sur divers accouchemens laborieux* (Brussels, 1782; cited in William Osborne, *Essays on . . . midwifery* (London, 1792), p. 117); Bland, *Some account*; J. Mulder, *Historia litteraria et critica forcipium et vectium obstetriciorum* (Leyden, 1794); of these I have consulted Bland.
8. Radcliffe, *The secret instrument*, pp. 30–34; J. de Visscher & H. van de Poll, *Het Roonhysiaansch geheim, in de vroedkunde ontdekt . . .* (Leyden, 1754), p. 19. The recipients were Rogier van Roonhuysen, Frederik Ruisch & Cornelius Boekelman: *ibid.*, preface, p. 38.
9. French surgeons known to possess the forceps were Jean Palfyn, before 1718; Guillaume Mauquest de la Motte from 1717; Gilles le Doux, around 1720; one Dusée, before 1733; and Grégoire the younger, in the 1730s. See Radcliffe, *The secret instrument*, pp. 32–5; Glaister, *Smellie*, pp. 155, 209; McClintock, *Smellie's midwifery*, ii, p. 250; L. von Heister ("Laurence Heister"), *A general system of surgery in three parts* (German original 1718; trans. anon., London, 1743), pp. 210–11, 231, and Table XXXII, Fig. 16, p. 230; La Motte,

Midwifery, pp. 529–30, 532–3, 533–4, 536; and A. Butter, "Description of a Forceps, etc.", *Medical Essays and Observations from a Society in Edinburgh* 3 (1733), p. 254.
10. On Dr Peter's instruments see Ch. 4. For the Dutch instruments see Glaister, *Smellie*, pp. 218–19, 223, 274; note that Rathlauw added a fenestration to the forceps, presumably in imitation of the English instruments that were well known by the time of his publication (1747). For the designs of different versions of Roonhuysen's lever, see also Visscher & van de Poll, *Het Roonhysiaansch geheim*, pp. 40, 68. The use of the forceps to dilate the maternal soft passages was seldom discussed in British midwifery, but was noticed by Groenevelt in discussing a case of Chamberlen's (presumably Hugh I) in 1679; by two British opponents of the forceps (William Cockburn & Henry Bracken); and by one English forceps user, Benjamin Pugh. See Bland, *Some account*, p. 15; W. Cockburn, *Symptoms... of Gonorrhoea* (London, 1713), p. 9, and *ibid.*, 2nd edn (London, 1715), pp. 11–12 (cf. Ch. 6 below); H. Bracken, *The midwife's companion, or, a treatise of midwifery; wherein the whole art is explained...* (London, 1737), pp. 133–4; B. Pugh, *A treatise of midwifery, chiefly with regard to the operation. With several improvements in that art* (London, 1754), p. 85.
11. Heister, *General system of surgery*, p. 211. Contrast the actions of William Smellie (Ch. 9 below).
12. La Motte, *Midwifery*, *loc. cit.*
13. See Ch. 10 below.
14. Quoted from Douglas's MS. notes by Helen Brock, James Douglas of the pouch, *Medical History* 18 (1974), pp. 162–72, at pp. 163–4. "Dr Johnson" was perhaps William Johnstone, MD, perhaps Nathaniel Johnstone MD; see their entries in Munk, *Roll*.
15. Douglas had practised midwifery for 27 years by December, 1726: James Douglas, *An advertisement occasion'd by some passages in Sir R. Manningham's diary lately publish'd* (London, 1727), p. 13 (for the context see Ch. 8 below).
16. See Ch. 4 above and Brock, James Douglas of the pouch.
17. See Ch. 6 below.
18. Dates of death: Hugh Chamberlen II, 17 June 1728 (Aveling, *Chamberlens*, p. 193); William Giffard, late 1731 (the last of his cases was on 17 October 1731); Middleton Walker, 16 November 1732 (*Historical Register*, 1732, p. 38). For a reference to Chapman at Halstead in 1711 see C. F. D. Sperling, An Essex pensioner in the days of Queen Anne, *Essex Review* 32 (1923), pp. 200–201. He took apprentices there in 1711 (James Skynner, premium £50) and 1724 (Robert Young, premium £105): see Wallis, *Medics*.
19. Wallis, *Medics*; Giffard, *Cases*, Case 177, p. 422. His London address in 1726 was apparently Norfolk Street: Royal Society Letters and Papers, Vol. 12 (ii), Item 30 (Giffard to William Rutty).
20. P. Portal, *The complete practice of men and women midwives... illustrated with a considerable number of observations* (French original 1685; trans. anon., London, 1705), pp. 26–242, comprised 81 "observations"; La Motte, *Midwifery*.
21. Giffard, *Cases*; see Ch. 7 below.
22. R. W. Johnson, *A new system of midwifery, in four parts* (London, 1769), p. 170.
23. Crossed handles and fenestrated blades were shown in Hody's illustration of 1734, in the frontispiece that Chapman added to the enlarged 1735 edition of his treatise, and (implicitly) in Wallace Johnson's description of Drinkwater's forceps. Yet Giffard sometimes described the blades of his "Eductor" as "cheeks", as if these were unfenestrated (Cases 42, 55, 133) – although he usually called them "sides" (e.g. Cases 48, 50, 59, 60, 61, 70).
24. However, none of Freke's six apprentices from 1724 to 1752 (listed in Wallis, *Medics*) ap-

pears to have practised midwifery. For his ingenuity see *Medical Essays and Observations from a Society in Edinburgh*, 6 (1747 edn), pp. 422–3; on Freke in general see S. Schaffer, "The consuming flame: Tory mystics and electrical showmen in the world of goods", in *Consumption and the world of goods*, J. Brewer & R. Porter (eds) (London: Routledge, 1993).
25. Chapman, *Treatise* (1735), pp. xxi, 21–2. A possible candidate for the second individual was Benjamin Pugh of Chelmsford, another early forceps user in Essex. But Pugh can almost certainly be ruled out as this "very ingenious practitioner, now living in the country", since he started practice not long before 1740. See Pugh, *Treatise of midwifery*, p. iv.
26. Hearne, *Remarks*, vol. VIII, pp. 147–8, 377 (12 June 1725) & vol. XI, pp. 271–2 (14 February 1726/7), 352–3 (3 October 1727); he sometimes calls him Woods, sometimes Wood. This was presumably Alexander Wood (1662–1749), known to have taken one apprentice (Richard Waldren in 1718): Wallis, *Medics*.
27. See Ch. 10 below.
28. See Giffard, *Cases*, as follows. Chamberlen and "forcing medicines": Case 140; cf. Case 101. "My Extractor": Cases 26, 30, 32, and *passim*. "My Eductor": Case 48. "This Instrument": Case 205.
29. Chapman, *Treatise* (1735), p. 5.
30. He had been apprenticed, probably before 1710, to the father of "Mr White of Ipswich"; he collaborated with Dr Beeston of Ipswich; and he inserted a long encomium to the memory of Dr Shapcote. See Chapman, *Treatise* (1735), Cases 31, 32, 38. These were probably John White (pre 1695–post 1729; his father unidentified); William Beeston, MD (1671–1732); and John Shapcote, MD (1675–post 1720), of Chelmsford. See Wallis, *Medics*, and for Shapcote, *Sloane index*.
31. Chapman, *Treatise* (1735), p. 5.
32. William Douglas asserted in 1748 that "Dr Walker pretended to improve Dr Chamberlen's forceps, but, in truth, spoiled them, by making them male and female": *A letter to Dr Smelle* (London, 1748), reprinted in Glaister, *Smellie*, pp. 74–89, at p. 77. This is interpreted by Aveling as referring to an English lock, for which there is some indirect support: see Aveling, *Chamberlens*, p. 193, and Radcliffe, *Milestones*, p. 32. It might, however, refer to a difference between the two blades: see *n*.48 to Ch. 11 below.
33. Aveling, *Chamberlens*, pp. 191–3; R. Trumbach, *The aristocratic family in England 1690–1780: studies in childhood and kinship* (PhD thesis, John Hopkins University, 1972), p. 31; Ch. 7 below.
34. Aveling, *Chamberlens*, p. 200 (Aveling's translation of Atterbury's Latin).
35. Giffard, *Cases*, Case 14, 8 April 1726, pp. 29–30.
36. *Ibid.*, Case 23, 28 June 1728, pp. 47–9.
37. *Ibid.*, Case 40, at pp. 86–7, shows that he was practising during the gap in his recording, and Case 71 suggests that he had been successfully using the forceps during the gap. See also Ch. 7 below.
38. Chapman, *Treatise* (1735), pp. xxi, 21–2 (cf. *n*.25 above).
39. See H. Collins, *Changing order: replication and induction in scientific practice* (London: Sage, 1985); S. Schaffer, "Glass works: Newton's prisms and the uses of experiment", in *The uses of experiment*, D. Gooding et al. (eds) (Cambridge: Cambridge University Press, 1989), pp. 67–104.
40. Ch. 4 above.
41. Schaffer, The consuming flame. Freke was associated in 1732–33 with Thomas Wilson, whose father had "much in him that was akin to the spirit of the Nonjurors". As soon as

NOTES

Wilson started to align himself with the Court, he apparently dropped his connection with Freke. See C. L. S. Linnell (ed.), *The diaries of Thomas Wilson, DD, 1731–37 and 1750, son of Bishop Wilson of Sodor and Man* (London: SPCK, 1964), pp. 1 (quoted), 67, 69, 94, 97 (links with Freke, the last in April 1733), 105, 109–11 (links with Court, starting October 1733).

42. See Ch. 8 below. According to Hody, Giffard contributed one of the associated pamphlets (Giffard, *Cases*, Preface, p. iv); this must have been anonymous.

43. Giffard, *Cases*, Case 154 (22 October 1730). George Wharton (1688–1739) subscribed to works by the Nonjurors Jeremy Collier (1721, 1727), Thomas Deacon (1721), John Blackbourne (1730), and to a book by Michael Maittaire (1725) who had Nonjuror associations at this time; his only other subscription of the 1720s (the first, in fact) was to a religious work by Randolph Ford (1720), whose allegiance I have not identified. Wharton's later subscriptions (some to books published after his death) suggest a move towards natural-philosophical interests and Court Whig allegiance: works by J. T. Desaguliers (1734, 1744), Richard Bundy (1740) and Roger Long (1742). For Wharton's subscriptions (and for those of other individuals below) see Wallis, *Medics* and Phibb, *Subscriptions*; for allegiances (here and below), see the respective *DNB* entries; for Maittaire, see Hearne, *Remarks*, vol. V, p. 179 and *DNB* entry for George Harbin.

44. Edward Milward (d. 1757) was, according to Chapman's dedication, already MD in 1733; Munk, *Roll* states that his first MD was from Leyden, but he has no entry in Innes Smith, *Students at Leyden*. One of this name was apprenticed in 1724 to the apothecary James Blackstone. Milward was delicately courting Sir Hans Sloane in June, November and December 1733 (BL, Sloane MSS 4053 ff. 76, 114; 4052 f. 373; 4059 f. 358; 4435 ff. 197–9), and this issued in the dedication to Sloane of his *Trallianus reviviscens* (London, 1734). From 1739 he becomes more visible, through book-subscriptions, his *Circular invitatory letter . . . concerning . . . an history . . . of the most celebrated British physical and chirurgical authors* (London, 1740); a Cambridge MD by Royal Mandate (1741), etc. See Wallis, *Medics*; Munk, *Roll*; *DNB*.

45. John Douglas, *A short account of the state of midwifery in London, Westminster, &c.* (London, 1736), pp. 63–4; E. Chapman, *A reply to Mr Douglas's short account of the state of midwifery in London and Westminster* (London, 1737), pp. 47–8. On this exchange see Ch. 8 below.

46. In addition, notice that one of the publishers of Chapman's posthumous edition (1753) was the Tory bookseller James Hodges, for whom see L. Colley, *In defiance of oligarchy: the Tory party 1714–60* (Cambridge: Cambridge University Press, 1982), p. 280. Chapman did, however, praise the Whig physician Sir Richard Blackmore: *Essay* (1735), pp. 101–2. But Blackmore was an old Whig of the 1690s; by the 1720s, when this case probably occurred, he was radically estranged from the Court party. See my "The politics of medical improvement in early Hanoverian London", in *The medical enlightenment of the eighteenth century*, A. Cunningham & R. French (eds) (Cambridge: Cambridge University Press, 1990), pp. 4–39, at pp. 29–30.

47. Both Chapman and Douglas at first elided the difference between the last two Chamberlen generations, and wrote as if Hugh Chamberlen I and Hugh Chamberlen II were the same person. This was only cleared up when Douglas briefly responded to Chapman's 1737 *Reply*, that is, in the Preface to his *Dissertation on the venereal disease. Part II* (London, 1737), pp. 22–3.

48. The testimonial for his episcopal licence was signed on 24 August 1694 by Samuel Packer, the local minister; Thomas Jackson (of Twickenham, licensed in 1690) and John Goslead,

surgeons; John Rees, apothecary; "and others". See Bloom & James, *Medical practitioners*, pp. 48, 33; Wallis, *Medics* gives 1697 as the year of Drinkwater's licence. For Packer see Venn, *Alumni cantabrigiensis*, I.iii.293.
49. N. Moore, *The history of St Bartholomew's Hospital* (2 volumes; London: C. Pearson, 1918), vol. II, p. 737; for the Tory character of St Bartholomew's Hospital, see C. Rose, "Politics and the London Royal Hospitals, 1683–92" in *The hospital in history*, L. Granshaw & R. Porter (eds) (London: Routledge, 1990). Bamber subscribed to 23 books between 1704 and 1719. His early subscriptions included works by William Nicholls, 1710; Simon Ockley, 1718; and Matthew Prior 1718, all Tories.
50. Bamber made no book-subscriptions between 1720 and 1726. For his medical realignment see Munk, *Roll*; S. Young, *The annals of the Barber-Surgeons of London, compiled from their records and other sources* (London: Blades, East & Blades, 1890), p. 345.
51. After 1726 the profile of Bamber's subscriptions became more complex, but he subscribed to works by the Nonjuror John Blackbourne 1730 and the Tory William Hawkins 1735, and subsequently to works by former clients of Lord Oxford (Conyers Middleton 1741, Michael Maittaire 1742). For Hawkins (admittedly earlier, in 1718) see Hearne, *Remarks*, VI. 126. In 1735 Bamber assisted at the delivery of Molly Wilson, whose husband had recently shifted towards the Court: Linnell (ed.), *Diaries of Thomas Wilson*, pp. 121, 123 (see n.41 above).
52. A dimension I have not explored is the identity of the instrument-makers employed by the early forceps users. Chapman's forceps was made by Thomas Swain in Bedford Street near Bedford Row: Chapman, *Treatise* (1735), Figs p. 29. Neither Giffard's nor Freke's instrument-maker was identified in the plate depicting their forceps in Giffard, *Cases*.
53. Hody's book-subscriptions at this time show a strong Whig profile (e.g. works by Richard Mounteney 1731, George Benson 1735 and Martin Clare 1735), in view of which his connection with John Freke is puzzling. It is not known how he obtained Giffard's manuscript; his motive for publishing it was perhaps to outflank Chapman (cf. Ch. 8 below). For his later eschewing the forceps see Glaister, *Smellie*, p. 92, and Ch. 11 below. Hody was the dedicatee of the 1752 treatise of George Counsell, whose obstetric allegiance is ambiguous (see n.52 to Ch. 12 below).
54. B. Exton, *A new and general system of midwifery* (London, 1751), 1766 edition, pp. 2, 5, 9–10; see also Ch. 11 below.

Chapter Six

The forceps contested: the London Deventerians

Just when Hugh Chamberlen II was distributing the midwifery forceps to selected Tory surgeons – that is, during the reign of George I – London medical practitioners of Whig allegiance were discovering an alternative to the forceps in the recent writings of the Dutch obstetric surgeon Hendrik van Deventer (1651–1724). These London "Deventerians" were contesting the forceps as early as 1716; and they went on doing so through the publication of the instrument in the 1730s, and beyond this until about 1750. Here I shall first examine the practical and conceptual resources that Deventer supplied, and then try to identify his London followers; the unfolding contest between Deventerians and forceps practitioners will be traced in Chapter 8.

Hendrik van Deventer and his obstetrics

In 1701 Deventer published at Leyden his *Manuale operatieen, nieuw ligt voor vroed-meesters en vroedvrouwen*.[1] This work – translated into Latin in the same year and subsequently into English, French and German – included the first account of the size, shape and obstetric significance of the female pelvis; appropriately enough, Deventer was also the first author to recognize in print the obstetric effects of rickets. His remarkably original approach to midwifery was religiously inspired. At the age of about 20 he had joined the Labadist brethren – the followers of Jean de la Badie (1610–74), a Huguenot *émigré* who split from the main body of Dutch Huguenots and attracted a small but devoted following. The Labadists, who numbered only a few hundred people, led a semi-peripatetic existence in the Dutch Republic and elsewhere during the later seventeenth century, settling in 1675 at Wieuward, near Leeuwarden. Despite its tiny size this sect

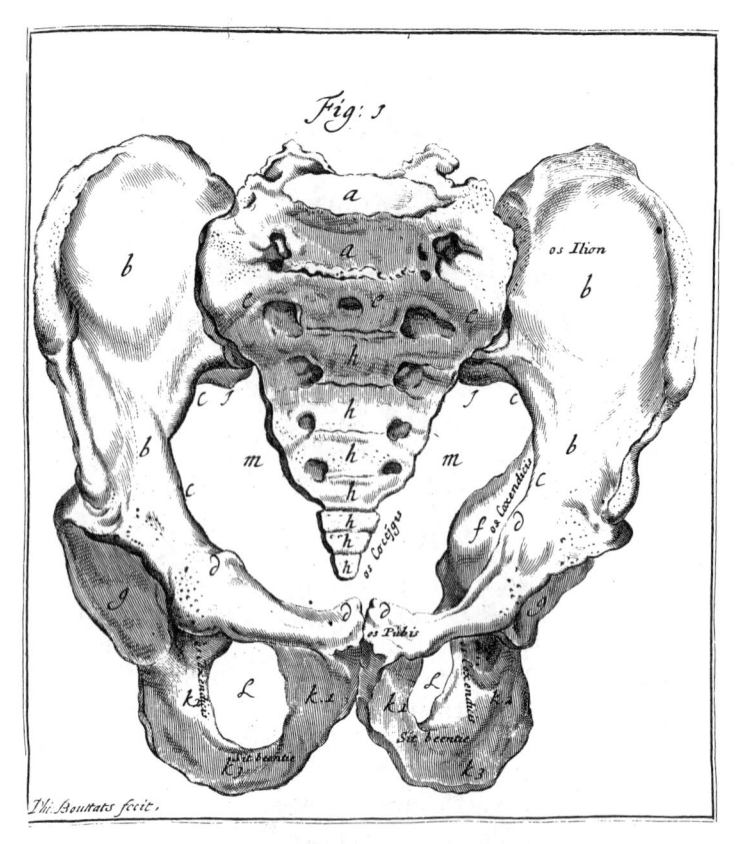

Figure 6.1   Female pelvis (Deventer, Operationes chirurgicae, 1701).

included three individuals who made important contributions to European culture — the religious writer Anna Maria van Schurman, the natural-philosophical artist Maria Sibylla Merian, and Deventer himself.[2] We may picture the Labadists as driven to intense creative efforts by their situation of internal exile, and supported in those efforts by their collective solidarity. Thus Deventer's very practising of medicine and surgery was a vocation acquired after his conversion to La Badie's sect.[3]

The "new light" that Deventer shed upon midwifery derived from a further conversion of a different kind, which apparently took place in about 1689, some 10 years after he began to practise obstetric surgery.[4] Here the key figure was probably his wife, who was a midwife and practised conjointly with him. She certainly gave him unusually early access to deliveries; and it may well have been she who alerted him to one of the cornerstones of his approach — the movement of the coccyx during birth. For we know from the testimony of Pieter van Foreest a century earlier that Dutch midwives (at least, those of Delft) adapted their practices to permit such movement. Perhaps Deventer's existing interest in diseases of the bones helped to sensitize him to such issues.[5] At all events Deventer swiftly developed a new theory and practice of obstetrics, practised this with great success in the 1690s, and published it as *New light* (*Nieuw ligt*) in 1701. (Perhaps the publication of this book at Leyden was partly inspired by the contemporary development of the Roonhuysen monopoly at Amsterdam.)[6] The aftermath was profoundly ironic. The success of his obstetric writings brought Deventer great wealth, which led him to contest the Labadists' insistence on communal property, and the resulting battle irrevocably divided the movement.[7]

Deventer's obstetric theory was based on seven concentric and interrelated zones: child, uterus, pelvis, mother, midwives, parents, the State.[8] The presentation of the *child* – on which previous authors had concentrated – Deventer reconceptualized as an aspect of its total bodily posture or "turning". The *uterus* could be oriented "directly", which favoured a natural birth, or "obliquely", producing difficulty; this was semi-independent of the child's "turning", so that the two could combine in complex ways. The *pelvis* might be too narrow to permit the child to pass (due chiefly to rickets), or it might be over-capacious, leading to obliquity of the uterus; it was largely rigid, but had one mobile part – the coccyx. And the mother's *posture* should be adjusted so as to promote delivery, whether by natural means or by manual operation. (Natural births were to be helped by a birth-stool, with an open seat to permit movement of the coccyx. If the child was ill-turned or the uterus oblique, this should be countered by so tilting the mother's body as to gain the assistance of gravity.) With this "new light" shed on midwifery, instruments should become almost unnecessary, and the management of childbirth would be revolutionized – but this required conscious civic effort. *Midwives* had a moral duty to learn the new theory and its associated practical methods – starting with the use of "touching" to diagnose the position of the child and the orientation of the uterus. *Parents* had both an interest and a duty to interrogate midwives to ensure that they had acquired the necessary understanding and diagnostic skill. And the *legislature* of the Dutch Republic ought to bring in laws to enforce such a raising of standards.

As to the methods of delivery, Deventer's approach had five practical implications.

1. Mildly unfavourable "turnings" of the child and "obliquities" of the womb could be corrected by manipulating the mother's posture, by applying external pressure with a hand on her abdomen, and by using the other hand "inwardly" to adjust the child's position.
2. More severe instances of "ill turning" and of uterine obliquity were to be delivered by the feet (that is, using podalic version with traction) very early in labour, assisted by the natural labour-pains. This applied not only to all malpresentations but also to some births by the head, particularly cases of face-to-pubis (occipito-posterior) presentation.
3. For obstructed births by the head, Deventer devised a new idea that can aptly be termed *Deventer's manoeuvre*. He would introduce his hand with the palm towards him, and the back of the hand against the mother's coccyx,

and by firm pressure outwards with the back of his hand he could force the coccyx to bend backwards (as it does naturally in normal labour), thereby slightly enlarging the diameter of the passage. The gain thus produced must have been very small, perhaps only about a centimetre – but this could give a huge advantage in the delivery. We may assume, therefore, that although this technique has apparently passed into oblivion, it worked. It should be noted that Deventer synchronized his manoeuvre with the mother's labour-pains, and that he accompanied it with encouraging exhortations to the mother – assurances that together she and he could effect the delivery.[9] The manoeuvre could also be used in breech-presentations, provided the uterus was "direct", not "oblique".

4. Although he criticized the use of instruments, Deventer nevertheless made occasional use of a bandage that closely resembled the *fillet* – apparently only in the delivery of a dead child.[10]

5. Finally, and seemingly inconsistently, Deventer permitted craniotomy under two sets of circumstances: in these cases, the child was to be "treated as dead" so as to save the mother's life.

(a) If there was gross disproportion between the child's head and the mother's pelvis, arising either from foetal hydrocephalus or from maternal rickety pelvis, delivery was physically impossible without opening the child's head.

(b) Certain combinations of the child's "turning" and the orientation of the uterus, if not correctly managed by the midwife, would lead to irreducible obstruction. Although such births did not in themselves require instrumental delivery, mismanagement (that is, failure to diagnose correctly and to deliver accordingly) would make the use of instruments absolutely necessary.

These two indications amounted to two escape clauses, each enabling a follower of Deventer to criticize craniotomy and yet to practise that operation.[11]

The use of Deventer in London

Deventer's approach was elegantly suited to its London role of serving as an alternative to the forceps, for it outflanked the forceps on several fronts. Early turning would take care of some labours in which the forceps might have proved useful. Others could be delivered by Deventer's own manoeuvre, which was based on a diametrically opposite conception to that underlying the use of the forceps: forceps practitioners reduced the size of the foetal head and supplied added traction, whereas Deventer enlarged the mother's pelvis and relied on the powers of the uterus.[12] And the remaining cases of obstructed births by the head could be dealt with by craniotomy (or perhaps with the fillet). The escape clauses not only rationalized such exceptional use of instruments; they also implicitly limited the possible achievements of the forceps, by positing that there were some births where craniotomy could not be avoided.

From the outset the London followers of Deventer were Court Whigs opposed to the midwifery forceps. Deventer's treatise was translated into English in two parts in 1716 and 1724; the translator, Robert Samber, was a minor Whig poet, his patron William Cockburn a prominent Whig physician.[13] Cockburn's anonymous preface of 1716 referred to a recent remark of his own, criticizing the use of "dilating instruments" in midwifery; Cockburn apparently had some inkling of the "Roonhuysen secret".[14] In 1724–25 another Whig, John Maubray, set himself up as a teacher of midwifery (despite his apparently limited practical experience) and produced his own plagiaristic treatises based on Deventer.[15] The association between Deventerian methods and Whig political allegiance persisted until mid-century. Some of its ramifications will be explored in later chapters; here it will be convenient to present an overview. Table 6.1 lists all the men-midwives I have identified as practising in London between 1700 and 1750, grouped by their political and obstetric allegiances where these are known. Those with known and

Table 6.1 Political and obstetric allegiances of London men-midwives, 1700–50.

	Whigs	Unknown/shifting	Tories
Anti-forceps			
Deventerian	Cockburn[b]		
	Maubray		
	Manningham		
	Exton		
Pro-fillet	John Douglas		
	Sandys		
?Pro-fillet	William Douglas		
Attitude to forceps unknown/shifting			
Unknown			
1. Fillet			Birch
2. Vectis	Cole	Middleton	
	Nesbitt	Morley	
3. Others	Hamilton	Brooke[a]	
	Macaulay	Beale[a]	
		Parsons	
		Layard	
Shifting	James Douglas		
	Hody		
	Smellie		
Forceps practitioners/supporters			
		Drinkwater	Chamberlen
		Walker	Chapman
		Bamber	Giffard
			Freke[b]

Notes: (a) For Jonathan Brooke (pre 1710–1735) and John Beale (d. 20 June 1724), both of whose allegiances (political and obstetric) are unknown, see Munk, *Roll*, ahnd Wallis, *Medics*. Other practitioners are named and discussed in Chapters 5–10. (b) William Cockburn and John Freke are not known to have practised midwifery, but were associated with public obstetric initiatives.

consistent political and obstetric allegiances comprise seven anti-forceps men, all Whigs, and four forceps practitioners, all Tories (the odds against this being a chance association are 120 to 1 if Hugh Chamberlen II is excluded, 330 to 1 if he is included). Next we may note that all the Deventerians belonged to the Whig, anti-forceps group. Further, two of the other three declared opponents of the forceps – John Douglas and the unrelated William Douglas – wrote polemical tracts, which although not explicitly Deventerian did not criticize Deventerian methods.[16] In short, political and obstetric allegiances in London were consistently associated. As we shall see, obstetric techniques were also connected with particular styles of practice, with geographical locations, and with gender.[17] Thus party politics was not the only cultural association of obstetric methods, and indeed politics may well have been secondary to religious allegiance in this respect. Moreover, both Tories and Whigs were far from homogeneous groups: each alignment was diverse both in politics and in religion. But the Whig/Tory split was the central axis of division in affairs of State at this time, and it is striking that the two main obstetric approaches were associated with these political parties.

Most of the uncertainties in Table 6.1 concern those other two Chamberlen instruments, the vectis and fillet. The vectis will be considered in Chapter 10. The fillet, which like the forceps could be used to deliver either a living child or a dead one, presents a complex and obscure picture in each of four respects.

1. *Origins:* As we have seen, it is unclear what relation obtained between the Chamberlen fillet and the various fillets that came into use in the early eighteenth century.
2. *Technical capacities:* In 1736 John Douglas wrote of the fillet as follows:

> I myself have seen eight or ten different sorts of them, contrived and used by different practitioners. Pray was not Dr Birch's fillet put up to be sold for £500 by the late excellent surgeon Mr Jos. Symonds? Has not Dr Sandys had one for many years?[18]

Widespread use, high price, and association with the successful Francis Sandys all suggest that the fillet was highly effective. Yet those who actually described the use of the fillet (La Motte, Chapman, Smellie, Pugh) found it an unsatisfactory device, and so far as I am aware it never received the candid discussion accorded to the forceps and, some decades later, the vectis.[19]

3. *Obstetric associations:* The fillet was used at times by the forceps practitioners Chapman and Smellie; yet there are several indications that it was chiefly an anti-forceps resource. As we have seen, it was among the suite of Deventer's methods. John Douglas vaunted it precisely as an alternative to the forceps: commenting on a case that Chapman had used to show the necessity of the forceps, he observed:

> supposing a man had been there who had no forceps about him, but was well acquainted with the use of Deventer's, Birch's, or any other fillet

... could not he have extracted the child with as much safety as he did with the forceps?[20]

And Francis Sandys, mentioned by John Douglas as using the fillet, was later named as an opponent of the forceps.[21]

4. *Political links:* Table 6.1 suggests some tendency for the fillet to be associated with Whigs, and this could be extended by noting that Richard Mead (not himself a man-midwife, and so excluded from the table) gave Smellie a whalebone fillet in 1743.[22] Yet we also have the contrary cases of Chapman and Birch; and to complete the confusion, Birch's associations were in fact more complex than Table 6.1 indicates.[23]

Whatever the significance of the fillet, the main line of contest was drawn between Deventerianism and the forceps, each connected with a specific political allegiance. Perhaps this politico-obstetric association merely reflected accidents of patronage – the fact that Hugh Chamberlen II was a Tory. Yet perhaps it had some deeper significance: this is suggested both by Deventer's own intensely religious motives, and by analogy with the other major practical medical innovation of the period, inoculation for smallpox, which was specifically a Court Whig project.[24] On the other hand, as we shall later see, the sharp division between Deventerians and forceps practitioners was specific to London, or rather to Westminster.[25] The two groups may also have had different styles of practice. Forceps practitioners mainly received emergency calls (see Chapter 7), but the Deventerian Whigs probably specialized in advance and onset calls with a midwife – just as Deventer himself had practised alongside his wife. Such was the practice of Francis Sandys in the 1730s and '40s.[26] In the 1730s both Sandys and Dr James Douglas received Court appointments in midwifery, which probably amounted to advance calls with a midwife.[27] And a similar practice is strongly suggested for the most visible of these individuals – Sir Richard Manningham, Hanoverian knight, Cambridge graduate, and founder of the first London lying-in hospital, which he set up for teaching purposes in 1739.[28] Manningham's methods are more easily identified than those of Sandys or James Douglas thanks to the Latin "syllabus" for his teaching which he published in 1739 (it was translated into English in 1744). This little treatise reveals that Manningham's teaching was strongly and plagiaristically Deventerian, yet with certain emphases of his own. In particular, Manningham promoted very early access to difficult births for the man-midwife.[29]

However, there was probably a further and associated niche of male practice: craniotomy work, the traditional staple of obstetric surgery. We have seen that Deventerian theory made craniotomy permissible. Did Manningham and his colleagues perform this operation? One Court Whig practitioner – not known to have been a Deventerian, but certainly an opponent of the forceps – apparently did so in a famous case. In 1738, Francis Sandys "was obliged to squeeze the child to death" in his attempt to deliver the Princess of Orange at The Hague.[30] Such cases would have been relatively rare – most advance and onset calls with a midwife resulted, of course, in normal birth – yet from time to time they would crop up. When practising in London, the Deventerians, most of whom were physicians, probably referred such craniotomy cases to surgeons, such as John Douglas, whom we shall meet in Chapter 8. Indeed such men may have practised as a physician–surgeon team.[31]

One of the most notable of the Court Whig men-midwives is for the historian the most elusive of them. This was James Douglas, John's brother, whom John described as "that consummate accoucheur", and whose involvement in midwifery is attested in a variety of other ways, including an allusion in Pope's *Dunciad*:

> To prove me Goddess clear of all design
> Bid me with Pollio sup as well as dine
> Where all the learned shall at labour stand
> And Douglas lend his soft obstetric hand.[32]

James Douglas had many activities; together with his brother John, he played a major role in the development of lithotomy, and he made important contributions to both anatomy and botany. Appropriately for a Scot who made his way in English polite society in the age of Addison and Steele, he produced in manuscript the first major work on English pronunciation.[33] But among his diverse interests, midwifery was certainly an important part of his practice; and his known obstetric associations began with an attempt to use the forceps around 1702 (as we have seen) and ended, 40 years later, with his teaching and helping William Hunter, supreme man-midwife of the following generation.[34] It is therefore frustrating to find that, save for the very early years of his practice, no record of Douglas's obstetric work survives among his numerous manuscripts; that although he planned a midwifery treatise, he never wrote it, not even in draft; and that references to him from other practitioners are vague and obscure.[35] But all the available indications suggest a shift away from his early, unsuccessful use of the forceps and towards the same Deventerian allegiance that characterized his Court Whig colleague and rival Manningham.[36]

The lucrative form of man-midwifery in early Hanoverian London, then, comprised onset calls with a midwife; the dominant practitioners were Whigs associated with the Court; and these men, where their obstetric allegiance can be identified, seem all to have been Deventerians. An aspiring young practitioner, if he wanted to enjoy the spoils of such practice, would have been well advised to trim his sails to the wind and to espouse Deventerian methods.

The importance of demonstrating one's correct obstetric credentials is illustrated as tragic farce by the actions of James Houstoun. Houstoun, endowed with much ambition but also with a certain clumsiness that repeatedly frustrated his high hopes in life, managed to get a trainee position at the Paris Hôtel-Dieu's "salle des accouchements" in 1718.[37] This gave him the experience, remarkable at that date, of perhaps 300 normal births; and he duly returned to London and approached the leading Whig man-midwife, Sir David Hamilton, in the hope of being eased into fashionable obstetric practice.[38] Hamilton spurned him, and Houstoun thereupon gave up the attempt – or so he told the world in his later autobiography. However, Houstoun also made at this time some further and equally fruitless efforts, not mentioned in the autobiography, to insinuate himself into London man-midwifery. In 1719 he produced a translation of Mauriceau's "Aphorisms", embellished with a few notes of his own experience at the Hôtel-Dieu, hoping to get this published and thus to advertise his own name. But before taking his manuscript to a publisher, Houstoun passed it to James Douglas, probably asking Douglas to contribute a preface or to accept the role of dedicatee.[39] At the last minute, Houstoun somehow found out that the way to win public support (and presumably Douglas's support in particular) was to align oneself not with Mauriceau but with Deventer. A wiser man would have sought a different patron or rewritten his treatise; but Houston clumsily tacked on to his existing text some "Additional Aphorisms" on the obliquity of the womb – the central concept of Deventer's theory – together with an unconvincing preface in which he assured the reader that he had indeed observed this obliquity many times while at the Hôtel-Dieu.[40] Evidently Douglas was unimpressed, for the work remained unpublished, although he preserved Houstoun's manuscript.

Houstoun's little effort suggests that the lines of London obstetric allegiance had been laid down as early as 1719. Fashionable practitioners were now to follow Deventer, not Mauriceau – just as learned physicians were turning for their rationale to Herman Boerhaave, in place of Cartesian iatromechanism.[41] Just when the forceps was spreading outwards from the Chamberlen family, among a select circle of Tory practitioners, Whig men-midwives were taking up Deventer as an alternative to the forceps. We shall take up the story of the conflict between these groups in Chapter 8.

Notes

1. H. L. Houtzager, "Hendrik van Deventer", *European Journal of Obstetrics, Gynaecology and Reproductive Biology* 21 (1986), pp. 263–70, at p. 267; for editions see *RCOG Catalogue*, pp. 22–3.
2. See T. J. Saxby, *The quest for the New Jerusalem: Jean de Labadie and the Labadists, 1610–1744* (Dordrecht: Nijhoff, 1987), *passim*. Labadie was trained by the Jesuits, but was from a Huguenot family who had outwardly followed Henri IV into Catholicism but privately "continued to respect their former allegiance" (pp. 1–2). On Anna Maria van Schurman see the entry for her in Todd, *Women writers*.
3. Houtzager, "Hendrik van Deventer", p. 265. Deventer's *Midwifery improv'd* frequently attested to his religious motives: see, for instance, pp. 266, 301–2.
4. See Deventer, *Midwifery improv'd*, p. 318.
5. On Pieter van Foreest (1522–97) see Garrison, *History of medicine*, p. 274, and E. Ingerslev, "Rösslin's "Rosegarten": its relation to the past (the Muscio manuscripts and

Soranos), particularly with regard to podalic version", *Journal of Obstetrics and Gynaecology of the British Empire*, **15** (1909), pp. 1–25, 73–92, at p. 6. G. Sarton, review of A. J. M. Lamers, *Hendrik van Deventer, medicinae doctor, 1651–1724* (Assen, 1946), *Isis* **39** (1948), pp. 182–4, at p. 182; cf. Deventer, *Midwifery improv'd*, pp. 22–3.

6. See Ch. 5.
7. Saxby, *The quest for the New Jerusalem*.
8. What follows is based on Deventer, *Midwifery improv'd* (i.e. *The art of midwifery improv'd*, London, 1716), which was translated from his *Operationes chirurgicae, novum lumen exhibentes obstetricantibus* (Leyden, 1701). The further work entitled *New improvements in the art of midwifery* (London, 1724) was translated from the new Part II, which had been added to the 1724 Latin edition of *Operationes chirurgicae*; this added only some changes of emphasis, slightly enlarging the scope for craniotomy and strengthening the argument for legislative intervention.
9. Deventer, *Midwifery improv'd*, pp. 126–36. The manoeuvre was endorsed by L. von Heister, *A General system of surgery in three parts* (German original 1718; trans. anon., London, 1743), pp. 209–10, 217–18, 219.
10. Deventer, *Midwifery improv'd*, p. 326.
11. *Ibid.*, Appendix (pp. 320–28).
12. Though Deventer suggested that the hand could apply some traction to the head in the course of performing his manoeuvre: *ibid.*, pp. 283–4.
13. *The art of midwifery improv'd* (1716) had a preface by an unnamed "eminent physician"; *New improvements* (1724) was dedicated to "Dr Cockburne" and made it clear that he had written the preface to Part I. For Robert Samber see D. N. Smith (ed.), *The letters of Thomas Burnet to George Duckett, 1712–1722* (London, Roxburgh Club, 1914), p. 221 and *passim*; *BL Catalogue*. For William Cockburn (LRCP 1694) see *DNB*; Munk, *Roll*; and H. J. Cook, "Practical medicine and the British armed forces after the 'Glorious Revolution'", *Medical History* **34** (1990), pp. 1–26.
14. Here Cockburn was referring to his own *Symptoms . . . of gonorrhoea* (London, 1713), p. 9; *ibid.*, 2nd edn (London, 1715), pp. 11–12. On the dilating use of the Roonhuysen instruments, cf. Ch. 5 above, at *n*.10.
15. For Maubray, see Ch. 8 below.
16. For John Douglas, see Ch. 8; for William Douglas, see Ch. 11.
17. A partial exception was that the Tory Giffard was for a time trying Deventer's manoeuvre and attending to the orientation of the uterus (Ch. 7 below, at *n*.21). For styles of practice see below, at *n*.26; for geographical locations, see Ch. 10; for gender, see Ch. 15 (Elizabeth Nihell).
18. John Douglas, *A short account of the state of midwifery in London, Westminster, &c.* (London, 1736), p. 60. For the context, see Ch. 8 below.
19. La Motte, *Midwifery*, p. 536; Chapman, *Treatise* (1735), *passim* and pp. 172–5; McClintock, *Smellie's midwifery*, vol. I, pp. 253–4; B. Pugh, *A treatise of midwifery, chiefly with regard to the operation. With several improvements in that art* (London, 1754), p. 91.
20. Douglas, *A short account*, p. 61. Smellie also described the fillet as an alternative to the forceps: McClintock, *Smellie's midwifery*, vol. I, p. 251.
21. W. Douglas, *A second letter to Dr Smellie and an answer to his pupil* (London, 1748), summarized in Glaister, *Smellie*, pp. 89–97, at p. 92 (see Ch. 11 below). To add to the confusion, Sandys's fillet appears to have been a double instrument, used both as vectis and as fillet: see Glaister, *Smellie*, pp. 43, 218, and cf. *n*.5 to Ch. 10 below. Francis Sandys (d. 1771): Admitted Fellow-commoner Emmanuel, Cambridge, 1726; matriculated, 1732;

MD (Lit. Reg.) 1739. Eulogized as Cambridge Whig man-midwife in 1735 by Edward Cobden. Around 1740 lectured on anatomy at Cambridge. Extensive fashionable practice in London, 1740s to probably mid-1750s. Physician-accoucheur to the Middlesex Hospital, 1747–49, subsequently man-midwife to the British Lying-in Hospital, Brownlow Street; variously associated with Manningham (1747) and Matthew Morley (1754). Retired to Potton, Beds., his London practice having been taken over by William Hunter. See Venn, *Alumni cantabrigiensis*; Ch. 11 below; A. Rook, "Medicine at Cambridge 1660–1760", *Medical History* 13 (1969), pp. 118–19, 252; *HMC Egmont* vol. II, p. 444–5, 463; ibid., vol. III, p. 86; Lady Llanover (ed.), *The autobiography and correspondence of Mary Granville, Mrs Delany* (3 volumes; London, 1861), vol. II, pp. 57–60, 203, 229, 252, 285; McClintock, *Smellie's midwifery*, vol. III, p. 222, Case 431; anon., *The trial of a cause* (London, 1754), p. 19; Brock, *William Hunter*, p. 8.
22. McClintock, *Smellie's midwifery*, vol. I, p. 255.
23. Birch's political allegiance may have changed towards the Court in the mid-1720s, and it is possible that his "fillet" was in fact a vectis. See Ch. 10 below.
24. See my "The politics of medical improvement in early Hanoverian London", in *The medical enlightenment of the eighteenth century*, A. Cunningham & R. French (eds) (Cambridge: Cambridge University Press, 1990), pp. 4–39.
25. Chs 8 & 10 below.
26. Llanover (ed.), *Correspondence of Mrs Delany*, vol. II, pp. 57–60, 203, 229, 252, 285; E. Cobden, *Poems on several occasions* (London, 1748), pp. 139–44, 145–8.
27. Both these appointments related to pregnancies of the Princess of Orange. For Douglas's appointment (1734) see C. H. Brock, "James Douglas of the pouch", *Medical History* 18 (1974), pp. 162–72, at p. 168; for that of Sandys (1738), see *HMC Egmont*, vol. II, pp. 318–19.
28. Sir Richard Manningham (1690–1759): Second son of Thomas Manningham, afterwards Bishop of Chichester. Born at Eversley, Hants., or in London. Cambridge (Magdalene) 1717, Ll.B. immediately (Com. Reg.); FRS 1720; LRCP 1720; knighted 18 February 1721/2; member of the Gentlemen's Society at Spalding from 24 December 1724; mandate (Royal?) for MD Cambridge 1725. Involved in the Mary Toft case, 1726; apparently an associate of Francis Sandys in 1747. See Munk, *Roll* (who lists his works); *DNB*; Venn, *Alumni cantabrigiensis*; Nichols, *Literary anecdotes*, vol. VI, p. 97; Ch. 8 below; McClintock, *Smellie's midwifery*, vol. III, p. 222, Case 431.
29. Sir Richard Manningham, *Artis obstetricariae compendium tam theoriam quam praxin spectans* (London, 1739); trans. anon. as *An abstract of midwifery for use in the lying-in infirmary* (London, 1744); see Ch. 8 below. A practice of advance and onset calls with a midwife would be consistent with Manningham's confidence that breech births would deliver naturally, provided the womb was situated normally. It would also explain his advocating cephalic version for transverse lie, which was unusual at this period and contrary to Deventer's precepts (cf. Ch. 12 below). See *Abstract of midwifery*, pp. 24, 17.
30. *HMC Egmont*, vol. II, pp. 318–19. The presumption that Sandys was a Deventerian arises from the support of John Douglas, discussed in Ch. 8 below.
31. See Ch. 13 below, at *n.*14.
32. Quoted in Brock, "James Douglas of the pouch", p. 170. For Douglas's various activities see this article, and also *idem*, "James Douglas (1675–1742), botanist", *Journal for the Society for Bibliography of Natural History* 9 (1979), pp. 137–45; K. Bryn Thomas, *James Douglas of the pouch* (London: Pitman 1964).
33. B. Holmberg, *James Douglas on English pronunciation c.1740* (Lund: C. W. K. Gleerup, 1956).

34. Ch. 5 above; R. Porter, "William Hunter: a surgeon and a gentleman", in *William Hunter*, Bynum & Porter (eds), pp. 7–34, at pp. 32–3; C. H. Brock, "The happiness of riches", in *ibid.*, pp. 35–54, at pp. 36–8; *HMC Egmont*, vol. I, p. 225.
35. Brock, "James Douglas of the pouch", pp. 164, 167.
36. These indications begin in 1719 with James Houstoun's actions, discussed below. They continue with Douglas's involvement in the Mary Toft case, 1726; the approval of his brother John, who opposed the forceps but endorsed Deventer and the fillet, 1736; and the fact that when Smellie went to London in 1739 (the year after Chapman's death) to learn about the forceps, "here I saw that nothing was to be learned". They conclude in 1748, six years after Douglas had died, with the opposition to the forceps of Douglas's ex-pupil, the unrelated William Douglas. (See Chs 8 & 9 below; McClintock, *Smellie's midwifery*, vol. II, p. 250.) In addition, Pope's phrase "his soft obstetric hand" suggests Deventerian methods (the hand rather than instruments); and like Deventer, Douglas worked on osteology (Brock, James Douglas of the pouch, pp. 164–5). Douglas's pupil James Parsons published a syllabus of his own midwifery teaching, but this did not make his methods clear: *Praelecturi Jacobi Parsons, MD, elenchus gynaico pathologicus et obstetricarius* (London, 1741).
37. James Houstoun, *Memoirs of the life and travels of James Houstoun, MD, collected and written by his own hand* (London, 1747), pp. 66–8, 73–4. Houstoun's predecessor was a "Mr Clayton" (p. 73); the only eligible Claytons identified in Wallis, *Medics* are: Robert, apprenticed 1724; Thomas of Manchester, master five times 1717–28; and Thomas of London, master 1717. Others later trained in midwifery at the Hôtel-Dieu included Henry Bracken, John Birch (cf. Ch. 10 below), Thomas Secker and Elizabeth Nihell: see *DNB* entry for Bracken; J. R. Guy, "Archbishop Secker as a physician", in *The church and healing*, W. J. Sheils (ed.) (Oxford: Blackwell, for the Ecclesiastical History Society, 1982), pp. 127–35, at p. 132; Ch. 15 below.
38. Houstoun, *Memoirs*, pp. 81–2.
39. So we must infer from the existence of Douglas MS 11.5, James Houstoun, "Aphorisms on childbirth", dated 1719, in Hunterian Library, University of Glasgow. Although Houstoun's autobiography did not mention writing his "Aphorisms" or sending them to Douglas, the book did attest that he knew Douglas, saying of Hamilton "that Dr Douglas told me that he never did a good office for any of his profession" (*Memoirs*, pp. 81–2).
40. Houstoun, "Aphorisms on childbirth", ff. ii–iv, 287–321.
41. A. Cunningham, "Medicine to calm the mind: Boerhaave's medical system, and why it was adopted in Edinburgh", in *The medical enlightenment of the eighteenth century*, A. Cunningham & R. French (eds) (Cambridge: Cambridge University Press, 1990), pp. 40–66.

Chapter Seven
The impact of the forceps

❧

William Giffard's case-series and his practice

Of all the early forceps practitioners, Giffard alone bequeathed a substantial case-series from which we might reconstruct his practice. His posthumous *Cases in midwifery,* edited by Edward Hody in 1734, contained 225 dated cases, presented in chronological order and supplied with such details as the patient's status or her husband's occupation, her location (sometimes by parish, usually by street), the way Giffard was called to the case, the activities of the midwife, the power relations and transactions in the lying-in room, the obstetric problems and Giffard's practical response. Yet this very rich record has been largely neglected, not only by historians but, long before them, by the obstetric writers of the eighteenth century. I cannot do justice here to the wealth of information that Giffard recorded; but it will be worth offering an overview of his treatise, his cases and his practice.

In all probability, this text was published very much as Giffard wrote it, that is, as a sequence of cases from January 1725 to October 1731. Edward Hody, who "revised and edited" it for publication, merely appended a "continuation" of a single case and provided no other annotation or commentary apart from numbers and headings to the 225 case-histories.[1] The nature of those histories is best conveyed by an example.

> On Sunday August the 14th 1726, I was fetched to a woman near Red-Lyon Square, who laboured under a violent flooding; I found her pulse very languid, and blood coming away upon every little pain: the midwife told me that she had been in that way for several hours, and had lost very much blood; I therefore passed up my forefinger into the vagina towards the inner orifice, which I found divided to the breadth of a crown

piece; it was thin, and would readily give way. I told the persons present, that upon consideration of the preceding great loss of blood, and the likelihood of its continuance (her pains being likewise so small that they would not force the child forward) I thought it highly advisable to attempt the delivery, whilst she had strength to undergo it, at the same time laying before them the danger the poor woman was in: both she and they readily submitted to what I thought fit; I therefore put her in a good posture and well greasing my hand, endeavoured to pass it, keeping my fingers close together; but I had some difficulty, for the outer orifice was very strait, it being her first child; after which, I gently dilated the inner orifice of the womb by spreading my fingers, and in a small time passed up my whole hand, where I found the child floating in the waters, with its head towards the birth: I gently pushed it backwards, and breaking the membranes with my fingers, took hold of a foot which I drew towards me; the other parts readily followed: When I had brought it to the shoulders, I passed up my hand and fetched down the arms, and then as usual, clapping one hand upon the breast to support it, and the other above the shoulders, I drew forwards, but finding the child stuck at the head, I put two fingers into the mouth, and pressing upon the lower jaw it readily followed. I then fetched the after-burthen, which gave me little or no difficulty. The child was born alive, and did well afterwards, and so did the mother.[2]

Here we see a specific rhetorical strategy: the argument is embedded in a wealth of detail, beginning with the date and location, which plunge the reader into a concrete reality. In this particular case there is no indication of how Giffard was summoned, although sometimes Giffard says that the patient's husband fetched him. But it is clear that most of the cases, like this one, were emergency calls. Giffard's first transaction is with the midwife, who gives him a history of the birth; he then investigates for himself by digital examination of the cervix (usually called "touching"), which enables him to make a more precise diagnosis than the humble midwife could achieve. All now seems ready for his own heroic intervention, but a further transaction is required: Giffard proposes a course of action – immediate delivery – to the mother and gossips, who "readily submitted". Only now is the purely obstetric drama enacted; and this is described in some detail, highly repetitive from case to case. Giffard's actions are successful, and this is all the more impressive because various difficulties are encountered along the way. Once the delivery is completed, the case-history is supplied with an ending, which varies from case to case. In this particular case we have the proverbial happy ending: mother and child "did well afterwards". Occasionally Giffard adds a separate paragraph that supplies a moral to the tale, and it is in these more reflective endings that the argument becomes most explicit. For instance, of another case (an emergency occasioned by arm-presentation), Giffard comments:

> This is one of the many inconveniences that occur from the ignorance of midwives: had I been sent for as soon as the membranes were broke, and before the waters were wholly run off, and the shoulder by reiterated pains so strongly locked between the bones of the pelvis, most of my trouble, and the child's life, might have been saved.[3]

The argument, then, was that male practitioners should be summoned to emergencies *much more quickly* than was usually the case; and that those who were to blame in this respect were midwives.[4]

In places the text reads as a body of instructions to an apprentice or pupil (e.g. "You are not always obliged to return the arm", when that part presents).[5] There are some reflections upon the ethical dilemmas of the obstetric surgeon, usually resolved by the slogan that "a doubtful attempt is better than none".[6] On a few occasions Giffard refers to other male practitioners: Dr Eaton assisted him with prescriptions in one case, Dr Wharton was responsible for his being called to another delivery.[7] Fellow obstetric surgeons are mentioned, for instance as having been summoned but not available ("not in the way"), and are occasionally criticized, but these practitioners are not named, save for a Mr Dowse who was the brother of one patient.[8] Some of the colleagues thus alluded to were physicians: "Dr—".[9] Strikingly, there are almost no references to existing obstetric treatises, nor indeed to other works of medicine or surgery.[10] "Dr Chamberlen" is commended for opposing "forcing medicines", that is, medicines to stimulate labour-pains; this probably referred to Hugh Chamberlen I in his translation of Mauriceau. A few midwives are named, but only those Giffard felt able to praise for their "good character and understanding" (Mrs Harrison); probably these were midwives who were more ready than most to send for him (for instance, Mrs Gooding).[11] In contrast with Willughby's case-histories from the Midlands some 60 years earlier, it is rare for more than one midwife to be present before Giffard was called.[12]

As a record of his practice, Giffard's case-series fell into three phases, shown in Table 7.1. In the first phase (January 1725 to August 1726), he seems to have recorded his cases only intermittently: many months are blank, and even those months for which cases are recorded usually only show one or two cases. Moreover, these cases were recorded selectively, for they include very few births by the head.[13] Then came a period of 20 months from the summer of 1726 to the spring of 1728, in which no cases were recorded at all. During this period Giffard was still practising in the area; as we saw in Chapter 5, the cessation of his case-recording probably reflects a period of further instruction in the use of the forceps.[14] Finally, Giffard resumed his case-recording in May 1728, and continued writing down cases until October 1731, around which time he died. In this third phase, his recording seems to have been continuous, for every month has at least one case, and most months have three or more. Correspondingly, obstructed births by the head were now the commonest type of case.[15]

The possibility thus arises that in the third phase Giffard was recording *all* his cases. Indeed for much of the time this was probably so; but this phase was also

Table 7.1 Chronological pattern of Giffard's cases.

	1725	1726	1727	1728	1729	1730	1731
Jan	2	–	–	–	1	12	6
Feb	–	1	–	–	4	5	9
Mar	–	1	–	–	5	1	5
Apr	–	2	–	–	1	5	3
May	–	–	–	2	2	6	3
Jun	–	1	–	4	4	2	7
Jul	–	–	–	3	4[b]	5	4
Aug	–	2	–	10	4	7	3
Sep	4	–	–	7[a]	4	6	6
Oct	3	–	–	3	3	6	8
Nov	–	–	–	7	7	8	
Dec	1	–	–	3	3	9	
Total	10	7	–	39	42	72	54

Notes: (a) Case 38 is described as 6 August [1728], probably in error for 6 September. (b) Case 75 repeats Case 72 and has therefore been excluded (whence total number of cases is 224, and not 225).

punctuated by intermittent returns to his earlier, selective mode of recording. In five separate months there were only one or two cases, and at least some of these months reflect a reversion to selective recording (for instance, there were no cases of obstructed births by the head in an interval of 70 days centring on the month of January 1729).[16] If so, Giffard's rate of practice would have been higher than the third phase suggests. In the calendar year 1730, he recorded 72 cases; in 1731, the final and incomplete year of the series, 54 cases in less than 10 months, suggesting a rate of 68 cases per year. Thus if we assess Giffard's rate of practice at around 70 per year, noting that it may have been a little higher than this, perhaps 80–90 per year, we shall not be too wide of the mark. It seems unlikely that the rate changed much over time: as early as August, 1728 he had received 10 calls in a single month.[17] Nor were there significant changes in either the geographical catchment area or the social profile of patients.

The cases reveal that Giffard's was predominantly an emergency practice, laced with a few onset calls and possibly, perhaps once or twice a year, a more lucrative advance call. His catchment area comprised roughly the West End of London, occasionally extending across the river to Southwark, westwards to Kensington and Chelsea, and eastwards as far as St Botoph's Bishopsgate. His patients were drawn from a very wide spectrum of the population, although there is indirect evidence that the very poorest people tended not to send for him because they felt they could not afford to pay for his services.[18] This catchment area would have comprised roughly a quarter of London's population at this time, producing perhaps 4000 births per year. Among this number of births, we should expect something of the order of 80 per year (2%) to produce emergencies, a number consistent with Giffard's probable rate of practice. Those emergencies comprised the expected mixture of obstructed births by the head (the commonest type of case), malpresentations and flooding. In addition, there were a few instances of the umbilical cord protruding alongside, or in front of, the presenting part; and some cases where Giffard was called to deliver a retained placenta. Giffard always delivered malpresentations by turning (podalic version with traction); in one case-description he inserted a digression against cephalic version. He also used turning for flooding and a prolapsed cord, even when the presenting part was the foetal head.[19]

It is of course for the management of obstructed births by the head that Giffard commands our attention, for he possessed his "Extractor", the midwifery forceps. Sure enough, we find many instances of the use of the forceps in the third phase of the case-series; and as we shall see, the instrument enabled him to deliver a living child. Yet three surprises await us amid Giffard's cases of obstructed births by the head. First, he sometimes tried to turn such births to the feet: not only before he had succeeded with the forceps (three cases), but also in the latter half of 1728, when he was perhaps still in the process of mastering the instrument (another three cases), and yet again, more surprisingly, in 1730 (two cases).[20] Secondly, in late 1728 and early 1729 we find four cases where he attempted Deventer's manoeuvre – pushing back the mother's coccyx with the back of his hand in order to widen the passage – and another four where he attended to the Deventerian theme of the orientation of the uterus.[21] This confirms that even after Giffard had begun to use the forceps with success, it still took him some months of further experience to acquire complete confidence in using the instrument. Thereupon, he abandoned his brief flirtation with Deventerian theory and practice – and on a subsequent occasion he expressed scorn for the Deventerians' claim to deliver without instruments.[22]

Thirdly, with regard to the forceps itself, we find that Giffard used the instrument not only in the way we would expect – inserting the two blades over the child's ears, grasping the foetal head, applying traction – but also in a very different mode: using a *single* blade of the forceps *as a vectis*. For example, on 18 February 1729 he used "one side of my extractor ... fixed ... on the lower part of the occiput near the neck". This adjusted the position of the head and gave some traction, which with the mother's bearing down resulted in the delivery of a living child. Giffard commented: "This is a further proof, that an infant presenting with the head, and sticking in the passage, may be brought out whole and alive, without hooks, or lessening the head".[23] Moreover, he deployed this improvised vectis in a further way, namely, to protect the mother's perineum from the risk of tearing.[24] But his main use of a single blade was to dislodge the head from the bones. In this he was possibly hampered by using a forceps blade, since a purpose-built vectis would perhaps have had a greater curvature for grasping the foetal occiput. Sometimes this approach failed, in which case Giffard withdrew the blade and then used both blades as a forceps. On other occasions the vectis method produced some success, but completion of the delivery required the use of the hand or forceps.[25] Nevertheless Giffard's cases show that more or less from the outset he was deploying *both* of the key Chamberlen methods – the forceps and the vectis. He probably learnt the single-blade technique from Hugh Chamberlen II in 1726–27, for he was using it as early as July 1728.

Remarkably, the use of a single blade of the forceps as a vectis passed immediately into oblivion, and remained there for over half a century. Giffard's London successor, Edmund Chapman, who came from Halstead in 1732 to fill the gap left by Giffard's death, also used the technique; and Alexander Butter, when publishing Dusée's forceps in 1733, drew attention to this way of using the forceps.[26] (Chapman and Dusée, like Giffard, had presumably learnt this method directly or indirectly from the Chamberlens.) Thus *all three* of the publications that announced the forceps in English mentioned the single-blade technique. Yet most subsequent users of the forceps were unaware of it; and neither of the two men who tried it in the next generation seems to have noticed that it had been recorded in the 1730s.[27] Indeed, it was not until 1790 that its use by Giffard, Chapman and Butter came to light – thanks to the emergence in Britain of the purpose-built vectis.[28] This underlines the point that the effective medium of instruction in practical obstetrics was not print, but face-to-face teaching.[29]

Mothers' expectations

Earlier we saw that traditional obstetric surgery was confined within a stable, self-perpetuating system, arising from the problem of obstructed births by the head, the use of craniotomy for such cases, and mothers' consequent fears of the male practitioner. Now let us imagine a man, such as Chapman or Giffard, who had acquired a forceps and the training to use it. In a typical obstetric emergency he would be called to deliver an obstructed birth by the head, after three days or so of labour, in the belief that the child had died. But sometimes the child would still be alive, as Cooke and Willughby had found; and on such an occasion the practitioner could try his new instrument. Sooner or later, therefore, he would achieve a miracle – delivering the child alive. Giffard in fact recorded his joy at the first occasion when this happened in his practice.[30] But if such an event gladdened the surgeon, it must have had a far more powerful effect on the mother, her husband, and the attending gossips – revealing to them that an emergency need not be so desperate as they had thought. Sooner or later, further emergencies of this kind would arise in the neighbourhood; at each of these deliveries there would be several women present; and before long there would occur such a birth attended by a woman who had been delivered by the forceps herself, or who had seen this happen to one of her friends or neighbours. Such a woman would reassure the mother that her child need not be killed, and thus, at some such occasions, the surgeon would be called slightly earlier than was usual. Sometimes it would still be too late, for the child was already dead. Sometimes the surgeon would be uncertain as to the child's condition; here he could operate immediately, without having to wait until the child was known to have died. And sometimes he would be able to perform again the miracle of delivering a living baby.

Thus the surgeon had begun to break the self-perpetuating cycle of fear, craniotomy and death. But to break this cycle was not just to stop it, but to *reverse* it. The more it was known he could deliver a living child, the less women would fear him; the less they feared him, the earlier they would call him; the earlier they called him, the more often he could deliver the child alive; and the more often this was so, the further it would be realized that he could achieve this. The "vicious circle" was replaced by a "benign circle": such a practitioner would be called progressively earlier, and would be able to deliver more and more living children. The logical stopping-point of this process was a profound switch of expectations, practices and possibilities: the male emergency practitioner *was now called to deliver a living child*. Previously, his task had been to save the mother's life; now it was his duty to save *both* lives. And this was the initial meaning of "man-midwife": a man who was expected – like the midwife – to deliver live births.

In some respects Giffard's cases are less than ideal for examining this postulated effect of the forceps. The gap in his case-series means that we observe the process not from the beginning but only after it had started; we can follow it for only a short period, 42 months at most; and we do not have many cases with which to work, since there were only about two obstructed births by the head each month. I shall compare an "early" group of cases (the first 13 relevant cases, spanning the seven months from August 1728 to February 1729) and a "late" group (the last 23 such cases, from November 1730 to October 1731). One could wish that the interval between the two groups was longer – on average it is only about 30 months – but this is the best we can do.

Despite the short time-scale it is clear that the forceps indeed exerted in Giffard's practice precisely the effect sketched above. The process had already started before our "early" group of cases, for Giffard observed on 4 June 1729, when forced to perform a craniotomy because the mother was severely rachitic:

> and that I could not think of without some reluctancy, having *for some years before* always been able to draw it out . . . by the use of my Extractor; but as the passage . . . was so very strait, and the head large, I was put under the necessity of lessening the head . . . for otherwise she must have died with the infant remaining in her.[31]

This implies that Giffard had been successfully using the forceps during the earlier gap in the case-series (even though, as we have seen, he was still in the process of mastering it in 1728). Correspondingly, even among our "early" cases most births by the head (around 75%) were delivered alive, and the median delay before Giffard was called was only 48 hours – in sharp contrast to the 3–4 days characteristic of traditional obstetric surgery. Our two groups of cases reveal that this shift continued between 1728 and 1731, in three linked ways. First, the median delay fell still further, from 48 to 36 hours. Secondly, and correspondingly, the proportion of stillbirths dropped from one-in-four to one-in-ten. Thirdly, we find that mothers and gossips were sometimes *surprised* when Giffard delivered a living child – and this was only half as common among the "late" cases as it had been in the "early" cases. Another way of bringing out these changes is to add together the cases where the child was stillborn and those where surprise was expressed at a live birth – for all of these were probably "traditional" emergency calls, made in the expectation that Giffard would deliver a dead child. Such calls comprised around half the early cases, but only a quarter of the late cases – a massive shift.

In a period of less than three years, then, Giffard's emergency calls shifted markedly towards the delivery of a living child. Had we been able to trace the process over a longer period, its effects would have been still more striking. As early as 1729 the need for craniotomy was becoming rare, not only because calls were coming much earlier, but also because the forceps could usually be deployed for a dead child just as for a living one.[32] It was this fact, of course, that created the opening for the dramatic social effects of the forceps – effects achieved not by argument, but by the repeated miracle of delivering a living child.

Male practitioners' attitudes

Success with the forceps in delivering a living child also transformed the male practitioner's perceptions of the midwife. This can be shown by comparing Giffard's views with those of Willughby, outlined in Chapter 4. Despite his criticisms of midwives' lack of skill, Willughby respected their office; as a result, he wanted to raise their standards of practice, enabling them to deliver all difficult births alive by turning the child. Had his writings had their intended effect, midwives would have become more skilled, not less, and the activities of male practitioners would have contracted, rather than expanded. But Giffard, starting from similar perceptions of midwives' skills, came to diametrically opposite conclusions. As we have seen, he believed that midwives should summon a male practitioner as soon as they encountered any difficulty in the birth; failure to do so he criticized as "self-sufficiency".[33] Midwives' ignorance and lack of skill were not contingent faults, but essential attributes: nowhere did he hint that these deficiencies might be improved by training. All skill resided in the male practitioner: the most that could be expected of the midwife was accurate diagnosis by "touching", the better to ensure that a man would be summoned promptly if need be, and the better to inform him when he arrived. The good midwife was the midwife who sent for Giffard and who could give him an accurate account of the state of the birth. Thereupon, the midwife was instantly subordinated, only reappearing in a case-history when he "ordered" her to cut the umbilical cord.[34] Both in his practice and in his treatise, power and skill went hand-in-hand and were male. The sphere of female practice should contract, the sphere of male practice should expand – precisely the opposite of Willughby's views.

This transformation of attitudes flowed from the use of the forceps. As long as the male practitioner deployed the crotchet or some other craniotomy device, the realm of live deliveries belonged to the midwife; this entailed an inviolable boundary between male and female competencies. As a result, medical men regarded the midwife's office with a certain implicit respect – whatever the weaknesses of real-life midwives, or some of those midwives. But once the male practitioner could deliver a living child, the boundary was broken; his critical attitude hardened and deepened, and his ambitions were transformed. In the moment of transition, exemplified by Giffard's practice, emergency calls comprised a mixture of "traditional" cases – the delivery of a dead child – and cases of the new kind, deliveries of living children. The natural desire of the male practitioner, doubtless founded on both self-interest and compassion, was to hasten the transition, to eliminate the "traditional" calls, to become pure man-midwife and no longer obstetric surgeon at all. Midwives were perceived as standing in the way of this development; hence the entire argument of Giffard's treatise. So too with both the other forceps practitioners who left explicit accounts of their attitudes – Edmund Chapman and, a little later, William Smellie.[35] And in all probability, much the same viewpoint had developed over a century earlier among the Chamberlens. This would make sense of the efforts of Peter Chamberlen II and of his son, Dr Peter, to regulate London midwives in 1617 and 1634, respectively.[36] Not until 1673 do we have any direct evidence on the attitudes of the Chamberlens, but that evidence, in Hugh Chamberlen I's translation of Mauriceau, suggests that they saw matters much as Giffard later did.[37] Presumably the wider social impact of the forceps (and vectis) in the Chamberlens' own practice was somewhat reduced by the secrecy of their methods, but its effect on their own ambitions was apparently consonant with its later effect on Giffard, Chapman and Smellie.

Limits of the effects of the forceps

So far I have been stressing the dissimilarities between traditional obstetric surgery and the new "man-midwifery" made possible by the forceps. On this account, the forceps brought about a discontinuity, a radical break with the past. Yet the effects of the forceps were contained within two important boundaries. First, different though the new practice was, it was profoundly rooted in the very realm which it superseded. Secondly, it may look as if forceps man-midwifery displaced the midwife – but this was far from being the case.

The thread of continuity between the forceps and craniotomy instruments such as the crotchet is variously shown by individual biography, practical obstetrics, and the structure of male practice.

1. At the individual level, virtually all of the early forceps users began as craniotomy practitioners. In the eighteenth century this is known from the personal testimony of Chapman, Giffard, Pugh and Smellie; and a century

earlier, it can surely be presumed for the Chamberlens themselves, since even the third-generation instruments of Dr Peter Chamberlen included crotchets.[38] The sole known exception is James Douglas, who "had not a hook" when he tried unsuccessfully to use the forceps in 1702 – and who subsequently abandoned the instrument.[39]

2. In the practical domain the forceps, although a more complex instrument than the crotchet, resembled it both in purpose (delivering obstructed births by the head) and in method (the double action of reducing the size of the head and enabling the operator to exert traction). So too the vectis can be described as a crotchet with a blade instead of a hook.

3. As to spheres of practice, we shall see shortly that forceps man-midwifery was associated with emergency work – once again, just like craniotomy. *It was precisely these resemblances and continuities that made the forceps so powerful.* The new technology was directly comparable to the old; it could be used in exactly the same cases; it was applied within the same sphere of practice; and while it dramatically enlarged the practical horizon (by permitting the delivery of a living child), it also preserved the traditional objective (the saving of the mother's life).

For all its effects, the forceps was not "the key to the lying-in room". It certainly did not confer on male practitioners the role of acting in lieu of the midwife, and there is almost no sign that it even stirred this ambition within them. The only hint of such an aim among this generation of practitioners is Chapman's assertion that some of his "brethren" wished to do away with midwives altogether. But this was probably a rhetorical strategy, the depiction of an extreme that would lend a milder cast to Chapman's own demand – identical to Giffard's – for earlier male access in difficult births.[40] (Chapman went on to explain that there were too many births for the men to attend, that most births were "natural", and that especially "in this metropolis" there were some very well-qualified midwives – a remark calculated to flatter his intended audience of London midwives.) And even if some forceps practitioners felt as Chapman suggested they did, there is nothing to indicate that they succeeded in such a project. For forceps practice was, and remained, strictly an emergency province. Whenever we know anything of the work of an early forceps practitioner – Giffard, Chapman, and subsequently Smellie – that work turns out to be dominated by emergency calls.[41] Conversely, men-midwives who enjoyed an "onset call" practice were opponents of the forceps or at least took pains to distance themselves from that instrument.[42]

This boundary to the social effects of the forceps is underlined by Giffard's attitude to midwives. Despite the vast distance between his approach and that of Willughby, even Giffard had no design to displace or eliminate the midwife. On the contrary, the midwife had an immense utility for him: she could take care of the slow tedium of normal labour, while also (so he hoped) acting as a rapid conduit to bring his own services into play when required. Chapman's view was identical, and subsequently Smellie actually hired midwives in precisely this capacity.[43] What the forceps dictated – both as practical reality and, reaching still further, male ambition – was not the displacement of the midwife, but rather a new equilibrium between midwives and male practitioners. The process of reversing the "vicious circle" had a natural stopping-point, namely, the summoning of the male practitioner after hours rather than days; but these were still emergency calls, which meant that midwives were still in charge of deliveries. The forceps did not displace the midwife; at the most, it was a precondition for this development. In short, while there was indeed an important break with the past, this was not yet the future: although forceps man-midwifery was radically distinct from craniotomy, it was equally distinct from the subsequent man-midwifery that involved primary responsibility for deliveries. That further transformation did not take place until mid-century. We will examine it in Part IV; but first we must attend to the unfolding contests and initiatives of the intervening generation.

Notes

1. Giffard, *Cases*, pp. 518–19 (continuation of Case 186). This case had occurred from 16 February to 6 March 1730/31. Hody's "continuation" extended for a year and a day, i.e. to 7 March 1731/32. Giffard had died in the interim: Hody gave no date for his death, but implied that this took place "a few months" after March 1730/31 (Case 186). Thus it is likely that he died soon after the final case (Case 225), which took place on 17 October 1731.
2. Giffard, *Cases*, Case 16, pp. 32–4.
3. Subjoined to Case 58 (7 February 1728), p. 134.
4. See also Cases 22, 24, 43, 77, 78, 79, 90, 126, 128, 142, 192.
5. Case 45; see also Cases 8, 44.
6. Case 120 (p. 289).
7. For Dr Wharton (Case 154) see *n*.43 to Ch. 5 above. Dr Eaton (Case 31) may have been Joseph Eaton (1655–post 1724: see Munk, *Roll*; Innes Smith, *Students at Leyden*; Wallis, *Medics*; *n*.19 to Ch. 10 below) or Robert Eaton (1688–1728: see Innes Smith, *Students at Leyden*).
8. Case 79.
9. Dr —: Cases 62, 113, 139. Mr —: Case 209 (p. 480). Others: Cases 5, 49, 105, 146 (on which cf. *n*.22 below).
10. For an unusual reference to "Mauriceau and others", see Case 205 (at p. 471).
11. For Dr Chamberlen, see Case 140 (and cf. Case 101). Mrs Harrison, Case 95; Mrs Gooding, Case 120. Other named midwives: Mrs Churchill at Chelsea, Case 73; Mrs H—s at Lambeth-Marsh, Case 123; Mrs Lucas (as patient), Case 160; Mrs Luddington, Case 154; Mrs Sexton, "a good sensible woman", Case 224; Mrs Weatherbone, Cases 90 (where she is praised), 160 (where her patient is her fellow midwife Mrs Lucas, above).
12. Exceptions include Case 63 (two midwives, arm); Case 65 (two midwives, footling); Case 113 (two midwives); Case 223 (four midwives, three of whom however "said that it was not a midwife's business").
13. Of the 17 cases in 1725–26, only three were births by the head; moreover, it is not clear whether these were emergency calls. (There were also two cases of births by the head with complications.)

14. Evidence from one of the later cases (Case 40, at pp. 86–7) shows that Giffard was practising during 1726–27 (cf. *n*.17 below). We also know that he was in London in December 1726, since he tried to see Mary Toft (Ch. 8 below, at *n*.9).
15. In fact the shift in types of cases recorded occurred three months after the start of the third phase, to be precise from 29 July 1728 – a month and a day after his first success with the forceps. Excluding cases involving complications as ambiguous, and cases from May–28 July 1728 as possibly transitional in the mode of recording, the difference between cases from 1725–26 and those from 29 July–September 1728 is associated with a probability of less than 1 in 50. For Giffard's cases in 1731 see Table 2.1 (Ch. 2).
16. These 70 days ran from 10 December 1728 to 17 February 1729.
17. However, a number of the later cases (at least 19) were deliveries of mothers Giffard had delivered earlier; this may imply that his rate of practice was expanding. Those I have noted, which may not be a complete list, are Cases 40 (cf. *n*.14 above), 105, 110, 126, 136, 137, 138, 142, 149, 150, 161, 166, 175, 177, 179, 188, 189, 191, 218. Sometimes Giffard recognized the mother, sometimes he had to be told that he had delivered her before; in no instance did he supply a cross-reference to the relevant case. It is not always easy to link these with deliveries earlier in the series. This aspect of the case-series would repay closer study.
18. Cases 22, 55, 126. But Giffard sometimes attended charitably: Case 38. See *n*.6 to Ch. 1 above for a sample list of trades and social status.
19. See Table 2.1 in Ch. 2 for a profile of Giffard's cases in 1731. Digression against cephalic version: Case 73. Protrusion of the umbilical cord: Cases 1, 20, 30, 57, 73 (here probably a by-product of severely rachitic pelvis), 169, 172, 181, 220, 222. Retained placenta: Cases 84, 87, 100, 111, 150, 163, 180 (on the significance of such cases see Ch. 12 below).
20. Turning: 1725, Case 10; 1726, Case 16; 1728, Cases 20, 48, 51, 54; 1730, Cases 122, 137.
21. Deventer's manoeuvre: 1728, Cases 32, 40, 47, 54 (and possibly also 1729, Case 90). Orientation of the uterus: 1728, Cases 28, 51; 1729, Cases 59, 60.
22. In Case 146, p. 350, Giffard observed: "This woman, in a former labour, had been obliged to make use of a person who pretends to perform any delivery without the use of instruments; but, upon enquiry, I found he had lessened the head before he could bring out the child". Cf. Chapman, *Treatise* (1735), p. 7.
23. Case 59; see also Cases 27, 36, 55, 61, 70, 81, 86, 103, 133, 146, 198, 199, 206, 216, 217.
24. E.g. Case 86 (19 September 1729).
25. Cases 26, 35, 48, 50, 60, 76, 83. Also Cases 30 and 71, where Giffard had to perform craniotomy with scissors (on the latter, cf. below at *n*.31).
26. Chapman, *Treatise* (1735), Case 23; A. Butter, Description of a Forceps, etc., *Medical Essays and Observations from a Society in Edinburgh* 3 (1733), p. 254.
27. These men were: William Clark, in a case-history of 1748 (at Box, Wiltshire) in his *The province of midwives in the practice of their art* (London, 1751), p. 32; and William Smellie, in 1750–51: see McClintock, *Smellie's midwifery*, vol. I, p. 257; vol. II, pp. 3–4 (note appended to preface), 324 (note appended to Cases 246, 247), 344 (part of a comment appended to a case of March, 1751). For discussion see Ch. 10 below (*n*.15 on Clark, text at *n*.25 on Smellie). The method was also noticed briefly by John Burton, *An essay towards a complete new system of midwifery* (London, 1751), pp. 219–20.
28. In R. Bland, *Some account of the invention and use of the lever of Roonhuysen* (London, 1790), p. 22, footnote.
29. See Ch. 5.
30. Giffard, *Cases*, Case 23 (28 June 1728); quoted in Radcliffe, *Milestones*, p. 33.

NOTES

31. Case 71.
32. Cases 55, 114, 143, 146; and for a child whose condition was unknown (Case 169). Note however that in two cases the forceps itself killed a child (Cases 105, 106), and that the forceps could injure the child's head (Cases 67, 83, 110, 117, 121, 203).
33. Case 89.
34. Cases 84, 216.
35. Chapman, *Treatise* (1735), pp. xi–xii and *passim*; McClintock, *Smellie's midwifery*, vol. III, p. 323.
36. Ch. 3 above.
37. Ch. 4 above.
38. Chapman, *Essay* (1733) and *Treatise* (1735); Giffard, *Cases*; Benjamin Pugh, *A treatise of midwifery, chiefly with regard to the operation. With several improvements in that art* (London, 1754), pp. 54, 121; McClintock, *Smellie's midwifery*, vol. II, Cases 277, 278, 282; vol. III, Cases 405, 406, 407 (for a complete list of Smellie's recorded Lanark cases, see Glaister, *Smellie*, pp. 359–60); *n.*46 to Ch. 4 above.
39. Chs 5 & 6 above.
40. For the argument that the forceps served as "the key to the lying-in room", see Radcliffe, *Milestones*, p.30; cf. Ch. 1 above. Chapman, *Treatise* (1735), p. x: "I am far from attempting or desiring with some of my brethren, that the practice of midwifery should be confined only to my own sex, and this for several reasons . . ."; for the quoted continuation see pp. x–xi.
41. For Smellie, see Ch. 9 below. A possible exception is Benjamin Pugh of Chelmsford, Essex: see Ch. 12 below, at *n.*49.
42. Ch. 6 above.
43. Chapman: *n.*35 above. Smellie: Ch. 9.

Part III

Whig and Tory men-midwives

Chapter Eight
Conflict and initiative in London, 1720–40

We have seen that London men-midwives were divided, from before 1720 until after 1740, between Tory forceps practitioners and Court Whig supporters of Hendrik van Deventer. It will now emerge that the various initiatives of the 1720s and '30s were reflections of the conflict between these two opposing camps, and not, as they seem at first to modern eyes, parts of a single movement towards fully-fledged man-midwifery or towards modern obstetrics.[1]

Early skirmishes

The contest between forceps and Deventerian man-midwiferies began in 1716, when Robert Samber translated Deventer's work into English. As we have seen, the associated remarks of William Cockburn show that this translation was precisely an anti-forceps move.[2] (The anonymous translation into English of Pierre Dionis's treatise three years later was probably a counter-blow, perhaps by Hugh Chamberlen II.[3]) So too in 1724–25, when John Maubray published his treatises based on Deventer, he opposed instruments, including the forceps – although he may have been referring to a craniotomy forceps.[4] Like James Houstoun a few years earlier, Maubray was an obscure Scottish practitioner newly arrived in London, and he too sought fashionable success in London by flying the flag of Deventer. Thus each time he went into print, and again on the eve of his public lectures on midwifery, he wrote to Sir Hans Sloane, President of the College of Physicians, to request that great man's patronage. These overtures had at least some success, for the College subsequently turned a blind eye to Maubray's unlicensed practice.[5] It is notable that Maubray coined a new term for the male practitioner of midwifery: "andro-boethogynist". Like Edward Baynard in 1715, who had proposed the term "midman", he was precocious in recognizing that male practice was changing from traditional obstetric surgery and thus required a new name.[6] Maubray also seems to have believed that stories associating childbirth with the marvellous and supernatural were becoming attractive, for he included in his treatise an elaborate account of the "Sooterkin", a fast-moving little monster that haunted deliveries in the Low Countries. In fact his "Sooterkin" was ably "dissected" by a pamphlet that exposed Maubray to ridicule.[7] Yet marvellous tales concerning childbirth were indeed of particular interest at Court in the mid-1720s, as became clear in the remarkable affair of Mary Toft, in which Maubray himself played a part.[8]

In the autumn of 1726 Mary Toft of Godalming, Surrey, gave birth to 17 rabbits, some in Godalming, others at Guildford under the eye of the local man-midwife, John Howard. Howard in turn notified his connections at Court, who moved Mary to London and lodged her in Lacy's Bagnio in the hope that she would produce further rabbits. There Mary became a spectacle for believers (Nathaniel St André), sceptics (Cyricaus Ahlers) and supposedly expert London men-midwives (Maubray, Limborch of the Royal household, James Douglas, Sir Richard Manningham). Strikingly, no part was played in this affair by any of the known or possible forceps practitioners in and near London (Hugh Chamberlen II, Middleton Walker, William Giffard, John Drinkwater, John Bamber and John Freke). In fact, they were deliberately excluded, for we know that Giffard was refused admission to Lacy's, along with "several other men of the profession".[9] Thus the Deventerian Whigs had a monopoly of Mary Toft; and it seems that they were predisposed to believe Mary's story. For as Gill Hudson has shown, the most notable of these men – Manningham and Douglas – were thoroughly taken in by Mary's brilliantly executed fraud.[10] Once the case was broken (chiefly by the discovery of a rabbit in the pocket of a porter at Lacy's), Manningham and Douglas published their own accounts of the story, in an attempt to extricate themselves. Manningham's *Exact diary* made the cunning aspersion that only Douglas had been taken in; Douglas's responding *Advertisement* was a delicate attempt to refute this insinuation.[11] But Douglas failed, for his neglecting to examine Mary's cervix was remembered long afterwards: it was recalled in a lampoon of 1738, and was being used in the 1760s as a warning to young practitioners by William Hunter.[12] Manningham and Maubray, on the other hand, managed to save their credit. A few years later (1730) Maubray became Chairman of the Charitable Corporation, and Manningham was not afterwards tainted by his association with the case.[13]

The publication of the forceps, 1733–35

At the very moment of the Mary Toft affair, Giffard was starting to acquire further instruction in the use of the forceps.[14] Meanwhile, the instrument was already being used with success by Chapman at Halstead, probably by Drinkwater at Brentford, and possibly by others in London and elsewhere.[15] Yet although some opponents were aware of the forceps, it remained in the private domain. Hence the fact that at this stage public controversy centred not on practical obstetric methods but on the theme of strange and monstrous births. The contest between Deventerianism and the forceps was potential rather than real as long as the forceps was in the private domain.

This equilibrium was bound to become unstable once the deaths of Hugh Chamberlen II and Middleton Walker had dissolved the pledge of secrecy that was keeping the forceps as private property. Sooner or later, someone in possession of the instrument would find it worth his while to publish it. In fact, the secrecy lasted for less than a year after Walker's death in November 1732. Perhaps Giffard would have taken that opportunity to publish his own treatise, but he had predeceased Walker by a year. These three deaths (Chamberlen, Giffard, Walker) within barely four years apparently created a vacuum in London forceps practice; and it was this which led to the publication of the forceps. For the man who took up this new opportunity – Edmund Chapman – naturally wanted to advertise his existence in London's West End, where he arrived in 1732. In Halstead, Essex, where he had previously been practising, he was well known, but in London he was a nonentity; and his London patron, Edward Milward, was a physician of impeccable obscurity.[16] Publishing the forceps was Chapman's way of placing himself in the public eye.

But Chapman had a potential rival, in the form of Edward Hody – possessor of the manuscript of Giffard's treatise. Learning that Hody was about to publish, Chapman tried to forestall the problem by adding this postscript to his own book:

> This essay, I confess, is much more imperfect than it would otherwise have been, because I was informed that there was a piece of midwifery in the press, which was expected to be published in a little time. It is highly probable there may be something mentioned in this work which is advanced in mine; and I should, after this, have incurred the censure of the town in publishing what was wholly my own. I chose therefore rather to let this make its appearance in a sort of undress, than run the hazard of being thought a plagiary by deferring it any longer.[17]

Chapman it was, therefore, who first published an account of the midwifery forceps and its use; his book, entitled *An essay towards the improvement of midwifery, chiefly with regard to the operation,* appeared in 1733.[18] The little detail wanting here was any illustration of the instrument; into this breach there swiftly stepped Alexander Butter of Edinburgh, and soon after this, early in 1734, appeared the rival treatise Chapman had feared – Giffard's text, edited by Hody, and supplied with a frontispiece depicting the forceps "as improved by Mr Freke". An instrument that had been a secret since its invention in the previous century was announced in print by three separate routes in a span of a few months.[19] It was doubtless the extinction of the Chamberlen family in November 1732 that had precipitated these developments.

This phase of activity was completed in 1735, when Chapman published a second edition of his book, now enlarged and called a *Treatise* and supplied with an engraving of the forceps.[20] The instrument was now fully in the public domain; the treatises of both Chapman and Giffard described its use in plentiful case-histories; they extolled its advantage over craniotomy; and Chapman announced that he was willing to teach its use, naming several men he had taught since 1733.[21] This was, of course, a dramatic moment in the history of obstetrics. Chapman in particular was aiming a powerful blow against both surgeons and midwives. Surgeons, he held, should henceforth abandon craniotomy; naturally he suggested that some practitioners were killing children with the crotchet, for this claim – which was doubtless true, but in only a tiny number of cases – dramatized the advantage of his own vaunted forceps.[22] As for midwives, Chapman's views were identical to Giffard's: he repeatedly criticized their alleged incompetence, and advanced the view that the suitably equipped male practitioner (himself and his pupils) should be called much earlier to difficult births.[23] Yet midwives were also the very audience he was seeking to persuade: hence his need to make some flattering remarks about London midwives.[24]

The publication of the forceps led to an unprecedented wave of printed interventions, of different provenance and types. From London came an attack on Giffard and Chapman by John Douglas in 1736 – which duly elicited a reply by Chapman in the following year – and then, in 1739, Manningham's treatise, associated with his new Lying-in Infirmary. In the provinces treatises or translations appeared from the pens of Thomas Dawkes of St Ives (1736), Henry Bracken of Lancaster (1737) and Thomas Jones of Norwich (1739); while Sarah Stone now moved from Taunton to London and published a treatise (1737) to advertise her own and her daughter's practice in the capital. This sudden new interest in midwifery suggests that the publication of the forceps turned it into a sphere of contest as never before.

John Douglas's intervention, 1736–37

John Douglas's *Short account of the state of midwifery in London and Westminster*, published in 1736, is of special interest – both as the first explicit London response to the forceps and for its remarkable contents.[25] To understand the vehemence of this work, one has to remember that its author was already a frustrated and embittered man, and had been so for many years. Before 1720 he had by his own researches and skill made a momentous innovation in lithotomy; for this he had received a certain recognition in some quarters (for instance, a free life-membership of the Company of Barbers and Surgeons), but he had also seen fame for lithotomy drift elsewhere – above all, to William Cheselden. By 1736

Douglas had long resented the fact that he had never been given the credit that he believed was his due.[26] Moreover, he was engaged in a series of contests over other aspects of surgery and medicine, centrally the use of salivation for venereal disease (which he opposed) and the wider remedial application of cinchona bark (which he supported). Indeed, he appeared at this time as a man for all battles.[27] Yet something about the treatises of Chapman and Giffard prompted him into a specific and well-directed anger. No doubt Douglas felt a particular pique at seeing Chapman profit from publishing a device (the forceps) that was not his own invention, in unpleasant contrast with Douglas's own lack of reward for real originality. But as we shall see, a more direct interest was also at work. What first concerns us is the content of Douglas's *Short account*; for this was a striking initiative on behalf of the midwife and against the male practitioner.

Douglas attacked not only Chapman and Giffard, but also Hugh Chamberlen I for the latter's claims in his 1673 translation of Mauriceau's treatise. All three were guilty of the same parcel of faults. They had gratuitously criticized midwives, and they had offered no means of help or instruction to those midwives; on the contrary, they had pushed themselves forward as the sole practitioners possessed of the skill to deliver difficult births. Douglas did not contest the claim that many midwives were seriously deficient in skill and knowledge – especially in the country, but even in London.[28] But from this premise he made precisely the opposite deduction from that of Chamberlen, Giffard and Chapman. Those authors had insisted that the sphere of midwives' practice be reduced, so as to encompass only easy natural labours: the domain of a midwife's activity should be narrowed down to the sphere of her competence. By contrast, Douglas wanted the competence of midwives enlarged so as to correspond with the scope of their activities – the scope dictated by both custom and propriety, that is, the delivery of almost all births. (*Almost* all, but not quite all: Douglas reserved a certain class of labours for male assistance, just as he acknowledged that despite the faults of Chamberlen et al., there were some male practitioners in midwifery who were "very learned and knowing men".) In short, Douglas was arguing for the better education of midwives. It was not the lack of native ability, but rather "the want of fit and full instructions in all the parts of their office" that produced unskilled midwives.[29]

Douglas accordingly produced a five-point plan, based on the Paris Hôtel-Dieu's *salle des accouchements* but incorporating further features of policing, and remarkable not least for its national focus in an age when all medical licensing was local.

1. A lying-in hospital should be erected, for instance in London or Westminster, "at the public expense", capable of receiving 200 or 300 mothers.
2. To attend these mothers, there should be appointed "a proper number" of midwives.
3. Two surgeons should be appointed to help the midwives "in all extraordinary cases", and to give them systematic teaching "in set lectures, at least three times a week".

4. It should be compulsory for any intending midwife to go through this course of education; to be examined afterwards by the two surgeons (along with "six or seven other persons, appointed by his majesty", this to prevent too much power falling into the two surgeons' hands); and, "if approved, to receive a certificate of their fitness to practise in London or anywhere else".
5. Until "fit hospitals" could be set up, a male practitioner should be appointed in every county town of England, to instruct the local midwives by means of lectures, "and demonstrate to them the truth of their doctrines on the poor of the neighbourhood".

Douglas concluded that if such a scheme could be implemented, "in a few years there would hardly be an ignorant [midwife] in England".[30]

All this was embedded in a specific rhetoric, designed to shift the terms of argument off the ground established by the forceps practitioners. Offended at the term "man-midwife", Douglas proposed for the male practitioner the term "midman" (already used by Edward Baynard in 1715) and so, correspondingly, "midwoman" for the midwife.[31] To support his contention that midwives were not wanting in capacity, merely in education, he repeatedly cited the 1677 treatise of Mme du Tertre, and announced on his final page that he would shortly be publishing an English translation of that work.[32] (In fact, Douglas did not carry out this plan.) Throughout his text he quoted liberally from his three opponents and ridiculed not only their main claims but also many points of detail: for example, Chamberlen was criticized as a "nostrum-monger", a man who trumpeted his possession of secrets rather than making new methods publicly available as he should have done.[33] The *Short Account* was indeed a remarkable document, a vigorous defence of the abilities of women – just as the plan it proposed for the education of midwives was well-conceived and potentially of radical effect. Equally significant is what Douglas did *not* say: he was completely silent on the pro-forceps and anti-craniotomy arguments of Chapman and Giffard.[34] Instead, he focused on the corresponding claims of Hugh Chamberlen I – which presented a softer target, for two reasons. First, since Chamberlen had kept his family's method secret, he was open both to the charge of being a "nostrum-monger" and to the insinuation that the method was of no account. Secondly, Douglas could and did exploit Mauriceau's anecdote of Hugh I's unsuccessful attempt to demonstrate his family's secret instrument.[35] But this was as near as Douglas came to addressing the claims made for the forceps – even though he implicitly endorsed Chapman's claim that the forceps was the Chamberlen secret.[36]

Although Douglas did not directly describe his own practice, his argument revealed several underlying interests. Centrally, he identified himself as a *surgeon:* thus he sniped back against certain condescending remarks about surgeons previously made by Hugh Chamberlen I from the viewpoint of a physician.[37] Further, Douglas saw midwifery as a part of surgery – his own profession – and it is clear that he practised obstetric surgery himself.[38] The operations with which he was familiar, as we would expect, were turning the child and craniotomy, and he asserted that there were some births where the use of the crotchet could never be avoided.[39] He praised some of the "midmen" – all Whigs: the deceased Sir David Hamilton, his own brother James Douglas, and Francis Sandys of Cambridge and London.[40] (Two Whig men-midwives, Sir Richard Manningham and the deceased Maubray, were excluded from such commendation, in each case probably for tactical reasons.[41]) Douglas also cited Deventer, and interpreted a case of Chapman's as an instance of difficulty arising from "the unnatural situation of the *os tincae*" (the cervix) – Deventer's "obliquity of the womb". And as we have seen, he characterized the fillet as an instrument of Deventer's that was used by many current London practitioners, including Sandys.[42] Thus all the indications are that Douglas was aligned with the London followers of Deventer. And this harmonizes with the political allegiance displayed in his dedication to Lady Walpole, which prayed "that God may continue to bless, with deserved honours, the person and conduct of your illustrious consort Sir Robert, your ladyship, and all your noble family". That is, the book began by waving the flag of a Court Whig.[43]

How are we to explain Douglas's sudden conversion in 1736 to the cause of education for midwives? The answer lies in the threat that the forceps posed to the existing balance between midwives and surgeons, a balance arising from the dependence of obstetric surgeons on craniotomy. Traditionally, midwives delivered living babies, surgeons delivered dead children; and the boundary between these two spheres of practice made for a certain harmony of interest between them. Forceps practitioners wanted to shift that boundary – thereby threatening both the midwife, who would be reduced to managing easy labours, and the traditional obstetric surgeon, who would surely lose practice to his new forceps rivals.[44] And the latter was the position of John Douglas. He had taken up the cause of midwives because the polemical threat to them from the forceps practitioners was part and parcel of a threat to himself. In contrast, Deventerian man-midwifery did not pose the same threat to surgeons – even though the Deventerians, too, wanted earlier access to difficult births. For despite his protestations against instruments, Deventer had permitted and practised craniotomy; and in London, Deventerian man-midwifery may even have promoted the work of traditional obstetric surgeons like John Douglas, since the Deventerian physicians probably referred craniotomy cases to surgeons.[45]

Moreover, Douglas was probably already being hurt by the practical effects of the midwifery forceps. We have already seen how rapidly Giffard's practice changed from calls to deliver a dead child to calls to deliver a living one, and that by the time of his death in 1731 these calls probably accounted for most of the difficult births in his catchment area. Similarly Chapman, who moved in 1732 into the heart of that area, rapidly gained a forceps practice himself, as was shown by case-histories he included in both the 1733 and 1735 editions of his self-advertising treatise.[46] It is thus likely that traditional obstetric surgeons such as Douglas were suffering a considerable loss of practice by the 1730s. By the same token, Douglas's book was not without effect on Chapman: he was stung into a *Reply* (1737) to Douglas's attack.[47] Douglas himself, when next going into print over one of his other battles, inserted a few paragraphs of scorn against Chapman's *Reply*.[48] There the controversy ended. Chapman died in 1738; none of his erstwhile pupils apparently bothered to enter the polemical fray; and Douglas himself lived only to 1743.[49]

Manningham's Lying-in Infirmary, 1739

Douglas's plan of instruction for midwives was never realized; yet only three years later, in 1739, Sir Richard Manningham set up in London the first Lying-In Infirmary.[50] The most remarkable feature of this new institution was its obscurity. Although his Infirmary was financed by voluntary subscriptions, and was thus dependent on support from the public, Manningham seems to have confined its printed publicity to Latin. Perhaps he wanted to restrict subscriptions to likeminded people; certainly his infirmary received no notice in the *Gentleman's Magazine*, which usually recorded the creation of new hospitals.[51] Naturally he wrote to his fellow Whig Sir Hans Sloane to inform him of the project and its progress, both in May 1739 and at the end of the year. Sloane himself had subscribed four guineas; by the end of the year almost £100 in subscriptions had been received, and some £118 expended on setting up "the apartment".[52] How long the infirmary lasted is a mystery. It was surely still active in 1744, when Manningham's treatise was translated into English (possibly without his consent); yet this is the last we hear of it. Indeed, its very existence seems to have been forgotten as early as 1747.[53] Probably the infirmary lapsed for want of subscribers; perhaps the use of patients as teaching material had proved unpopular; and Manningham's high fees may have deterred prospective students, especially as William Smellie was offering much cheaper teaching from 1740.[54]

It is instructive to compare Manningham's infirmary with John Douglas's earlier proposal. Not surprisingly, the scale was far smaller: Manningham's institution probably had about 30 beds, whereas Douglas had proposed 200 or 300 beds.[55] This reflected the voluntary subscription method of finance: all the voluntary hospitals began on a modest scale, aiming to expand thereafter (usually with limited success). But the important contrast concerned teaching – the main reason behind both Douglas's projected hospital and Manningham's actual Infirmary. Douglas's aim was to teach midwives, not male pupils, and he saw the role of surgeons in the planned institution as being to help midwives, not replace them, in the management of difficult births. As we shall now see, Manningham's infirmary offered a precise travesty of this scheme. He taught both midwives and male practitioners; the fees he charged them were unequal; and the reason for this was that he taught the male practitioners more, restricting the midwives to managing easy, natural labours. The chief lesson to be imbibed by the midwives, in fact, was to send for a male practitioner as soon as difficulty arose – turning Douglas's ideas on their head.

Manningham's teaching was to be provided in the infirmary; but to avoid the "inconveniences" arising in "foreign hospitals" (probably the Paris Hôtel-Dieu) from having students delivering patients, the students were to be instructed first on a "glass machine" – presumably a glass model of the pelvis.[56] Midwives would be taught the management of normal deliveries, for a fee of 10 guineas; male practitioners would learn about both normal births and difficult cases, paying 20 guineas for this double instruction. The content of Manningham's teaching was clearly Deventerian: criticism of instruments, especially of the forceps; emphasis on the mobility of the coccyx (as he put it, of the sacrum); awareness of the "variety of pelvis[es] in different bodies"; and an overwhelming stress on the importance of the situation and "obliquities" of the womb.[57] Obstructed births by the head were to be delivered by "our own invention" – left secret in the published treatise.[58] This was probably an adaptation of Deventer's manoeuvre (Manningham's only known pupil, Brudenell Exton, later emerged as a straightforward Deventerian).[59] The first lecture, illustrated on the "glass machine", argued that midwives were to be interrogated – apparently by the attending women – on the position of the uterus, the situation of the child, and the prospects for the labour. If the midwife was evasive she was to be deemed ignorant; if she did not answer satisfactorily, "better assistance" was required. All this was taken almost directly from Deventer, but with two modifications. Deventer had written that in such a case, "a skilful midwife, or a surgeon that practises midwifery, is to be sought"; but Manningham's "better assistance" was specifically that of "a man midwife". And Manningham dropped Deventer's argument that legislative action was needed to raise the standards of midwives' practice.[60]

Manningham's reworking of Deventer's argument aimed to drive a wedge between midwives and gossips, creating a space for the earlier intervention of a male practitioner. The midwife remained the central figure in the management of childbirth, and correspondingly, the male practitioner was specifically concerned with difficult births – in the Lying-in Infirmary just as in Manningham's intentions for private practice.[61] Nevertheless, the midwife's office was to be redefined, in such a way as to get the man-midwife called both earlier and more frequently. The requirement for *earlier* calls was no different from the arguments of Giffard and Chapman, published just a few years earlier and associated with the forceps. But the *frequency* of summoning the male practitioner was a different matter, for Manningham was redefining the criterion of difficulty. According to his precepts, a birth was implicitly guilty until proven innocent: the delivery could only be regarded as normal if everything proceeded aright (the situation of the child, the position of the uterus, the progress of the labour) *and* if the midwife could assure the gossips on these points; otherwise, a male practitioner should be summoned at once. Such a shift, if implemented, would have massively increased the opportunities for male practice. As we have seen, the experience underlying these precepts was probably advance and onset calls with a midwife.[62] The social sphere of such practice was very restricted; but the opportunities were surely expanding at this time with the increasing wealth and commercialization of London.

Manningham was thus making a bid to expand the opportunities for male practice, within the limits suggested by his own experience. In addition, he believed that there was scope for greater male practice in the disorders of pregnancy – traditionally probably managed by midwives.[63]

Thus Manningham's aims ironically converged with those of the forceps practitioners: the two parties agreed that the male practitioner should be given much easier and earlier access to difficult births. They differed, of course, as to who were the right male practitioners for this role. But there was also another difference, a difference of strategy, of persuasive technique. It is striking that the forceps practitioners did not propose or create lying-in institutions – and equally striking that Deventerians did not produce treatises illustrated with case-histories.[64] That is, each obstetric allegiance generated its own distinctive type of initiative. Forceps practice issued in treatises of the case-history type, of which the limiting instance was Giffard's treatise – consisting entirely of histories. Anti-forceps practitioners produced either no texts at all (James Douglas, Francis Sandys), or a text devoid of case-histories (Manningham). What stood in place of such histories was the lying-in infirmary, where the nature of birth could be demonstrated. This corresponded to a difference in spheres of practice. Forceps practitioners mainly received emergency calls; it was precisely for these cases that the forceps was of such dramatic value; and case-histories demonstrated the miraculous effects of the instrument. Deventerians chiefly received onset calls with a midwife; their methods for difficult births depended on very early intervention; and the lying-in infirmary, where early male access to difficult births could be guaranteed, made it possible to show both male and female pupils exactly where the boundary lay between their respective spheres of practice.

The specificity of the London pattern

We have seen that the wave of publications unleashed in the 1730s emanated not only from London but also from elsewhere. Such initiatives would repay closer study, attending to their various local contexts, which is beyond my scope here, but one general observation can be made: all the works that issued from other localities departed from the London pattern of allegiances. As the following brief summary will show, the provincial practitioners who went into print either distanced themselves from both London parties of man-midwifery (Henry Bracken, Sarah Stone) or in some way bridged the divide between them (Thomas Dawkes, Thomas Jones).

1. Thomas Dawkes of St Ives based his *The midwife rightly instructed* (1736) on Deventer, and did not discuss the forceps; yet he made a point of praising Chapman as well. This eirenic posture sets him apart from the London men-midwives. The available indications are that Dawkes was a Whig and perhaps a Dissenter.[65]

2. Henry Bracken of Lancaster was a Tory, but no supporter of the forceps. Instead he practised a method of manual rectification of the foetal head, claiming in *The midwife's companion* (1737) that this must have been the famous Chamberlen secret. Distancing himself both from Deventer and from the forceps, Bracken may perhaps be seen as the complementary case to Dawkes.[66]
3. Sarah Stone published her *Complete practice of midwifery* (1737) to advertise her practice on her move to London, but she was an outsider to the capital, having practised successively in Bridgwater (where she started around 1702), Taunton (c.1705?–21) and Bristol (1721–37). Thus she had specific provincial roots, as well as bringing the distinctive perspective of a midwife who practised emergency obstetric surgery. As we have seen, Mrs Stone could deliver obstructed births by the head without instruments, using her own manoeuvre.[67] Her method was very different from that of Deventer, and she duly criticized Deventer along with other male authorities – even though her patron John Allen was a supporter of Deventer. And while she did not mention the forceps, her whole argument was an implicit critique of that instrument.[68]
4. Thomas Jones of Norwich published in 1739 a translation of Mauriceau's *Aphorisms*. This would seem to align him with the forceps practitioners, who tended to follow Mauriceau as against Deventer. Yet Jones appended "a vindication of Deventer's opinion" both on the thickness of the gravid uterus (one of the points at issue between Mauriceau and Deventer) and on the "obliquity of the womb". In this Jones was behaving very like James Houstoun 20 years earlier, but a more relevant comparison is probably with Dawkes of St Ives, discussed above: each in different ways combined approaches that in London were deeply divided.[69]

Finally, we must mention the two other capital cities of the British Isles – Edinburgh and Dublin. In each of these important centres we find a pattern of early eighteenth-century initiatives in midwifery that differs once again from the London story. Edinburgh witnessed the publication of McMath's treatise as early as 1694; the appointment of Joseph Gibson as city professor of midwifery, that is, official instructor to the town's midwives, in 1726; in 1733, the publication by Butter of an engraving of Dusée's forceps; and on 29 June 1737, a Caesarean section on the living mother performed by a surgeon called Smith.[70] Dublin presents a particularly striking picture, which can conveniently be followed here into the 1740s.[71] Its College of Physicians, when refounded by William and Mary in 1692 (incidentally as a national Irish institution, not merely a Dublin corporation) enjoyed the chartered power to examine, supervise and license both male and female practitioners in midwifery.[72] In the early eighteenth century we find practising there both Chamberlen Walker (brother of Middleton Walker, and a cousin of Hugh Chamberlen II), and Johannes van Lewen.[73] By the 1740s there were several Dublin men-midwives, including Matthew Carter, George Maconachy, Bartholomew Mosse, Fielding Ould, Thomas Southwell, and possibly John

Harvie.[74] These men generated at least two important public initiatives: Ould's treatise of 1742 (which included the first notice in print of the rotation of the foetal head in labour), and Mosse's lying-in hospital of 1745 (the first permanent hospital of this kind in the British Isles, post-dating Manningham's short-lived infirmary but preceding the enduring London institutions to be outlined in Chapter 11). It is certain that some underlying conflict was involved here, just as in London: Ould's treatise was immediately attacked by Thomas Southwell, who extended his anti-Ould *Remarks* in an enlarged edition published in London in 1744.[75] Meanwhile, in 1743, a Dublin Professorship of Midwifery was created (by an Act of Parliament administering the proceeds of Sir Patrick Dunn's estate).[76] The lines of battle here overlapped with those in London, since Ould used the forceps whereas Southwell supported Deventer; yet they were also distinctive, for the Ould/Southwell argument also concerned the theme of Caesarean section on the living mother, which was not debated in London at this time.

Thus the London association between political and obstetric allegiances was locality specific. No doubt we can generalize the point that public initiatives were generated by conflict between rival interests. And it was probably true not only in London but also elsewhere that particular obstetric methods were associated with specific politico-religious allegiances. But the form of the latter association, and the structure of the associated conflict, differed from place to place. The picture would surely become still more variegated if we were to widen our focus to other European polities. In the next three chapters we shall see that the London pattern extended into the next generation of man-midwifery, that of the 1740s; and yet that "London" as I have been referring to it actually comprised only Westminster and the West End, for the City tells a different story altogether.

Notes

1. Dorothy George, *London life in the eighteenth century* (first published 1925; Harmondsworth: Penguin, 1966), p. 62.
2. See Ch. 6 above.
3. Dionis wrote, probably against Deventer: "Though instruments are never to be made use of but when there's an absolute necessity for it . . . yet . . . there's no doing without them; and therefore those who are forced to use them themselves, but will not allow others to do it, are very much to be blamed". The only clue as to the provenance of the English translation is provided by the booksellers (Bell, Bettesworth, Pemberton, Rivington, Hooke, Cruttenden, Cox, Clay, Battley & Simon); their book-list appears to be Hanoverian Tory, but I have not investigated this closely. See P. Dionis, *Traité general des accouchemens* (Paris, 1718), p. 303; idem, *A general treatise of midwifery* (London, 1719), p. 247 (quoted), final leaf (book-list).
4. Deventer himself had included forceps in his list of instruments for delivering a dead child: *Midwifery improv'd*, pp. 325-6. See J. Maubray, *The female physician* (London, 1724), *passim*; idem, *Midwifery brought to perfection by manual operation* (London, 1725),

pp. 28–30 (see also p. 36 on obliquity of the uterus). John Maubray (d. 27 October 1732): Three book-subscriptions: the two I have identified were by John Ayliffe 1726, ardent Whig, and James Anderson 1732, Presbyterian minister (Wallis, *Medics*; Phibb, *Subscriptions*). Obituary, from *Monthly Intelligencer*, in *Gentleman's Magazine*, 1 (1731–32), p. 627.

5. BL Sloane MSS 4059 f. 321, 4047 ff. 284, 297; Clark, *College of Physicians*, vol. II, p. 502. For Houstoun see Ch. 6 above.
6. E. Baynard, Appendix to the 1715 edition of Sir John Floyer, *The history of cold bathing, ancient and modern*, at p. 345; Spencer, *British midwifery*, p. 7.
7. Philalethes [pseud.], *The sooterkin dissected. In a letter to John Maubray, MD, alias Dr Giovanni. By a lover of truth and learning* (London, 1726, reprinted 1727). This was attributed by John Douglas to Dr Archibald Mitchell, and the attribution was endorsed by his opponent Edmund Chapman. See John Douglas, *A short account of the state of midwifery in London, Westminster, &c.* (London, 1736), p. 55; E. Chapman, *A reply to Mr Douglas's short account of the state of midwifery in London and Westminster* (London, 1737), pp. 37–8. I have discovered nothing more about Dr Archibald Mitchell.
8. G. Hudson, *The politics of credulity: the Mary Toft case* (MPhil dissertation: Cambridge, 1987).
9. Thomas Braithwaite, *Remarks on a short narrative . . . as published by Mr St André, anatomist to His Majesty. With a proper regard to his intended recantation* (London, 1726), p. 32. According to the later (1734) testimony of Edward Hody, Giffard contributed one of the associated pamphlets (Giffard, *Cases*, Preface, p. iv); perhaps this was Lemuel Gulliver [pseud.], *The anatomist dissected* (London, 1726).
10. Hudson, *The politics of credulity*.
11. Sir Richard Manningham, *An exact diary of what was observed during a close attendance upon Mary Toft* (London, n.d.); James Douglas, *An advertisement occasion'd by some passages in Sir R. Manningham's diary lately publish'd* (London, 1727). It was later said that in response to Douglas's *Advertisement*, Manningham "printed a reply in 24 pages, 8vo; but did not think proper to publish it" (Nichols, *Literary anecdotes*, vol. I, p. 346). A nice verse satire on the disparity between Douglas's account and his earlier role in the affair was Flamingo [pseud.], *A shorter and truer advertisement by way of supplement, to what was Published the 7th Instant: or, Dr D–g–l–s in an Extasy, at Lacey's Bagio, December the 4th, 1726* (London, 1727).
12. *The lady's decoy: or, the man-midwife's defence* (London, 1738), Canto vii, p. 4 ("Up stairs she was led,/And laid on a bed, /But now to refute an objection, /I vow and declare, /And safely may swear, /I never made use of *inspection*."); Hunter, lectures, p. 54 (the "eminent professor" in question was tactfully unnamed).
13. On the Charitable Corporation (where Maubray had perhaps been placed as court agent to root out alleged Jacobites/embezzlers) see *Commons Journals* 21 (1727–32), pp. 788, 792, 795–6; CUL, Cholmondeley (Houghton) MSS 73/19, 80/314/1–6, 91/126, P/314/1–6; *Gentleman's Magazine*, 1 (1731–2), pp. 497, 578–9, 627, 773, & 3 (1733–4), pp. 235, 429; *HMC Egmont*, vol. I, pp. 35–6, 219–25, 242–4, 250, 254, 257–8, 260–62, 296, 368, 371.
14. The 20-month gap in his case-series began in September 1726: see Table 7.1 and Ch. 7 above.
15. Ch. 5 above.
16. For Chapman at Halstead and for Milward see *n.*18 & *n.*44 to Ch. 5 above.
17. Chapman, *Essay* (1733), p. xxiv.
18. Chapman, *Essay* (1733).
19. Ch. 5 above.

20. In the *Treatise* (1735), p. xxvii, Chapman praised Maubray's book, of which he claimed he had been unaware when writing the *Essay* (1733). His praise was doubtless insincere, since Maubray had opposed instruments and followed Deventer, and indeed elsewhere Chapman criticized both Deventer and Maubray (pp. 7, 89, 122). The praise for Maubray was presumably inserted with a view to winning some favour in London. But in view of the earlier controversy over the "sooterkin" this was a tactical error, which exposed Chapman to scorn from John Douglas (see *n*.41 below).
21. Chapman's named pupils were John Page of Lutterworth, from whom he inserted a letter attesting to the way the forceps had enhanced his practice; Dr W. Weltden; Mr Smither of Reading; and Mr Philip Haste, Jr, of Coggeshall, Essex. See Chapman, *Treatise* (1735), pp. 23–5, 186. In addition, Brudenell Exton later claimed to have been taught by Chapman, but added that he then went over to Manningham, whose doctrines he espoused (Ch. 5 above).
22. See Chapman, *Treatise* (1735), pp. xvii–xviii, xxi; compare and contrast p. 156, where Chapman supported this practice to save the mother's life.
23. Ch. 7 (Giffard); Chapman, *Treatise* (1735), *passim*, e.g. pp. xi–xii, 143.
24. Chapman, *Treatise* (1735), pp. vii, x–xi; Ch. 7 above.
25. John Douglas, *A short account of the state of midwifery in London and Westminster* (London, 1736).
26. See BL, Sloane MS 4048, f. 267 (John Douglas to Sloane, 17 March 1726/67); and cf. *A short account*, p. 20, where Douglas observed that "any private man who . . . makes any considerable discovery in manual operations . . . ought to be handsomely rewarded". For John Douglas's contribution to lithotomy see the (not impartial) testimony of his brother: James Douglas, *The history of the lateral operation* (London, 1726), pp. 5–6.
27. John Douglas, *A dissertation on the venereal disease* (London, 1737); *A dissertation on the venereal disease. Part II* (London, 1737); *A dissertation on the venereal disease. Part III* (London, n.d.).
28. Douglas, *A short account*, pp. 5–6, 66, 68.
29. *Ibid.*, quoted from pp. 72, 71.
30. *Ibid.*, pp. 73–5.
31. *Ibid.*, p. [vii]; *n*.6 above.
32. Douglas, *A short account*, pp. 25–6, 41–2, 46, 47, 48, 49, 56–7, 59, 61, 75.
33. *Ibid.*, pp. 11, 14, 24. At p. 18 Douglas acknowledged that "secrets . . . may be really useful in some cases", but he added "yet they are not so in all".
34. At *ibid.*, p. 53, Douglas digressed to commend consultations, in such a way as to imply that the obstetric branch of surgery was peculiarly divided into separate camps in London at this time.
35. Ch. 4 above.
36. Douglas, *A short account*, pp. 10–12.
37. *Ibid.*, pp. 6–8, 20–23.
38. 53. *Ibid.*, pp. 1, 21, 72.
39. *Ibid.*, pp. 13, 22–3, 30, 32–3, 36, 42–3, 45–6, 49, 57–8, 69–70.
40. *Ibid.*, pp. 10, 75. James Douglas was to be the dedicatee of his proposed translation of du Tertre. See also *A dissertation on the venereal disease. Part III*, dedication, which described Sandys as "the very worthy and unbias'd judge . . . accurate anatomist, and consummate accoucheur . . . my good old friend".
41. Manningham he omitted to mention, surely because of his rivalry with Douglas's brother James in the Mary Toft case 10 years earlier. Maubray he ridiculed as superstitious (citing

NOTES

The sooterkin dissected), doubtless because Chapman had insincerely and unwisely inserted a few words of praise for him in his own second edition. See *A short account*, pp. 53–6; cf. *n*.7 & 20 above.

42. Douglas, *A short account*, pp. 60 (Deventer, fillet, Sandys), 47 (difficulty from "the unnatural situation of the *os tincae*"); see also pp. 58, 64–5, 69. For his remarks on the fillet see Ch. 6 above.
43. *Ibid.*, p. [v].
44. See Ch. 7 above.
45. See Ch. 6 above & Ch. 13 below, at *n*.14.
46. By the 1735 edition Chapman could claim that he had used the forceps in London about 30 times: *Treatise* (1735), p. 176. Giffard had about two forceps cases a month. Chapman had come to London in 1732; if his 30 forceps cases were evenly spread over two and a half years, his rate of practice would be about half Giffard's; but surely his practice would have increased over time, suggesting that by 1735 it was close to the rate Giffard had experienced.
47. Chapman, *A reply to Mr Douglas's short account*.
48. Douglas, *A Dissertation on the venereal disease. Part II*, pp. 21–4.
49. Chapman's date of death is given as 22 November 1738 in a biographical card in RCSL.
50. In BL Sloane MS 4034, f. 65 is a similar plan to that of Douglas (not, however, in his hand, cf. Sloane MS 4048, f. 267); here it was envisaged that "none be admitted but women" to the lectures on midwifery to be held in the proposed infirmary.
51. Contrast Manningham's restricted publicity with the Foundling Hospital, set up in the same year, for which Thomas Coram sought and obtained a Royal Charter. Dorothy George suggested that Manningham's infirmary was located in the workhouse infirmary of St James Westminster: *London life in the eighteenth century* (first published 1925; Harmondsworth: Penguin, 1966), pp. 60, 67. This seems not to have been the case, for Lord Egmont, who was on the St James vestry in the 1730s, included in his diary many references to its meetings, including discussions of the infirmary, but without mentioning a lying-in ward: *HMC Egmont, passim*. See also Spencer, *British midwifery*, pp. 15–16.
52. BL Sloane MS 4056, ff. 84, 85v.
53. Manningham, *An abstract of midwifery for use in the lying-in infirmary* (London, 1744), pp. 28–30; *Gentleman's Magazine*, 1747, p. 211; James Houstoun, *Memoirs of the life and travels of James Houstoun, MD* (London, 1747), pp. 66–7.
54. See Ch. 9 below.
55. Manningham's infirmary had room for 300 deliveries in a year; allowing five weeks per delivery (a week before birth and a month's lying-in afterwards), this implies 29 beds.
56. Manningham, *Abstract of midwifery*, pp. 15, 21, 33.
57. Criticism of instruments, especially forceps: *ibid.*, pp. vii–viii, 35; mobility of the sacrum p. 2 (and cf. p. 13, "How to enlarge the pelvis"); "variety of pelvis's" [*sic*] p. 13 (and cf. p. 9); situation and "obliquities" of the womb, pp. 3, 11, 13, 15, 16–18, 19, 22–5.
58. *Ibid.*, pp. 35 (fees), viii ("our own invention").
59. B. Exton, *A new and general system of midwifery* (London, 1751); for details see *n*.25 to Ch. 11 below.
60. Manningham, *Abstract of midwifery*, pp. 16, 21–6; cf. Deventer, *Midwifery improv'd*, pp. 305–15, and *New improvements in the art of midwifery*, pp. 58–81.
61. Manningham, *Abstract of midwifery*, p. 34.
62. Ch. 6 above.
63. Manningham, *Abstract of midwifery*, p. 32; cf. Ch. 3 above.

64. A partial exception was Exton, *A new and general system of midwifery*. Deventer himself had included a very small number of case-histories: see *Midwifery improv'd*, pp. 316–19, 324–5; *New improvements in the art of midwifery*, pp. 30–32, 33–6. On the obstetric associations of lying-in hospitals, see also Ch. 11 below.

65. T. Dawkes, *The midwife rightly instructed* (London, 1736). Thomas Dawkes of St Ives: one apprentice, 1730 (Wallis, *Medics*); author of *Prodigium Willinghamense* (London, 1747) which has various hints of a Whig and Dissenting orientation.

66. H. Bracken, *The midwife's companion, or, a treatise of midwifery; wherein the whole art is explained* (London, 1737). On Bracken, see D. Harley, "Honour and property: the structure of professional disputes in eighteenth-century medicine", in *The medical enlightenment of the eighteenth century,* A. Cunningham & R. French (eds) (Cambridge: Cambridge University Press, 1990), pp. 138–64, at pp. 148, 155, 161–4, and Harley, "Ethics and dispute behaviour in the career of Henry Bracken of Lancaster, surgeon, physician and manmidwife", in *The codification of medical morality in the eighteenth and nineteenth centuries,* R. Baker et al. (eds) (Dordrecht, 1993), pp. 47–71.

67. Stone, *Complete practice*; see Ch. 4.

68. J. Allen, *Synopsis medicinae* (2 volumes; 1749 edn), vol. II, pp. 259–70; Stone, *Complete practice*, pp. 156–7.

69. François Mauriceau, *Aphorisms . . . Translated by Thomas Jones* (London & Norwich, 1739). For James Houston see Ch. 6 above.

70. See Innes Smith, *Students at Leyden* (McMath); Spencer, *British midwifery*, p. 91 (Gibson); Ch. 5 above (Butter); Young, *Caesarean section*, pp. 36–7 (Smith).

71. John Ringland, *Annals of Midwifery in Ireland* (Dublin, 1870); S. A. Brody, "The life and times of Sir Fielding Ould: man-midwife and master physician", *Bulletin of the History of Medicine* 52 (1978), pp. 228–50.

72. Ringland, *Annals*, p. 10.

73. Chamberlen Walker: Radcliffe, *The secret instrument*, p. 72; Radcliffe, *Milestones,* p. 32. Johannes van Lewen: Innes Smith, *Students at Leyden*; Laetitia Pilkington, *Memoirs of Mrs Laetitia Pilkington* (first published 1748; reprinted, 3 volumes in 1; London: Routledge, 1928), vol. I, pp. 30, 36, 110–21, 433.

74. Matthew Carter & Fielding Ould: Brody, "The life and times of Sir Fielding Ould", pp. 231, 238, *passim*. George Maconachy and John Harvie: Innes Smith, *Students at Leyden*. Bartholomew Mosse: Ringland, *Annals*, pp. 14–16. Thomas Southwell: see below.

75. T. Southwell, *Remarks on some of the errors both in anatomy and practice, contained in a late treatise of midwifry, published by Fielding Ould, man-midwife* (Dublin: Thomas Bacon, 1742); *idem, A continuation of remarks on Mr Ould's Midwifry* (London: Thomas Meigham, 1744).

76. Ringland, *Annals*, p. 11.

Chapter Nine

A new synthesis: William Smellie

We come now to the most famous of the men-midwives. William Smellie initiated the large-scale teaching of midwifery in London; he realized the potential of the midwifery forceps; and he produced a *Treatise on the theory and practice of midwifery* that dominated published obstetrics for a generation and beyond. And Smellie towers even higher over historical images of this subject: he has received two full-scale biographies, his three-volume treatise was reprinted with copious notes in 1876–78, and his name even finds its way into history books and into the *Dictionary of scientific biography*.[1] A rounded picture of Smellie's midwifery would require a book in itself; here I shall examine him from a few selected angles, paying particular attention to the development of his methods, chiefly in the 1740s.

Life and writings

In the 1720s Smellie was a surgeon and apothecary in Lanark; among the cases in his local practice was emergency obstetric surgery of the traditional kind.[2] His chief techniques were craniotomy and turning the child – although at some point he acquired a fillet from his local colleague Dr Inglis, and a blunt hook from Dr Gordon of Glasgow. Neither of these instruments altered the basic constraint that he was usually called to deliver a dead child, and his obstetric surgery was merely part of a wider general practice, for which he was well equipped by his earlier experience as a naval surgeon.[3] But in 1737, having become aware of the recently published forceps, Smellie began to concentrate on midwifery, embarking on a mission to acquire the instrument and to realize its potential for saving the lives of children.[4] Although married, he had no children of his own and could therefore travel in pursuit of this goal. In 1739 his quest took him first to London and then to Paris, where he attended the forceps classes of Grégoire. Returning to London in the following year (1740), Smellie set himself up as a teacher of midwifery; in the next 10 years he taught over 900 male practitioners, and an unknown number of "female pupils". Like Grégoire in Paris and Manningham in London, Smellie used "machines" that simulated the female pelvis and the unborn child. In a remarkable innovation that both imitated and outflanked Manningham's lying-in infirmary, he induced poor mothers to be used as teaching material by setting up a fund for their maintenance during lying-in. This inverted the prevailing relations between practitioner and patient; and the gossips, the mother's female friends, were replaced by the pupils, Smellie's mostly male friends.[5] The lying-in fund (to which his pupils contributed) was a large-scale initiative, encompassing 1150 mothers within 10 years, i.e. more than two deliveries a week.[6] Smellie made his teaching cheap – three guineas as against Manningham's 10 or 20 guineas; he offered further courses at a discount rate, enabling a pupil to deepen his or her knowledge; and he issued certificates of attendance, which gave his former pupils quasi-licences. All these arrangements Smellie seems to have developed in the early 1740s.[7]

To judge by the selected cases he subsequently published, Smellie's practice at this time chiefly comprised emergency calls (about 70% of his cases), with a substantial minority of onset calls but none of the more lucrative advance calls. This is in line both with Smellie's style (he lacked the grace and polish required to secure advance calls) and with his extensive teaching activities (which made him too busy to accept such calls, but supplied a handsome alternative source of income). The dominance of emergency calls fits with what we have seen of other forceps practitioners: the new instrument was associated with an entirely traditional "path" to childbirth. The corollary was that Smellie's experience consisted chiefly of difficult births.[8] Moreover, this was the central focus of his teaching – despite the opportunities presented by his lying-in fund. By placing deliveries within Smellie's power, the fund potentially gave him and his pupils a vastly enlarged experience of normal labour; yet he chiefly used such deliveries to teach the management of *difficult* births. To take care of normal labours among these mothers Smellie hired a midwife; if the birth became difficult she "assembled" some of "the gentlemen", among whom the "senior pupil" would manage the delivery; only if it proved especially difficult was Smellie himself summoned.[9]

Subsequently Smellie reached an even wider audience with his *Treatise on the theory and practice of midwifery*. The main text appeared in late 1751, two supplementary volumes containing numbered "collections" of case-histories in 1754 and 1764, and an accompanying volume of illustrations (*Anatomical tables*) in 1754. Meanwhile Smellie retired "from business" in 1759, and returned to his native Lanark; he died in 1763, aged 66, so that the final volume was published posthumously. All three volumes were seen through the press, and possibly rewritten, by his close friend and ally Tobias Smollett.[10] From the publication of the first volume onwards, Smellie was the biggest name in midwifery in Britain, and possibly in Europe; no-one could discuss the subject without referring to his book. The text at once became the object of attack, both by rival practitioners (John Burton of York) and by opponents of man-midwifery (Elizabeth Nihell, Philip Thicknesse).[11] But it received highly favourable notices not only in Smollett's own *Critical Review* (as was predictable), but also in the rival *Monthly Review*.[12] For this praise there was good reason: Smellie's work took midwifery onto a new and higher plane.

The development of Smellie's methods

Smellie's quest for improved methods in midwifery started and ended with the forceps, and from 1751, thanks to his *Treatise*, he was identified with the instrument by friend and foe alike. Yet that very text reveals that his attitude to the instrument had gone through a series of changes in the 1740s. The most suitable way to approach this theme is to start with Smellie's own autobiographical account of his methods for the management of obstructed births by the head, an account he appended to one of his cases.[13] The picture he offered can be divided into four stages.

As a country practitioner at Lanark in the 1720s, he tried to deliver such cases by turning to the feet, but found that this could not always be used and that even when it succeeded it often destroyed the child. The only alternative was craniotomy. The consequent "loss of children", Smellie recalled, "gave me great uneasiness".

Then, from 1737, he embarked on his quest for the forceps, first using those published by Butter, then travelling to London to find out about the Chapman–Giffard instruments, and finally (on the advice of Alexander Stuart) going to Paris to study under Grégoire.[14] At each step of this pilgrimage Smellie was dissatisfied. Butter's forceps were "ill contrived" and "by no means answered the purposes for which they were intended"; in London, "nothing was to be learnt" (Chapman had died in 1738, leaving no teacher of the forceps there); and in Paris, although Grégoire offered systematic instruction, Smellie was "very much disappointed" by Grégoire's "machine", and found that "as for the forceps, he taught his pupils to introduce them at random, and pull with great force".

Now came the crucial third stage, apparently on his return to London in 1740:

> Little satisfied with his [Grégoire's] method of instructing, I considered that there was a possibility of forming machines, which should so exactly imitate real women and children as to exhibit to the learner all the difficulties that happen in midwifery; and such I actually contrived, and made by dint of uncommon labour and application.
>
> I endeavoured to reduce the art of midwifery to the principles of mechanism, ascertained the make, shape, and situation of the pelvis, together with the form and dimensions of the child's head, and ex-

plained the method of extracting, from the rules of moving bodies, in different directions.

But what was Smellie teaching at this stage? What was "the method of extracting"? The answer is enfolded within Smellie's next sentence, which recalls that his efforts at this stage were only partially successful:

> Nevertheless, I had still some occasion to perceive that children were lost, and the mothers endangered, *by turning*, when the head was large and presented, or even *by leaving the head to stick long at the lower part of the pelvis* . . .

Thus in the third stage Smellie was systematically attempting to deliver all cases of obstructed births by the head without instruments – apparently either by turning or by the natural pains.[15] That was the aim of his mechanical studies, of his new machines, of his "uncommon labour and application", and of his initial teaching. His "method of extracting, from the rules of moving bodies, in different directions" *was designed to do away with instruments altogether*: Smellie was now *opposed* to the forceps. Indeed, he may even have been at this stage a follower of Deventer. On this point clear evidence is wanting as to his methods of practice, since Smellie was never to discuss Deventer's manoeuvre with the hand on the coccyx – an omission that is suspicious in itself. But both his theoretical focus on pelvic anatomy and his practical determination to deliver without instruments suggest a Deventerian inspiration at this time. Indeed, that would be precisely the direction in which to turn after the repeated disappointments he had experienced with the forceps.[16]

As we have seen, Smellie's retrospective account stresses the limited success of his efforts at this stage. His next sentence delineates the transition to stage four, the final phase of Smellie's development as he recounted it:

> *To obviate these misfortunes, I was sometimes obliged to have recourse to* the fillet or forceps; with which last I frequently succeeded so as to save the child; though the use of them was sometimes attended with a laceration of the external parts of the woman, until I contrived an alteration in their form, and gave new directions for using them; by which this inconvenience is prevented.

Thus in stage four Smellie returned to the forceps – but he did so with reluctance. He used it only because his previous plan to deliver without instruments was failing, and even then only as an alternative to the fillet. In fact, this single sentence summarized a very complex series of developments. What must be stressed here is that the meaning of stage four arose from its relation to the preceding stage, when Smellie had sought to deliver without instruments.

Smellie's autobiographical story implies that his return to the forceps took place in the 1740s, but gives no precise date. Further clues are supplied by the relevant cases – births by the head – in volumes II and III of Smellie's *Treatise*. Suspiciously, there was only one such case from 1740 and 1741, the first two years of his London practice and teaching. It was doubtless during this period that Smellie had been attempting to deliver all births by the head without instruments, using turning or the natural pains, and perhaps also Deventer's manoeuvre.[17] By the time he wrote his treatise and compiled his retrospective case-series, he no longer believed in this approach, and he therefore suppressed such cases from inclusion. Indeed the sole exception confirms the rule: the one birth by the head that Smellie included from these two years (an emergency call, in which the child presented by the face) was inserted for the purpose of retrospective self-criticism. He had left the birth to Nature, and the child had died; when reporting it over a decade later, he observes self-critically that he should have used the forceps.[18]

Subsequent cases show that Smellie's reluctant readoption of the forceps spanned the three years from 1742 to 1744: of 26 recorded births by the head during this time just five were delivered by the forceps, 21 by other means. One case from 1742 continued the pattern of 1740–41: Smellie insisted on leaving the delivery to Nature, and did not even consider using the forceps, even though the mother had been three days in labour and the midwife wanted to deliver her. In the event the natural powers effected the delivery, but this took another day and the child was dead.[19] Another 1742 case led to the same result by a different route: this was an onset call, and here Smellie's not intervening arose from the mother's fear of him (induced, so he claimed, by the midwife) rather than from his own choice. On this occasion, the child "appeared to have been but a very little time dead". It was directly after his account of this case that Smellie inserted the autobiography summarized above – and we can guess at the reason. By the time the child's life was in danger, the head was low in the pelvis, which would have made turning difficult or impossible, and therefore only the forceps could have saved this child. Perhaps this experience provoked Smellie to view the forceps in a more positive light.[20] A further case from 1742 (which involved three or more of Smellie's pupils) provides his first recorded use of the forceps in London. Here Smellie used the instrument to save the life of the mother, not the child – though, as a bonus, the child was born alive.[21]

In the following year – 1743 – Smellie made some further, hesitant use of the forceps. He tested them in a delivery where the child was already known to be dead; and he used them on a living child, but only after trying unsuccessfully to use the whalebone fillet that he had just been given by Richard Mead.[22] Even though the forceps saved this child's life, Smellie was still reluctant to use the instrument, as is clear from his cases in 1744. In that year he used turning to the feet for two cases of face-presentation, in one of which the mother died (Smellie was later to prefer the forceps for such births).[23] And in a case where the child's head presented face-to-pubis he used the forceps with some success, but only after trying first manual rectification and then turning.[24] A final case from 1744 is of particular interest. This was an emergency call, to a mother with an apparently rickety pelvis. Smellie postponed acting, but eventually delivered with the forceps in the hope of saving the child's life. In the event, the forceps "slipped several times", ripped the mother's perineum and left a deep mark on the child's forehead – although happily both mother and child recovered. This confirms that Smellie was still inexperienced with the forceps, and fits with the earlier testimony of Douglas, Heister, Chapman and Giffard as to the difficulty of using the instrument. But what interested Smellie himself about this case was the mark on the child's skull – for this taught him that the head had not been positioned in the pelvis as he had thought:

> I at that time imagined, with others, that in labours the forehead was mostly to the sacrum, and the ears to the sides ... [But] from [the] indentation on the os frontis, by a blade of the forceps, which had been fixed on that and the occiput, I discovered that the ears were not to the sides as I imagined.

This case demonstrated something that he could in fact have learnt from the recent treatise of Fielding Ould (1742), but that he had evidently not noticed in that work, i.e. that the child's head rotates in the course of delivery.[25] However, Smellie still drew no practical inference from this discovery.

Smellie's pivotal experience was a related case in the next year, 1745. In an early emergency call where the presentation was occipito-lateral, Smellie tried to deliver by the forceps but without success. Then,

> While I paused a little, considering what method I should take, I luckily thought of trying to raise the head with the forceps, and turn the forehead to the left side of the brim of the pelvis where it was widest, an expedient which I immediately executed with greater ease than I expected. I then brought down the vertex to the right ischium, turned it below the pubes, and the forehead into the hollow of the sacrum; and safely delivered the head. . . . This method succeeding so well, gave me great joy . . . my eyes were now opened to a new field of improvement on the method of using the forceps in this position, as well as in all others that happen when the head presents.[26]

What Smellie had learnt was the practical corollary of his earlier discovery that the foetal head rotates during labour. *Using the forceps he could produce this same rotation artificially*. It was this discovery that converted him to the forceps, and its effect was immediate. In 1745, the ratio of forceps deliveries to other types became 5 to 10; in 1746, it reached 7 to 9; and the increase was entirely due to his new practice of forceps-rotation. The non-rotation forceps cases continued to appear at the same low rate of 0–2 per year, just as in 1740–44. Thus in the three years from 1745 to 1747, there were in all 15 recorded forceps deliveries, 12 of which used rotation.[27]

Smellie's new confidence in the forceps was swiftly translated into a new *teaching* message: from 1746 onwards, 9 of the 10 recorded births by the head involving his pupils were forceps deliveries. Moreover, he now decided "to commit my lectures to paper for publication" – that is, to start writing his *Treatise*.[28] And at the same time Smellie set in motion a public refutation of the methods of Deventer. The way he went about this was to get Thomas Tomkyns, doubtless one of his pupils, to translate into English La Motte's French obstetric treatise of 1722. Smellie clearly attached much importance to this project: according to Tomkyns, he "did me the favour all along to compare the translation with the original, and carefully examined that nothing useful might be left out, and nothing useless retained".[29] The Tomkyns–Smellie translation was duly published in 1746. At first sight this seems an odd initiative for Smellie to take at this time, since Guillaume Mauquest de La Motte had been an entirely traditional obstetric surgeon. Although La Motte opposed the crotchet and advocated turning for births by the head, he performed craniotomy with scissors, and when he began to use a forceps (after 1717) this was solely for the delivery of a dead child.[30] But the puzzle is resolved by La Motte's remarks on the maternal coccyx. "If any one consider the figure, use and articulation of the *os coccygis*," wrote La Motte (as translated by Tomkyns), "he will soon be persuaded that it can be no obstacle to the coming forth of the child." The coccyx "could never resist the impetuous rushing forth of the child", and even if it did, the child "would nevertheless force its way out, suffering . . . an impression from it upon its face or some other part of its body".[31] Thus Deventer's manoeuvre was nugatory; nothing was to be gained by forcing back the coccyx. And this was why La Motte was a valuable resource for Smellie in 1746: as a weapon against Deventer, who had to be displaced now that Smellie endorsed the forceps.

Remarkably enough, Smellie soon changed his methods yet again. For although the forceps henceforth predominated among his teaching cases, in 1747–48 he made much less use of it in his private practice – only twice in 17 recorded births by the head. Moreover, around this time he made a series of experiments with the instrument. First, in 1748, he devised a forceps made of *wood* in place of metal, and delivered three mothers with this new instrument. This promptly led to a skirmish in print: the instrument was roundly attacked by William Douglas, who went on to criticize Smellie's teaching and methods in general, and one of Smellie's pupils replied on his behalf.[32] Then, in 1748 or 1749, Smellie discarded the wooden forceps (perhaps because of Douglas's attack, or perhaps because wood was "not so durable"), and instead added a leather covering to the metal blades. Finally, in 1749, he shortened the handles and devised "new directions" for applying the instrument. By now he was satisfied, for from 1749 onwards the forceps resumed its importance in his private practice. But why had he become ambivalent about the forceps for his private practice in 1747? In a letter to his friend Gordon in Glasgow, apparently written in 1748, he explained that the purpose of the wooden forceps was "to make them appear less terrible to women". And this was also why, on reverting to steel blades, Smellie introduced the leather covering – to mask their metallic feel. Here we have a strange paradox: the very instrument that had saved lives and had broken and reversed the vicious circle of craniotomy and fear, had now itself become "terrible". The reason for this will emerge in Chapter 12.

Smellie's synthesis

By 1751 La Motte, who in 1746 had been such a valuable resource against Deventer, had outlived his usefulness to Smellie. Now, in his *Treatise*, Smellie bracketed La Motte and Deventer together – a nice irony, this – as men whom he had once "determined to follow" in their attempt to deliver without instruments, but whose ideas he had found to be wrong since "sometimes . . . it is absolutely impossible to bring [the foetus] along without the help of instruments". And he claimed that both La Motte and Deventer had "suppressed those unsuccessful cases which must have happened to men of their extensive practice".[33] With these neat strokes Smellie discarded La Motte; he mentioned Tomkyns's translation, although not its date of publication nor his own role in producing it. As for Deventer himself, Smellie's published comments were suspiciously incomplete and indirect. He discussed Deventer's "book on midwifery", but did not mention that it had been translated into English, nor that Deventer had English followers. He criticized Deventer's theory of the oblique uterus, but gave no hint that this had been part of a larger theoretical framework.[34] When commenting on Deventer he omitted to mention his focus on the mobility of the coccyx, yet three years later, very early in his second volume (1754), he took some trouble to prove that a rigid coccyx did not retard labour, without naming Deventer as his target:

> I have of late, in a particular manner, examined the os coccygis, especially in laborious cases, and in women who were turned of thirty before the birth of their first child; and have found it actually ossified in two patients . . . but in neither of these cases could I perceive that this rigidity retarded the labour; for, in both, when the head of the child came down to the os externum, it passed along, and the women were as easily delivered as those in whom the coccyx is moveable, though both children were of an ordinary size.[35]

And although he devoted a detailed critical discussion to Deventer's method of delivering the *aftercoming* head in breech and footling cases, he never mentioned Deventer's more important manoeuvre with the hand on the coccyx for delivering difficult births that *presented* by the head.[36]

The reason for Smellie's lack of candour towards Deventer was precisely that he was aiming to displace him. In this he succeeded brilliantly, for in due course Deventer's theoretical framework and practical methods were forgotten. What

Smellie had in fact achieved was a remarkable synthesis of the opposing viewpoints of the previous generation. In using the forceps he was inheriting the practical mantle of Chapman and Giffard. In supplying a rationale he was taking over Deventer's role as theorist – all the more so because his central resource, the anatomy of the maternal pelvis, was itself derived from Deventer. This double legacy was captured in the very title of his *Treatise on the theory and practice of midwifery*. No doubt Smellie's coming to London as an outsider helped him to transcend the existing dichotomy of obstetric allegiances; and to judge by his association with Smollett, his allegiance seems to have been Country Whig, a position that was perhaps analogous in the political sphere. Nevertheless, as we have seen, his synthesis was only achieved by a protracted struggle, involving a long period of antipathy and ambivalence towards the forceps.

To our eyes, Smellie's synthesis appears magisterial. Yet his apparent hegemony at mid-century is the product of a distorting hindsight, arising from the long-term triumph of the forceps and the later canonical status of his *Treatise*. For during his own working lifetime, Smellie was far from holding uncontested sway in London man-midwifery, as we shall see in the next two chapters.

Notes

1. McClintock, *Smellie's midwifery*; Glaister, *Smellie*; R. W. Johnstone, *William Smellie, the master of British midwifery* (Edinburgh: Livingstone, 1952); D. George, *London life in the eighteenth century* (first published 1925; Harmondsworth: Penguin, 1966), p. 62; *DSB*, vol. III, pp. 37, 38, vol. VI, p. 568.
2. Smellie's recorded Lanark cases are listed in Glaister, *Smellie*, pp. 359–60.
3. J. Butterton, "The education, naval service and early career of William Smellie", *Bulletin of the History of Medicine* 60 (1986), pp. 1–18.
4. Contrast Smellie's response to the forceps with that of Heister over 15 years earlier (Ch. 5 above, at *n*.11). Heister was sufficiently interested to modify the design in response to the inevitable initial difficulties, but not to persevere when these difficulties recurred. Smellie's intense motivation suggests that attention should be paid to his religious convictions, a topic I have not pursued.
5. McClintock, *Smellie's midwifery*, vol. III, Case 502, p. 298.
6. *Ibid.*, vol. I, p. 27.
7. A convenient summary is the Memoir in McClintock, *Smellie's midwifery*, vol. I, pp. 1–23. For evidence that Smellie's teaching arrangements were in place by 1741, "soon after I began to teach midwifery", see *ibid.*, vol. III, p. 207, Case 415. For advertisements for his courses, including a brochure of 1742, see Johnstone, *William Smellie*, p. 22 and Figs 1 & 2 (facing pp. 24–5). For an attendance certificate, see P. H. Nankivell, "Certificate of attendance at William Smellie's lectures, 1757", *Medical History* 1 (1957), pp. 279–80.
8. See my William Hunter and the varieties of man-midwifery, p. 355.
9. Midwives: Mrs Moore, now Simpson, Case 398 (1749); for his private practice, Mrs Maddox ("my midwife") Case 411, (1753). Senior pupils: Mr Potter and Mr Chapman, Case 286 (1747); Mr Chapman again, Case 287, August 1749; Mr Prosser, Case 418

(1752); Mr Mackenzie, Case 387 (1753).
10. See Johnstone, *William Smellie*, pp. 39, 120–25.
11. J. Burton, *A letter to William Smellie, MD, containing critical and practical remarks upon his treatise* (London, 1753). For Nihell & Thicknesse see Ch. 15 below.
12. *Monthly Review*, December, 1751, pp. 465ff. (review of vol. I, reprinted in Glaister, *Smellie*, pp. 130–31); 1754 (2), p. 318 (review of vol. II); *Critical Review* (founded in 1756), 18 (1764), pp. 444–6 (review of vol. III).
13. McClintock, *Smellie's midwifery*, Case 186; my emphases throughout.
14. Alexander Stuart (1673–1742): MD Leyden 1711; FRS 1714; LRCP 1720; MD Cambridge (Com. Reg.) and FRCP 1728; see *DSB* (where he is included for his iatromechanical researches on muscular motion). Also apparently author of *New discoveries in surgery* (London, 1738). This treatise, its author and his connection with Smellie would repay further study.
15. Contrast McClintock, *Smellie's midwifery*, vol. I, pp. 251–2, where Smellie gave an account that omitted any mention of turning in his development; yet he redressed this in a coda (pp. 252–3). Cf. also vol. I, pp. 71–2 (on which see the following note).
16. Compare McClintock, *Smellie's midwifery*, vol. I, p. 71, where Smellie says that "when I first began to practise, I determined to follow the method of those gentlemen" – that is, "the method" of Deventer and of La Motte, whom he has just discussed as opponents of instruments. Taken literally, this should refer to the 1720s, but it may be a cryptic allusion to the early 1740s. There is certainly something odd about the statement, since La Motte opposed Deventer. For this and for Smellie's attitude to Deventer, see below. Cf. also *ibid.*, vol. I, p. 243; vol. III, p. 131.
17. One contrary indication should be mentioned. It was in just these years (1740–41) that William Hunter was living with Smellie and presumably learning from him; yet Hunter's own early practice seems to have been forceps-based, and in his lectures of the 1760s he depicted Smellie entirely as a forceps practitioner; see Ch. 13. However, (a) it is clear that Hunter and Smellie had many dealings after 1741 (see Glaister, *Smellie*, pp. 120–22; McClintock, *Smellie's midwifery*, vol. II, p. 252), so that Hunter could have learnt the use of the forceps from Smellie after 1741; and (b) in the interim Smellie's *Treatise* had been published, establishing him as the leading exponent of the forceps.
18. Case 134 (1740).
19. Case 180.
20. Case 186.
21. Case 235.
22. Cases 280, 236. For Mead's giving Smellie the whalebone fillet in 1743, see McClintock, *Smellie's midwifery*, vol. I, p. 255.
23. Cases 324, 389.
24. Case 257. (The forceps brought the head only partly out, and to complete the delivery Smellie employed "a blunt hook, that had a round button on the end for that purpose . . . above the chin". This was "the common method" in such cases at this time, but it had the effect of damaging both the child and the mother. I know of no other discussion of this "common method".)
25. Case 251. (McClintock here observed "that even so late as the year 1744 . . . Smellie was still imperfectly acquainted with the proper mode of applying and using the midwifery forceps".) F. Ould, *A treatise of midwifery* (Dublin, 1742), quoted in Radcliffe, *Milestones*, pp. 42–3. Another case from 1744 was managed successfully with the forceps: here delivery was retarded by the shortness of the umbilical cord (Case 174).

NOTES

26. Case 258.
27. There were four such cases in 1745, five in 1746 and three in 1747.
28. McClintock, *Smellie's midwifery*, vol. I, Preface, p. 26.
29. La Motte, *Midwifery*, translator's preface, pp. xi, xii.
30. See Ch. 5 above.
31. La Motte, *Midwifery*, pp. 152, 156. Compare Dionis, writing at about the same time (see Ch. 8 above, at *n*.3).
32. McClintock, *Smellie's midwifery*, vol. I, pp. 22, 258–9; vol. II, p. 359. For William Douglas see Ch. 11 below.
33. *Ibid.*, vol. I, p. 72; cf. *n*.16 above.
34. *Ibid.*, vol. I, pp. 69–70. Smellie here acknowledged that "there are some very useful hints in his book, particularly that about floodings ... and his method of dilating the os externum". In fact, he also drew on Deventer for the posture for turning: see Cases 357 (1745), 285 (1746), 376 (1749), 372 (1752).
35. *Ibid.*, vol. II, Collection I, Number 2, Case 3.
36. On Deventer's method for the aftercoming head see *ibid.*, vol. I, pp. 308–9, and McClintock's note, p. 318. For Deventer's manoeuvre see Ch. 6 above.

Chapter Ten

John Bamber, the vectis, and the City of London

As we have seen in Chapter 5, the vectis was another Chamberlen instrument that, like the forceps, could deliver a living child in an obstructed birth by the head. It will also be recalled that in Amsterdam the vectis was used in secret by Roonhuysen and his successors from the 1690s until about 1750.[1] Now throughout the English controversies that we have been reviewing, the vectis was never mentioned. Thus either Hugh Chamberlen II – who passed on the forceps in England – did not sell the vectis in England, or those to whom he sold it guarded this secret with extreme care. In fact, there is reason to suspect that Hugh II did sell the vectis to one or more English practitioners; that one of these recipients, at least, used it in perfect secrecy from the 1720s to the 1740s; and that subsequently the instrument was passed on to a wider circle, who preserved its secrecy for another generation, until the 1780s. I shall argue here that the man who thus transmitted the vectis from the Chamberlen family to a select group of inheritors was John Bamber. This episode is difficult to reconstruct, since we depend on later evidence; I shall begin by surveying what is known of Bamber's remarkably long career.

John Bamber and his associates

Born in 1667, Bamber practised for many years as a surgeon in the City of London, receiving a naval appointment in 1693 and the post of co-lithotomist to St Bartholomew's Hospital in 1721. In the mid-1720s, when almost 60 years old, he made both a political and a medical realignment, exchanging his former Toryism for a Whig allegiance and transferring from surgery to the more lucrative practice of physic. To achieve the latter, he obtained a dismissal from the Company of Barbers and Surgeons and then a licentiateship of the College of Physicians (1724), a Cambridge MD by Royal mandate (1725), and finally a Fellowship of the College of Physicians (1726).[2] This shift from surgery to physic would have been assisted by a practice in midwifery, which potentially spanned the two professions, and it is likely that Bamber was already practising midwifery at this time. For just a few years later, in October 1731, Bamber had (according to the subsequent testimony of one of his associates, Starkey Middleton) "great experience and judgement in midwifery", which with his other abilities "made him unquestionably the most proper person to be consulted" by a midwife confronted with a difficult labour near Bishopsgate. Subsequently, in 1733–35, Bamber began to involve Middleton in the deliveries of this particular mother, and thereafter Middleton inherited her as a patient.[3] No mention here of the Deventerians (Manningham, Douglas), nor of the forceps practitioners (Giffard, Walker, Chapman): the Bamber–Middleton nexus was an independent centre of obstetric practice. And it was differentiated geographically as well: Bamber lived in the City, whereas Manningham, Douglas, Giffard and Chapman worked in Westminster and Walker resided in Southwark.[4] Other sources show Bamber acting as man-midwife to Mrs Molly Wilson in 1735 (in an onset call with the midwife Mrs Gates of Gower Street), and as physician to the pregnant Mrs Delaney in 1744.[5]

Bamber next comes to light in 1751, when he had passed the age of 80 and was doubtless retiring from practice. He was now given an important role in two linked sets of satirical attacks on Fellows of the London College of Physicians: the writings of Frank Nicholls against man-midwifery, and one of the anonymous poems published in support of Isaac Schomberg's efforts to become a College Fellow.[6] Nicholls and Schomberg had common enemies, centrally Robert Nesbit; and they both depicted Bamber as handing on his medical methods to a select group comprising Nesbit and others. In the pro-Schomberg poem *Iatro-Rapsodica*, "Dr B—r" was made to speak first; his 13 lines concluded:

> Be here transcribed the recipes I wrote,
> My recipes shal C—le and N—t quote!
> Mor—ey and Han—de when females groan
> My bills shall read, and make my bills their own![7]

Of these four alleged recipients of Bamber's methods, at least three (Joshua Cole, Matthew Morley and Robert Nesbit) practised midwifery; whether Clifford Handeside did so I have not ascertained, although *Iatro-Rapsodica* was implying that he did.[8] The picture portrayed soon afterwards by Frank Nicholls in *The petition of the unborn babes* and two further satires was different, yet compatible.[9] Here the chief targets were Morley ("Dr Maulus") and Nesbit ("Dr Pocus"), both depicted as murderers of unborn children through the rash practice of man-midwifery. Their erstwhile "tutor" was "Dr Barebones" – whom readers of *Iatro-Rapsodica* would recognize as "Dr B—r", that is, John Bamber.[10]

The Schomberg–Nicholls claim, then, was that Bamber was passing on his methods, chiefly in midwifery, to a select group of practitioners. But the nature of those methods is by no means clear from these attacks. *Iatro-Rapsodica* referred only to prescriptions; Nicholls portrayed "Pocus" and "Maulus" as craniotomy practitioners, yet he would certainly have known that there was nothing new about craniotomy, and we cannot take this as an accurate depiction of their practice. Whatever Bamber's obstetric methods were, it appears that he passed them on to a circle comprising Joshua Cole, Robert Nesbit, and Matthew Morley; perhaps Clifford Handeside (according to *Iatro-Rapsodica*); and probably also Starkey Middleton (since Bamber had handed a patient to him in 1733–35, and Middleton publicly praised Bamber in 1747). Presumably these men continued to use Bamber's techniques after Bamber's own death in 1753.

Bamber and the vectis

In fact Bamber's method was probably the vectis, as we learn from the much later testimony of Thomas Denman. Since Denman had come to London as a student around 1750, he may have had some inkling of the workings of the Bamber circle at this time; certainly he later acquired some connection with that group.[11] In the 1801 edition of his *Introduction to the practice of midwifery*, Denman referred to Bamber as an earlier practitioner in midwifery who was known for concealing his instruments.[12] And elsewhere in the same book he wrote (my emphases):

> When the vectis was very much used, and highly esteemed, at Amsterdam, as an invaluable improvement in the art of midwifery, the forceps was the favourite instrument in this country, especially as altered by Smellie, who was then the principal *teacher* of the art in London. But the chief *practice* in this city was successively in the hands of Drs Bamber, Griffith, Middleton, Nesbit, and Cole, some, if not all of whom, except Dr Bamber, whose forceps I have seen, preferred the vectis to the forceps.[13]

Thus Denman, independently of Nicholls and Schomberg, and from a very different perspective, linked Bamber with a circle including Nesbit and Cole. He depicted these as the most eminent practitioners because they favoured the vectis – like Denman himself, who had gone over to that instrument from the forceps. (Hence Denman's extraordinary omission of William Hunter, who was a far more eminent man-midwife than any of the men Denman named, but was unaware of the vectis.[14]) And Denman was asserting that the vectis had been secretly used in London in Smellie's time (that is, before 1760) and independently of its use in Amsterdam.

Denman's testimony strongly suggests that Bamber had passed the vectis on to his circle of pupils. The only contrary indication is Denman's observation that

Bamber possessed a forceps; but he could have had *both* a forceps and a vectis, and Denman's wording does not rule this out. All other considerations suggest that Bamber had the vectis and passed it on to a select group of pupils.[15] First, Bamber was, on Denman's testimony, equipped with some secret obstetric instrument(s): neither the forceps nor the fillet was secret any longer, leaving the vectis as the most likely possibility. Secondly, three of the five men who were during Bamber's lifetime identified as his pupils or professional heirs also appear in Denman's later list of four vectis practitioners. (The various links are summarized in Table 10.1.) Thirdly, there must have been some route of transmission for the Chamberlen vectis between Hugh Chamberlen's death in 1728 and the circle of London vectis practitioners listed by Denman; and Bamber is the only eligible candidate for this role.[16] The only other known man-midwife practising in London from before the extinction of the Chamberlen line in 1732 until the apparent wider release of the vectis around 1750 was Sir Richard Manningham. His Deventerian allegiance makes him an unlikely candidate, and he had no known connection with any of the vectis practitioners on Denman's list.

Table 10.1 The associates of John Bamber according to four different sources.

Source	1	2	3	4
Middleton	●			●
Nesbit		○	●	●
Cole		○		●
Handeside		●		
Morley		●	(●)	
Griffith				●

Key to sources (for references, see text): (1) Starkey Middleton, *Philosophical Transactions of the Royal Society*, 1747; (2) *Iatro-Rapsodica*, 1751; (3) *Petition of unborn babes* and other satires by Frank Nicholls, 1751–52; (4) Denman's *Midwifery*, 1782/1801. Key to links: ○ – link; ● – link specifying midwifery; () – link indirect (Bamber was described as tutor to "Pocus" (Nesbit), who in turn was associated with "Maulus" (Morley).

From whom did Bamber get the vectis? Probably not from Roonhuysen or his successors, since he is not known to have visited the Dutch Republic, nor from Hugh Chamberlen I, given Bamber's Tory allegiance during Hugh I's lifetime.[17] This leaves Middleton Walker and Hugh Chamberlen II, of whom Hugh II seems the more likely candidate to have possessed the instrument since he was in the direct line. When did Bamber receive it? Probably before his transition from surgery to physic in the mid-1720s – a move that would have been assisted by practising man-midwifery as distinct from traditional obstetric surgery, and would thus have been helped by having the vectis.[18] Certainly well before 1731, by which date he had "great experience" in midwifery according to Starkey Middleton's later testimony. It thus seems likely that Bamber got the vectis around 1720 – that is, at about the time when Hugh II was distributing the forceps. Since Bamber also had a forceps, he may have purchased both instruments from Hugh II, just as members of the Roonhuysen circle obtained them both from Hugh I in the 1690s.

There may have been another recipient of the vectis around 1720: John Birch.[19] Unlike Bamber, Birch died young (in his mid-thirties, on 26 January 1729/30); after his death, according to the slightly later testimony of John Douglas (1736), "Dr Birch's fillet" was "put up to be sold for £500 by the late excellent surgeon Mr Jos. Symonds".[20] Now £500 would have been a very high price for a fillet, since that instrument was neither unusual nor particularly efficacious. But it might have been a realistic price for a vectis at this time; and John Douglas may well have been confused about the identity of the instrument. The possibility thus arises that Birch's instrument was a vectis rather than a fillet. It is therefore intriguing to find several parallels between the careers of Birch and Bamber. Like Bamber, Birch gained remarkable advancement in the London College of Physicians in the mid-1720s: both these promotions would surely have required the support of its President, Sir Hans Sloane, and in Birch's case we know that Sloane made active efforts on his behalf. (Sloane put Birch forward for an Honorary Fellowship, but this was at first "carried in the negative"; after a further attempt, involving a change of the rules, Sloane got his way.[21]) Like Bamber, Birch began as a Tory, and like Bamber, he seems to have transferred to a Whig allegiance in the mid-1720s.[22] And like Bamber, Birch practised in the City of London – as did Josiah Symonds, the surgeon who after Birch's death "put up" his instrument "to be sold".[23] Perhaps, then, Hugh Chamberlen II sold the vectis to two City practitioners – Birch at Bow Lane off Cheapside, Bamber half a mile to the east at Mincing Lane, near the Tower.[24] Certainly it would be worth exploring the actions and motives of Sir Hans Sloane in promoting both Bamber and Birch in the mid-1720s: was he, for instance, building politico-medical bridges with selected Tory or ex-Tory surgeons?

One other fragment of information is consistent with the inference that there was a London vectis associated with Dr John Bamber. William Smellie was unaware of the vectis until 1753, after the publication of the "Roonhuysen secret". (In that year its existence was forcefully brought to his notice by de Preville, the French translator of his own *Treatise*, who added a description and a print of the Roonhuysen vectis to his translation of Smellie's first volume. Smellie duly inserted a brief report of this into his Preface to volume II (1754), saying that de Preville had "obliged the world" with this print.[25]) However, some two or three years earlier Smellie had twice tried to use a single blade of the forceps as a vectis – first in December 1750 and then in the following month, January 1751.[26] Both these attempts were unsuccessful, suggesting that Smellie had no previous experience with the method. Smellie could conceivably have derived this idea from the writings of Chapman, Butter or Giffard, since, as we have seen, these men had all described the technique in the early 1730s.[27] Yet this is unlikely, for Smellie never mentioned their use of the single-blade technique; and in any case it would not explain why he took up the idea for the first time in late 1750. In short, it would seem that in 1750 Smellie got some inkling of the vectis, and duly experimented as best he could – that is, with a single blade of the forceps.[28] How did he learn about the vectis at this time? Perhaps he heard about the Roonhuysen instrument from Peter Camper of Amsterdam, who would soon be assisting him with his *Anatomical tables* (published in 1754). But perhaps Smellie's information pertained to the London vectis and derived from the Bamber circle. In particular, we may suspect that his informant was Robert Nesbit, since a few years earlier, in 1747, Nesbit had helped Smellie improve the forceps.[29] Thus Smellie's experimenting with the single-blade technique in late 1750 and early 1751 was perhaps a further and indirect reflection of John Bamber's passing on the London vectis to a wider circle of practitioners around this time.

The vectis and the City of London

The story of the vectis provides an ironic counterpoint to the battles reconstructed in previous chapters. Forceps man-midwifery and Deventerian man-midwifery were in more or less open contest from 1716 until about 1750; the significance of the fillet was relatively shadowy, but its presence was at least acknowledged by some participants in the unfolding struggle. Yet it seems that the vectis was meanwhile being quietly used by John Bamber, and from about 1733 by Starkey Middleton, without anyone else suspecting that there had been another Chamberlen secret apart from the forceps. In the early 1750s some slight awareness flickered of the existence of the vectis or of Bamber's passing the instrument on to a wider circle, but this soon died away. Even after 1754, when the Roonhuysen vectis was mentioned in Smellie's preface, most British observers remained unaware of the vectis; and Bamber's heirs, like Bamber himself before them, kept their secret and avoided public contests. Just as the use of a single blade of the forceps by Chapman, Butter and Giffard had been forgotten, so too the purpose-built vectis attracted no public interest: it was not mentioned, for instance, by Elizabeth Nihell or Philip Thicknesse in their attacks on man-midwifery in the 1760s, by William Hunter in his lectures at this time, by Wallace Johnson in his forceps-based *New system of midwifery* of 1769, nor again by William Perfect in his treatise of 1783.[30]

In the 1780s this long silence was finally broken: the vectis at last became public knowledge in England, competing openly with the forceps, and thereafter the respective merits of the two instruments were keenly debated, as were different designs of the vectis itself.[31] But what accounts for the earlier silence, so sharply contrasting with the history of the forceps? It may be relevant that vectis practitioners received both emergency calls, like forceps practitioners, and onset calls with a midwife, like the Deventerians.[32] But the most notable point is that the different techniques had distinctive *geographies*. The vectis was specifically associated with practitioners in the City of London: first Bamber, then Cole, Griffith,

Middleton, Morley and Nesbit, later Thomas Cogan, Jonathan Wathen and John Ford.[33-41] By contrast, the battle between the forceps and Deventerian midwifery – both in its early phase and then between Smellie and his rivals in the 1740s – was waged in the West End and in Westminster. It was here that Giffard, Chapman and Smellie practised; that Manningham and Douglas lived; and that in 1747, as we shall see in the next chapter, the Middlesex Hospital opened a lying-in ward staffed by men-midwives opposed to the forceps. Thus "London" is too broad a category: the metropolis needs to be broken down into smaller units. Perhaps the reason for the intense conflicts of the Westminster area was the fact that here were to be found the richest pickings of practice – attendance at the delivery of aristocratic ladies, who lay in "in town" and expected to spend 100 guineas on a man-midwife. Again, the City had a distinct political tradition: until the 1740s the Court Whigs had no hope of capturing it in Parliamentary elections.[42] Whatever the reason, the silence surrounding the vectis stands in remarkable contrast to the sound and fury over its sister instrument, the midwifery forceps, in the early eighteenth century.

Notes

1. See Ch. 5 above.
2. *Ibid.*
3. *Philosophical Transactions of the Royal Society*, No. 484 (1747), pp. 617–21; cf. *ibid.*, No. 475 (1745), pp. 336–40, at pp. 338–9.
4. Manningham lived in Jermyn Street, Douglas from probably c.1719 in Covent Garden (previously however in the City), Walker in Great Suffolk Street, Bamber in Mincing Lane. See BL Sloane MS 4056, ff. 84, 85v; C. H. Brock, "James Douglas (1675–1742), botanist", *Journal for the Society for Bibliography of Natural History* 9 (1979), pp. 137–45, at p. 138; Aveling, *Chamberlens*, p. 193; *DNB*, entry for Sir Crisp Gascoyne (1700–1761). (The mother in Bamber's case of 1731 was "Mrs Ball, without Bishopsgate"; see previous note.)
5. C. L. S. Linnell (ed.), *The diaries of Thomas Wilson, DD, 1731–37 and 1750, son of Bishop Wilson of Sodor and Man* (London: SPCK, 1964), pp. 121–3; Lady Llanover (ed.), *The autobiography and correspondence of Mary Granville, Mrs Delany* (3 volumes; London, 1861), vol. II, pp. 247, 249, 253, 257.
6. See Clark, *College of Physicians*, vol. II, pp. 503–5, 547–51.
7. *Iatro-Rapsodica: or, a physical rhapsody* (London, 1751). The copy in WIHM, 29904/C/1, has all the various names filled in in pencil. Another pro-Schomberg verse satire at this time was *The Battiad* (London, 1750), which attacked William Battie and "Pocus" (Robert Nesbit).
8. For Matthew Morley, see anon., *The trial of a cause between R. Maddox, plaintiff, and Dr M—y, defendant* (London, 1754); for the identity of Morley as the defendant, rather than George Macaulay who was the other possible candidate, see Glaister, *Smellie*, p. 322. For Joshua Cole, see A. E. Clark-Kennedy, *London Pride: the story of a voluntary hospital* (London: Hutchinson, 1979), p. 17; for Robert Nesbit, see McClintock, *Smellie's midwifery*, vol. II, p. 252 (Case 186).

9. *The petition of the unborn babes to the Censors of the College of Physicians* (1751); *A Defence of Dr Pocus and Dr Malus against the petition of the unborn babes to the Censors of the College of Physicians of London* (1751); *A vindication of man-midwifery, being the answer of Dr Pocus, Dr Malus, and Dr Barebones, and others, their brethren, who, like Legion, are many, to the petition of the unborn babes, &c. In a letter to the President and Censors, and The Elect, of the College of Physicians, London* (1752). There was also a set of "satirical proposals for publishing the art of midwifery", of which I know of no copy; this was summarized in *Gentleman's Magazine* (December 1751), p. 563.

10. Pocus was surely Nesbit. Barebone(s) was certainly Bamber: *A vindication of man-midwifery* was signed "E. Schola Bareboneana prope Turrim Feb 14th, 1752", i.e. "from the school of Dr Barebone near the Tower" (Bamber lived in Mincing Lane). The identification of Maulus/Malus as Morley is less sure, but would fit with *Iatro-Rapsodica* and with the fact that Maulus, like Pocus, was a Fellow of the College (*A defence of Dr Pocus and Dr Malus*, p. 5). In "Biographical memoirs of Frank Nicholls, MD" (*Gentleman's Magazine*, 50:1, 1785, pp. 13–15), and subsequently elsewhere, Maulus was identified as Dr Maule, Barebone as Dr Barrowby. But neither of these is identified as practising midwifery in any source known to me, and the identification of Barebone as Barrowby is certainly in error.

11. Thomas Denman (1733–1815): see *DNB*.

12. Thomas Denman, *Introduction to the practice of midwifery* (first published 1782; third edition, London, 1801), vol. I, p. xlv.

13. *Ibid.*, vol. II, p. 118.

14. Hunter, lectures, *passim*.

15. Two other individuals are worth investigating in this regard. (1) Francis Sandys: It seems that his "fillet" (Ch. 6 above) served both as fillet and as vectis; and in 1753 he was called as a witnesss in the defence at law of Matthew Morley, whom *Iatro-Rapsodica* had associated with Bamber (*The trial of a cause*, p. 19; *n*.8 above). (2) William Clark (1698–1780), who in 1747 moved from London to Bradford, in his native Wiltshire, on at least one occasion there used a single blade of the forceps as a vectis: see his *The province of midwives in the practice of their art* (London, 1751), pp. 20, 32. Published on midwifery and on the passions; retired 1772 to Colchester, where the known vectis practitioner Moses Griffith had retired 1768 (*n*.35 below); published a religious work there in 1779. See Innes Smith, *Students at Leyden*; Munk, *Roll*; CUL Catalogue.

16. However, some of Bamber's associates might have received the vectis directly from Hugh Chamberlen II (d.1728). Nesbit was born *c*.1697, Morley 1701, and Handeside (not known to have practised midwifery except on the evidence of *Iatro-Rapsodica*) 1694. In this respect Cole, born 1706, is a marginal case, as is Starkey Middleton, MD (d.1768), perhaps born *c*.1710. (Middleton was born before 1715, probably *c*.1710 since he was practising with Bamber in 1733. Wallis, *Medics*, indicates that the namesake of St Botolph Bishopsgate who received a bishop's licence in 1720 was his father, d. 1755). Moses Griffith was born in 1724 and thus could not have got the vectis from Chamberlen. Dates of birth are from Wallis, *Medics* except Nesbit (Innes Smith, *Students at Leyden*).

17. See *n*.49 to Ch. 5 above.

18. Cf., a generation later, Samuel Wathen and William Hunter, both of whom also used midwifery to make the transition from surgery to physic: Brock, *William Hunter*, pp. 7–9, 35. (Wathen was probably a vectis practitioner: see Ch. 11 below.)

19. John Birch: born Cheshire *c*.1694; studied medicine at Leyden (1714–16), where the dedicatees of his MD thesis included Joseph Eaton, MD (1655–1724 or later; also from Cheshire; former nonconformist clergyman). At some point between 1718 and 1720 stud-

NOTES

ied midwifery at the Paris Hôtel-Dieu under Grégoire the elder (father of Smellie's later teacher); also "a pupil of Dr Woolhouse, physician to the hospital of blind men at Paris". Died 26 January 1729/30; his books were auctioned on 30 April 1730. See Wallis, *Medics*; Munk, *Roll*; Innes Smith, *Students at Leyden*; John R. Guy, Archbishop Secker as a physician, in *The church and healing*, W. J. Sheils (ed) (Oxford: Blackwell, for the Ecclesiastical History Society, 1982), pp. 127–35, at p. 132; BL, Sloane MSS 3172, 3182, notes at beginning of volumes.

20. John Douglas, *A short account of the state of midwifery in London, Westminster, &c.* (London, 1736), p. 60 (quoted in Ch. 6 above).
21. Royal College of Physicians, Annals, 22 March 1724/5; 22 December 1725; 7 January 1725/6.
22. Birch's political allegiance, as indicated by his book-subscriptions, was Tory (works by Simon Ockley 1718, Richard Fiddes 1724, George Smalridge 1724, Thomas Hearne 1728 and 1729), yet two of his subscriptions were distinctly Whig (Gilbert Burnet 1724, Richard Mounteney 1731). Sloane's patronage in 1725 suggests that Birch turned his coat before that date; some of the subscriptions may have been arranged several years before the books were published. See Wallis, *Medics* and Phibb, *Subscriptions;* for allegiances of authors, *DNB*.
23. Birch was of Bow Lane (Munk, *Roll*), Symonds of Fenchurch Street (Wallis, *Medics*).
24. Admittedly, Birch could have got his instrument from Grégoire *c.*1719 (*n.*19 above); if so, this was probably a fillet, since the vectis seems to have been unknown in France until 1753.
25. See McClintock, *Smellie's midwifery*, vol. II, pp. 3–4 (Smellie here referred to his own use of a single blade of the forceps, discussed below).
26. *Ibid.*, vol. II, p. 324, note appended to Cases 246, 247. See also p. 344 (part of a comment appended to a case of March, 1751). Smellie's only other reference to this use of the forceps was a single sentence in vol. I, p. 257.
27. Ch. 7 above.
28. McClintock made only one passing comment on this subject: "from [Smellie's] general silence with regard to the vectis ... we may suppose he set very little value upon it" (*Smellie's midwifery*, vol. II, p. 325); see however *ibid.*, vol. I, pp. 218, 260.
29. *Ibid.*, vol. II, p. 252.
30. For Nihell & Thicknesse see Ch. 15 below. R. W. Johnson, *A new system of midwifery, in four parts* (London, 1769); Hunter, lectures; W. Perfect, *Cases in midwifery, with references, quotations, and remarks* (2 volumes; Rochester, n.d. & 1783).
31. The silence seems to have been broken in 1783 by both William Dease and Thomas Denman; in addition William Lowder is said by Radcliffe to have played some role. See R. Bland, *Some account of the invention and use of the lever of Roonhuysen* (London, 1790), pp. 42–4; *DNB*, entry for Thomas Denman (1733–1815); W. Osborn, *Essays on the practice of midwifery in natural and difficult labours* (London, 1792), pp. v–x; Radcliffe, *Milestones*, pp. 48, 62. In the mid-1780s there was still no mention of the vectis in *Chambers's cyclopaedia* (Abraham Rees (ed.) 4 volumes; London, 1783–86): see its entries for "forceps" (recommending Smellie's instrument, mentioning that Hunter seldom used forceps); "vectis" (cross-referring to "lever"); and "lever" (in its mechanical sense only, with no obstetric application).
32. John Bamber's known cases were an emergency call in 1731, a call of unknown type in 1734, and an onset call with a midwife in 1735; Starkey Middleton's known cases, in 1735–41, seem to have been onset calls with a midwife; Matthew Morley's known case was

an emergency of 1753. See *Philosophical Transactions of the Royal Society*, No. 484 (1747), pp. 617–21; Linnell (ed.), *Diaries of Thomas Wilson*, pp. 121–3; *The trial of a cause* (cf. *n*.8 above).

33. Bamber: of Mincing-Lane; retired to Barking, Essex. See Munk, *Roll* and *DNB*, entry for Sir Crisp Gascoyne (1700–1761).
34. Joshua Cole: apothecary to, and one of the founders of, the London Hospital, 1740 (Clark-Kennedy, *London Pride*, p. 17).
35. Moses Griffith: of Mincing Lane, 1752 (*An account of the City of London Lying-in Hospital for Married Women*, 1752, p. 6); retired to Colchester 1768 (cf. William Clark, *n*.15 above).
36. Starkey Middleton: his namesake, presumably father, was of St Botolph, Bishopsgate, in 1720; attended deliveries of Mrs Ball, without Bishopsgate, 1735–41; attended wife of Richard Maddock, City lawyer, in 1753, after Morley's failure to deliver her; subscription(s) however from Hoxton. See *n*.16 above; *Philosophical Transactions of the Royal Society*, No. 484 (1747), pp. 617–21; *The trial of a cause*, p. 14; Wallis, *Medics*.
37. Matthew Morley: of Lincoln's-Inn Fields, 1752; of St Bride's, Farringdon Without, 1753; some subscription(s) however from Kennington. See G. Ballard, *Memoirs of several ladies of Great Britain*, Oxford, 1752; complaint of Richard Maddock: Glaister, *Smellie*, p. 322; Wallis, *Medics*.
38. Robert Nesbit: of King Street, Cheapside, 1739 (R. H. Nichols & F. H. Wray, *The history of the Foundling Hospital*, London, 1935, p. 348). Clifford Handeside, Bamber's other associate, not included in Denman's list, was of Red-Lion Square when he died in 1772 (Munk, *Roll*).
39. For Cogan, Wathen, Ford and others as vectis practitioners of the next generation see Denman, *Introduction to the practice of midwifery*, pp. 118–19. Dr Thomas Cogan (1736–1818): of Paternoster Row from *c*.1772; had strong religious associations, a peripatetic life including a period in the Dutch Republic, and three successive careers of which midwifery was the second. In 1767 dedicated his Leyden thesis to John (Jonathan) Wathen, fellow vectis practitioner; around this time a governor of Leake's lying-in hospital at Lambeth; in 1776 had a position at the Lying-in Charity; translated Camper's works on anatomy and the plastic arts (1794). See *DNB;* Innes Smith, *Students at Leyden*; *account of the Lying-in Charity* (London, 1776); *BL Catalogue*; P. Rhodes, *Doctor John Leake's Hospital: a history of the General Lying-In Hospital, York Road, Lambeth, 1765–1971* (London: Davis-Poynter, 1977), pp. 30–31; Chs 11 & 15 below.
40. Jonathan Wathen (fl. 1760s–1780s): of Bartholomew Lane in 1769, as subscriber to the Lying-In Charity (*An account of the Lying-In Charity . . . instituted 1757*, London, 1769, p. 51); dedicatee of Cogan's thesis in 1767 (see previous note); see Ch. 11 below.
41. John Ford (c. 1736–1806): of Old Jewry in 1769, as physician and man-midwife to the Lying-In Charity and one of its governors (*Account of the Lying-in Charity*, 1769). Not the John Ford to whom Philip Thicknesse ironically dedicated an anti-man-midwifery tract of 1790; for both men, see Munk, *Roll*, and Ch. 15 below.
42. See Ch. 11 below, at *n*.42.

Chapter Eleven
New institutions: the London Lying-in Hospitals

An overview of London's lying-in hospitals

Since the mid-seventeenth century Paris had its *salle des accouchements* at the Hôtel-Dieu; but there was no parallel in London, for the old endowed hospitals of St Bartholomew and St Thomas excluded lying-in women, as did Guy's new endowed hospital (1725) and the first three of the capital's new voluntary hospitals – Westminster Infirmary (established in 1719), its offshoot St George's Hospital (1733), and the London Hospital (1740).[1] Various individuals proposed that there should be some London provision for lying-in women, both for their charitable relief and for the teaching of midwifery; but all that came of these suggestions was Manningham's apparently short-lived lying-in infirmary of 1739.[2] In the 1740s the success of Smellie's lying-in fund revealed the potential demand for help, yet by 1747 the metropolis still had no institutional provision for lying-in women.[3] Thereupon a very rapid change set in: within five years, London had three lying-in hospitals, and a fourth was added in 1767. In sharp contrast with Manningham's infirmary, all these institutions proved permanent – probably because they acquired a broader base of initial support.

The starting-point was London's fourth voluntary hospital, the Middlesex, founded in 1745 – and perhaps also the example of Dublin's lying-in hospital, which was set up in the same year (and after a later rebuilding was known as the Rotunda Hospital).[4] The Middlesex, which had a strong Whig complexion, may have been established by Sir Hugh Smithson (later Earl of Northumberland) and his associates to win favour among the Middlesex electorate in the next general election, held in 1747.[5] Somehow the governors of the Middlesex, or some of them, came to feel that the hospital should include a lying-in ward, and such a ward was duly added in 1747. It was from this beginning that the whole lying-in hospital movement took its origin. In 1749 a rift developed in the Middlesex, with some of the governors wanting to enlarge the lying-in ward, and others being opposed to this. The first group split off, taking with them the men-midwives Francis Sandys and Daniel Layard, and established a separate new hospital entirely devoted to lying-in mothers. Thus was founded the British Lying-in Hospital at Brownlow Street.[6] Next year a second hospital of this kind was created in the City of London (1750) and two years later a third, the General Lying-in Hospital, in Westminster (1752).[7] Like other voluntary hospitals, these institutions had a high public profile yet were very small in scale: between them they delivered only a tiny minority, perhaps 5%, of London births around 1760. An overview of the founding of these new institutions is shown in Fig. 11.1, which also specifies the early men-midwives and the particular regulations of the various institutions. Geographically, these hospitals were dispersed in an arc parallel to the Thames, as is shown in Fig. 11.2. At this stage there was no lying-in hospital in London's Surrey outpost of Southwark and Lambeth. But in 1767 this was redressed by Dr John Leake and his associates, who set up the "Westminster New Lying-in Hospital" at Lambeth. The siting, at least, of this later hospital (which I shall not be discussing systematically) was no doubt partly prompted by the fact that Lambeth was now on the eve of rapid commercial development, thanks to the recent building of Westminster Bridge (1750) and the impending opening of Blackfriars Bridge (1769).[8]

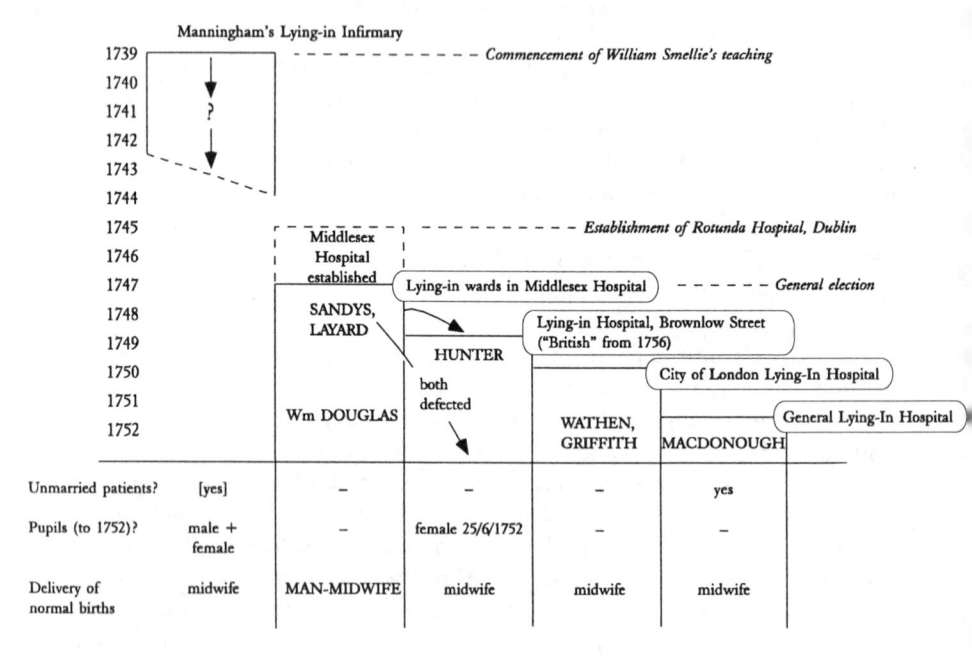

Figure 11.1 Overview of the foundation of lying-in wards and hospitals in London to 1752, with NAMES of men-midwives, variations of practice, and *possibly related events.*

Each lying-in hospital had to confront three central policy issues. Should it admit unmarried mothers? Should it allow its man-midwife or men-midwives to use patients as teaching material? And should normal delivery be handled by a midwife or by a man-midwife? As Fig. 11.1 shows, these questions were answered in different ways. The delivery of *single women* posed a dilemma: the unmarried mother stood most in need of help, yet her admission raised local opposition, for delivery would give her child a "settlement" in the parish where the hospital stood, making that parish liable for the child's indefinite support.[9] In the event the Middlesex, British and City of London hospitals all decided not to admit unmarried mothers (indeed, the very name of the last proclaimed that it was "for Married Women"). This created a vacuum that was filled by Felix Macdonough's "General Lying-in Hospital" – so named because it took in mothers irrespective of their marital status.[10] Yet the topic remained hot thereafter. In 1754 the British Lying-in Hospital, having found that "several persons" refused benefactions because it excluded single women, issued a public statement to justify its policy. Subsequently, Leake's hospital had to wrestle with the issue in its first few years, and it was apparently as a result of this problem that an Act of Parliament was passed in 1773, requiring lying-in hospitals to secure licences from Quarter Sessions.[11] The issue of *teaching* seems also to have been contentious. The idea was attractive: a lying-in hospital offered unrivalled opportunities for the practical teaching of midwifery, whether to female pupils, male pupils, or both; the Paris example had long been cited as worthy of imitation in this respect; and, of course, Manningham's Lying-in Infirmary had been set up for just this

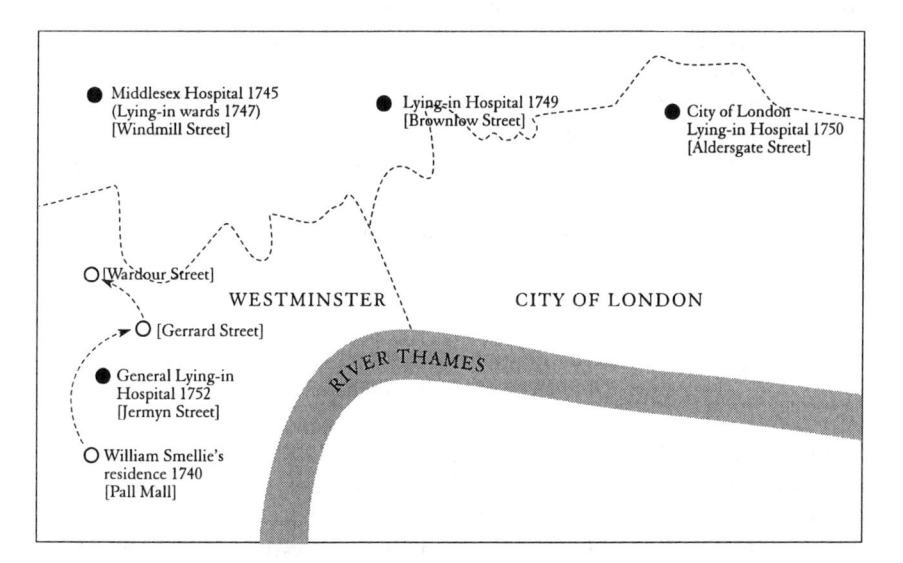

Figure 11.2 Locations of lying-in hospitals (and wards) in London, to 1752; except for Manningham's Lying-in Infirmary (1739–?) (location unknown) and adding the known residence of William Smellie, 1740–c.1759.

purpose. Yet women doubtless disliked being used in this way, and they must have made their objections felt, for in 1748 the Middlesex announced that "no pupils are permitted to attend the lying-in ward" (in contrast with its general wards).[12] However, mothers may have found midwife-pupils more acceptable; thus the Brownlow Street Hospital began to take female pupils from 1752, and the Middlesex Hospital soon followed suit.[13]

Finally, the issue of *midwife or man-midwife* for normal births initially differentiated the lying-in ward of the Middlesex from the lying-in hospitals proper. For at first, delivery in the Middlesex was performed by the hospital's honorary man-midwife in ordinary – Daniel Peter Layard until the 1749 split, then William Douglas. By contrast, each of the lying-in hospitals employed a midwife-matron who delivered "natural and easy labours", restricting their male practitioners to emergency work. (There were also different ways of implementing the latter policy. Both the City of London and the General had a three-tier system, with midwife, man-midwife-in-ordinary, and man-midwife-extraordinary; but in the City of London the man-midwife-in-ordinary attended charitably, whereas at the General this position was a salaried and residential one, denominated "house surgeon".[14]) However, in this respect the hospitals soon converged: by 1761, normal births were delivered by the midwife in the Middlesex just as in the lying-in hospitals.[15] (So too Leake's hospital, even though founded by a man-midwife with particular methods of his own, appointed a matron-midwife and two assistant midwives from the outset.[16])

We should expect that behind the creation of the lying-in hospitals there lay both obstetric and party-political interests. Man-midwifery was still divided: to what camp or camps did the hospital men-midwives belong? And the subscribers inhabited a world split by party-political allegiances: were the lying-in hospitals Whig or Tory, or did they represent an eirenic intervention, an attempt to bridge the long-standing battle of political factions? Like other voluntary hospitals, they announced themselves as disinterested philanthropic initiatives – but this may have been propaganda.[17] Charity bought votes, particularly in large and keenly contested electorates such as the three London ones of the City (four MPs), Middlesex and Westminster (two MPs each).

Obstetric allegiances

Until at least 1760 the men-midwives who staffed these institutions included few if any forceps practitioners, and several declared opponents of the instrument. We may conveniently review this theme hospital by hospital.

When the Middlesex Hospital created its lying-in ward in 1747, *Daniel Peter Layard* was man-midwife-in-ordinary, while *Francis Sandys* was the man-midwife extraordinary, called "in all dangerous or doubtful cases".[18] Sandys was certainly opposed to the forceps, as we shall see below. Layard's methods are unknown, but since his task was to deliver the normal births, and given that he worked in tandem with the anti-forceps Sandys, it is most unlikely that he used the forceps.[18] After these men defected to the Brownlow Street Hospital in 1749 they were replaced at the Middlesex by *William Douglas* – who in the previous year had published a blistering attack on Smellie, starting with the wooden forceps with which Smellie was then experimenting, and going on to criticize his manner of teaching, the low price of that teaching, and the forceps in general.[20] Of the forceps Douglas had written:

> Steel forceps have been used heretofore by very good professors, but as practice and industry has discovered safer and easier methods, every man that knows them is right to use what serves his purpose best . . . for my part, I have entirely excluded all forceps out of my practice, and so have some others of my acquaintance; and I find that what I use never fails, when the forceps would be ineffectual. This, Sir, I don't pretend to call a nostrum, because there are some few that I know, use the same method; and I am ready, for the public good, to teach anyone that will put himself a proper time under my directions. There are several better ways to extract head-births than the forceps, which you appear to be quite a stranger to; I know there are some gentlemen of the profession who decry instruments entirely, but that must arise from a want of the proper knowledge upon the use of them.[21]

In a subsequent pamphlet, Douglas revealed that the "others of my acquaintance" who "entirely excluded" the forceps were Francis Sandys, Sir Richard Manningham and Edward Hody; "Two of those gentlemen always publicly declare against the use of forceps, and the third makes use of no such thing."[22] Presumably these were also the "some few that I know" who "use the same method" as Douglas himself; that method was probably some variant of the fillet.[23] Moreover, Douglas was proud to announce that he had spent five years under the "immediate care for anatomy and midwifery etc." of the unrelated James Douglas, who had died in 1742. Thus William Douglas was both aligned and connected with the Deventerian practitioners of the previous generation.[24] So too was his successor at the Middlesex, *Brudenell Exton*, who was man-midwife there by 1757 and continued until 1760. Like Douglas, Exton had gone into print before his appointment, publishing in 1751 *A new and general system of midwifery*, where he announced that he was a recent convert away from the forceps. In the late 1730s he had been a pupil of Edmund Chapman, who taught the forceps, but in 1747 he had learnt from Manningham, and he now assailed the reputation of the forceps by claiming that it was not the Chamberlen secret after all. As we would expect from a pupil of Manningham's, Exton's approach and methods were straightforwardly Deventerian, including the use of the fillet and, in exceptional cases, craniotomy.[25] In 1761 the pattern at the Middlesex may have changed, for Exton was succeeded by *Dr John D'Urban*, a pupil of Smellie's who had been using the forceps in 1752.[26] This would seem to imply a change of policy on the part of the Middlesex Hospital, yet it might equally reflect a change of obstetric allegiance by D'Urban, after the pattern of his predecessor Exton.

At Brownlow Street the first men-midwives were Sandys and Layard, who had come from the Middlesex, and *William Hunter*. As we have seen, Sandys was an opponent of the forceps and Layard probably did not use the instrument. Hunter is a very ambiguous case. His initial training in midwifery may have been along Deventerian lines – in 1740–41 as a living-in student of Smellie in the latter's anti-forceps phase, then possibly in 1741–42 with James Douglas, who employed him as a dissector and may also have taught him midwifery. (It was perhaps a legacy of these years that in his later lectures Hunter paid some respect to Deventer.[27]) Subsequently, however, he learnt the use of the forceps – probably from Smellie in the late 1740s, at which time Hunter would have found the forceps useful since he was practising as a surgeon. Thus when he joined the Brownlow Street Lying-in Hospital in 1749, it would seem that he was a forceps practitioner – unlike his colleagues Layard and Sandys. Yet in the very next year he changed his private practice from surgery to physic (getting a Glasgow MD for the purpose); and since he now began to specialize in midwifery, he may have been moving away from the forceps at just this time. As we shall later see, Hunter's subsequent trajectory was away from the forceps; but it is difficult to ascertain his obstetric views and methods at the moment of his appointment.[28] By 1752 Sandys and Layard had retired as men-midwives (although they remained as subscribers) and Hunter had acquired two new colleagues at the Brownlow Street Hospital – *George Macaulay*, MD, and the surgeon *John Torr*.[29] I have not established what methods either of these men followed. (Macaulay had only recently moved to London; he was married to the famous historian Mrs Catherine Macaulay.[30]) In due course they moved on, but Hunter continued his association with the hospital until at least 1767.

The most intriguing case is the City of London Lying-in Hospital, which was served for at least its first 17 years by Moses Griffith – who was also one of its governors – and by Samuel Wathen.[31] For according to the later testimony of Thomas Denman, discussed in the previous chapter, Moses Griffith used the vectis. Indeed, his name was the next after that of John Bamber on Denman's list of City vectis practitioners, and in 1752 he resided in Mincing Lane, whence Bamber had just retired.[32] Samuel Wathen's methods are not known to me, and he was not on Denman's list.[33] But it is suggestive that his namesake and contemporary Jonathan Wathen was another City vectis practitioner, whom Denman described – with a glowing tribute to his skill – as the successor to Griffith, Middleton, Nesbit and Cole.[34] Given that Samuel Wathen practised side by side for over 15 years at the City Hospital with one known vectis practitioner (Moses Griffith), and shared an unusual surname with another (Jonathan Wathen – probably his brother), there is good reason to presume that he too used the vectis. Thus the strong association between the vectis and the City of London, discussed in the previous chapter, extended also to the City's Lying-in Hospital.

The obstetric alignment of the General Lying-in Hospital is obscure, since its man-midwife and founder Felix Macdonough – a member of the Company of Surgeons who claimed the title of "Doctor" – avoided public obstetric controversy. But Macdonough surely had some specific obstetric allegiance, for he was offering lectures on midwifery at the Hospital in 1753, and in 1768 it was stated that he had taught both the Hospital's matron (i.e. midwife) and its house-surgeon. He also had an original mind: his 1768 *Account* tabulated the numbers of women delivered not only by year, as was customary in such publications, but also by their parishes of origin, their social circumstances and marital status, and the numbers of easy and difficult deliveries.[35]

With the opening of John Leake's New Westminster Lying-in Hospital in 1767, we find for the first time a clear association between a lying-in hospital and forceps man-midwifery. Yet even this exception in certain ways confirmed the prevailing rule. In the first place, Leake's forceps was of a new kind, incorporating a third blade based on the vectis.[36] Moreover, one of the Hospital governors, Dr Thomas Cogan, was a man-midwife who used the vectis.[37] Secondly, the fact that Leake's hospital was located at Lambeth, combined with the unique nature of his forceps, extends the previous pattern of association between distinctive obstetric methods and particular places.[38]

Political orientations

An adequately detailed political study of these institutions would require a book in itself, but it is possible to give a general picture: at least the first three of them had strong Whig associations. In the 1747 general elections there were eight Whig candidates, all of whom were or shortly became subscribers to the Middlesex Hospital or to a lying-in hospital;[39] and six Tory candidates, only two of whom had any connection with a lying-in hospital in the 1750s.[40] This suggests that lying-in hospitals and wards had a strong Whig complexion when first founded.[41] (As it happened, all the Whig candidates were elected and the Tories defeated.) Yet this allegiance had two distinct meanings. The Whigs standing for the seats of Middlesex and Westminster, and serving as governors of the corresponding hospitals (the Middlesex and the British Lying-In), were aligned with the Court; but the City Whigs, including Slingsby Bethell, the first president of the City Lying-in Hospital, were allied with the opposition. This befitted the City's strong earlier tradition of opposition to Walpole's ministry: in effect, while the 1747 election gave the Whigs their first victory in the City constituency for many years (thanks to the defeat of the '45 and to Pelham's placatory moves), the City electorate was so suspicious of the ministry that even a Whig MP had to take up at least a partly oppositional stance.[42] Hence the fact that the City of London Hospital had a broader political base: one of its vice-presidents was the Tory bookseller James Hodges, and its preachers in 1752 and 1753, Samuel Doughty and Thomas Church, seem to have been Tories.[43] The political complexion of the hospital reflected the politics of the City itself.

The General Lying-in Hospital probably also began as Whig – since Tories tended to be less sympathetic to unmarried mothers – but its initial profile of subscribers is unknown, for not until 1768 did it issue an appeal for further funding.[44] It must have started on a very small scale: in its first three years it delivered only 359 women, suggesting fewer than 10 beds. But from 1755 it began to expand, and in the hard times of the Seven Years' War it was delivering hundreds of women each year (apparently over 1500 in 1761). In response to this demand, the Hospital began an out-patient service in 1762. Its vast expansion must have been financed by a growing roll of subscribers; by 1768, these comprised a mixed political bag. On the one hand, there was a prominent Whig presence – chiefly of aristocrats with a military career – including most of the 16 vice-presidents whose names were blazoned at the top of the list of subscribers. On the other hand, the political leader of this group, Lord Rockingham, was not on the list, and the mass of subscribers included several prominent Tories. (Conspicuous by their absence were the clergy and the medical professions.[45])

In the case of the Middlesex Hospital there is reason to suspect an active connection between its Court Whig politics and its anti-forceps man-midwifery. The Whig cleric Edward Cobden, who in 1749 preached a charity sermon for the Middlesex, referred in that sermon to his own recently published *Poems on several occasions*; and these showed a lively awareness of medical issues.[46] One poem attacked Edmund Massey, "a clergyman who", as a footnote explained, "preached against inoculation of the smallpox". Inoculation was a Court Whig project promoted in the 1720s by Sir Hans Sloane and opposed by Tories such as Massey.[47] Two other poems, both from the 1730s, had lavished praise on the Whig man-midwife Francis Sandys.[48] The lines "To Mr Sandys at Cambridge", dated 20 June 1735, included an attack on his rivals:

> These qualities extend your fame
> And above titles raise a name:
> While W—, C—, and the rest
> Whose blunders hardly bear a jest
> . . . Are doomed for ever to be quacks.

The metre suggests that "W—" was Middleton Walker (who in fact had died four years earlier) and that "C—" was Edmund Chapman – both forceps practitioners.[49] The poem went on to eulogize Sandys's attendance on the Duchess of Portland, thus linking him firmly with the Court Whigs. Cobden's own Court credentials were impeccable (he was Chaplain to George II) – hence the invitation in March 1748/49, shortly after the publication of these poems, to preach for the Middlesex Hospital, where Sandys served as "man-midwife extraordinary". Cobden's sermon, entitled *The parable of the talents,* specifically praised the new lying-in ward established at the Middlesex 16 months earlier. Hospitals in general were "a happy means of improving the skill of physic and surgery"; such skill was particularly needed in the management of childbirth. The dangers of childbirth were "an affliction ... peculiarly entailed on women ... the daughters of Eve, for their mother's fatal transgression in paradise", which was "as evident a monument of the Fall, as the disorders on the face of the earth are of the universal Deluge". Though God-given, these dangers could be mitigated by man. Skill was needed in deliveries, to enable mothers to escape "dismal consequences ... from forward empirics in this business", such as the "wounds and bruises they receive from unskilful hands". It was here that Cobden referred to one of his recently published *Poems*; the reader who followed up this reference would find that skill meant Sandys, "forward empirics" meant forceps practitioners. In the context of the late 1740s, this was a coded criticism of Smellie – and subsequent appointments at the Middlesex Hospital suggest that its leading governors shared Cobden's views. Shortly before Cobden preached his sermon, William Douglas had published his two *Letters to William Smellie* (1748), attacking both Smellie and the forceps. Eight months or so after Cobden's sermon, Douglas was chosen as man-midwife at the Middlesex (to replace Layard and Sandys, who had seceded to the Brownlow Street Hospital). Another two years later Brudenell Exton published his frankly Deventerian and anti-forceps *New and general system of midwifery*, and also became a subscriber to the Middlesex; when Douglas retired in turn, it was Exton who succeeded him. Thus when the governors of the Middlesex appointed their men-midwives, they knew who they were getting – declared opponents of the forceps.

The significance of the lying-in hospitals

In an important essay, Margaret Versluysen has suggested that it was the lying-in hospitals which were chiefly responsible for promoting man-midwifery at the expense of the traditional midwife. The hospitals, Versluysen argues, gave male practitioners access to normal births; they served in this respect as exemplars to the wives of subscribers; they conferred on childbirth a new medical aura; and they emphasized the subordination of the midwife to the male practitioner.[50] The latter point indeed has force: in each lying-in hospital the consultant men-midwives had power and status, whereas the matron-midwife was firmly placed in the role of a servant. But the wider argument does not stand up, for the lying-in hospitals simply reproduced the traditional demarcation between midwife and male practitioner, namely the line between normal and difficult births. The way that line was drawn was indeed changing, in the direction of earlier male access in cases of difficulty, but this had been in progress since the 1720s: at most the hospitals reinforced an existing trend. From the outset, *all* the lying-in hospitals employed a midwife for normal births. Only in the lying-in ward of the Middlesex Hospital were normal births delivered by the man-midwife; and that ward was

NEW INSTITUTIONS: THE LONDON LYING-IN HOSPITALS

even smaller in scale than the lying-in hospitals themselves. (In the first nine months it delivered just 16 mothers; and even after the lying-in facility was expanded in 1755 it could only handle about 140 births a year, less than half the number then being delivered at Brownlow Street.[51]) And by 1761 the Middlesex had fallen in line with the lying-in hospitals by employing a midwife-matron to deliver normal births.

Rather than contributing to the displacement of the midwife, the hospitals attested to the battles *within* early Georgian man-midwifery – that is, the continuing contest against the forceps. Edward Cobden, preaching for the Middlesex in 1749, knew what was at stake. He raised the issue of obstetric skill and methods, not to promote male practice at the expense of midwives – despite the fact that the Middlesex itself was then using a male practitioner (Layard) to deliver normal births – but instead to fire a subtle salvo against Smellie and the forceps. It was indeed remarkable that the Middlesex Hospital at first entrusted normal births to its man-midwife, even though this experiment was small in scale and persisted for only a few years. But this was a reflection, not a cause, of the contemporary change in the role of the man-midwife – the unprecedented shift by which he came to be called in lieu of a midwife. It is to that momentous change that we will now turn.

Notes

1. For comments on this chapter I thank Bronwyn Croxson, whose forthcoming doctoral thesis will examine this subject in detail. On voluntary hospitals in general see my "The politics of medical improvement in early Hanoverian London", in *The medical enlightenment of the eighteenth century*, A. Cunningham & R. K. French (eds) (Cambridge, 1990), pp. 4–39, at pp. 24–34; D. E. Owen, *English philanthropy 1660–1960* (Cambridge, Mass.: Belknap, 1965), pp. 43–4; J. Woodward, *To do the sick no harm: a study of the British voluntary hospital system to 1875* (London: Routledge & Kegan Paul, 1974); D. Andrew, *Philanthropy and police: London charity in the eighteenth century* (Princeton, NJ, 1989); S. Cavallo, "The motivations of benefactors: an overview of approaches to the study of charity", in *Medicine and charity before the Welfare State* J. Barry & C. Jones (eds) (1991); R. Porter, "The gift relation: philanthropy and provincial hospitals in eighteenth-century England", in *The hospital in history*, L. Granshaw & R. Porter (eds) (London: Routledge, 1990), 149–78; and K. Wilson, "Urban culture and political activism in Hanoverian England: the example of voluntary hospitals", in *The transformation of political culture: England and Germany in the late eighteenth century*, E. Hellmuth (ed.) (Oxford, 1990), pp. 165–84.
2. For instance, William Petty (before 1687), Mrs Cellier (1687), John Maubray (1725) and John Douglas (1736). See G. McLachlan & T. McKeown (eds), *Medical history and medical care* (London, 1971), p. 84; John Maubray, *Midwifery brought to perfection by manual operation* (1725), pp. 19–23; Chs 3 & 8 above.
3. For Smellie's lying-in fund, see Ch. 9.
4. On the Rotunda Hospital see J. Ringland, *Annals of midwifery in Ireland* (Dublin, 1870), pp. 14–16 (cf. Ch. 8). For a summary of the London lying-in hospitals, see Donnison,

Midwives, pp. 25–8.
5. The political character of the Middlesex is inferred from the identities of its leading governors, traced in *DNB* and in R. Sedgwick, *History of Parliament: the House of Commons 1715–1754* (2 volumes; London: HMSO, for the History of Parliament Trust, 1970).
6. J. Donnison, "Note on the foundation of Queen Charlotte's Hospital", *Medical History* 15 (1971), pp. 398–400, at pp. 399–400.
7. See, respectively, *An account of the City of London Lying-in Hospital for Married Women at Shaftesbury-House in Aldersgate-Street, instituted March 30, 1750* (London, 1752) and *An account of the rise, progress, and state of the General Lying-in Hospital, the corner of Quebec-Street, Oxford-Road* (London, 1768).
8. See P. Rhodes, *Doctor John Leake's Hospital: a history of the General Lying-In Hospital, York Road, Lambeth, 1765–1971* (London: Davis-Poynter, 1977), Ch. 3; *DNB*, entry for John Leake; J. Summerson, *Georgian London* (3rd edn, London: Barrie & Jenkins, 1978), p. 277.
9. A "settlement" in a specified parish was an entitlement to poor relief there, usually derived from birth or apprenticeship but also secured in other ways. See D. Marshall, *The English poor in the eighteenth century: a study in social and administrative history* (London: Routledge, 1926), pp. 237–9; W. E. Tate, *The parish chest: a study of the records of parochial administration in England* (Cambridge: Cambridge University Press, 1969), pp. 192–3, 217; G. W. Oxley, *Poor relief in England and Wales 1601–1834* (London: David & Charles, 1974), pp. 19–21; R. Porter, *English society in the eighteenth century* (Harmondsworth: Penguin, 1982), p. 143.
10. How the General Lying-in Hospital resolved the settlement problem I have not ascertained; perhaps its location ("the corner of Quebec-Street, Oxford-Road") was extra-parochial. By 1768 the issue must have been acute, with hundreds of deliveries taking place there each year (see below).
11. *An account of the rise, progress, and state of the British Lying-in Hospital for Married Women . . . Brownlow-Street* (London, 1756), pp. 18–19; Rhodes, *Doctor John Leake's hospital*, pp. 27, 31–2, 34, 39, 44.
12. *An account of the Middlesex-Hospital*, appended to E. Cobden, *The parable of the talents. A sermon* (London, 1749), p. 2.
13. *Account of the . . . British Lying-in Hospital* (1756), p. 12; Clark, *College of Physicians*, vol. II, p. 505; Donnison, *Midwives*, p. 27.
14. *Account of the City of London Lying-in Hospital* (1752), pp. 4, 6; *Account of the rise, progress, and state of the General Lying-in Hospital* (1768), p. 1.
15. *An account of the Middlesex-Hospital . . . to 24 June 1761*, appended to C. Dodgson, *A sermon . . . St James Westminster . . . April 28, 1761* (London, 1761), p. 2.
16. Rhodes, *Doctor John Leake's Hospital*, pp. 28–9.
17. The issue of politics in the voluntary hospitals at large is at present unresolved. The very first voluntary hospital, the Westminster Infirmary, was created in 1719 by Tories; in sharp contrast, the infirmaries of Wakefield and Huddersfield, founded well over a century later, drew their support from the whole political spectrum; in between, particularly in the 1790s, tensions within voluntary hospitals reflected the developing conflicts of class and faction. See my The politics of medical improvement; H. Marland, *Medicine and society in Wakefield and Huddersfield 1780–1870* (Cambridge: Cambridge University Press, 1987), p. 144; J. V. Pickstone & S. V. F. Butler, "The politics of medicine in Manchester 1788–1792: hospital reform and health services in the early industrial city", *Medical History* 28 (1984), pp. 227–49.

18. *Account of the Middlesex-Hospital*, appended to Cobden, *The parable of the talents*, p. 2. For a list of men-midwives to the various hospitals see Spencer, *British midwifery*, pp. 179–81; this is incomplete and has some inaccuracies, e.g. James Douglas for William Douglas on p. 181.
19. Layard was of both Huntingdon and London: see Munk, *Roll*.
20. *An account of the Middlesex-Hospital,* appended to J. Dalton, *A sermon . . . St Anne's, Westminster . . . April 25, 1751* (London, 1751), p. 15; *An account of the Middlesex-Hospital*, appended to J. Thomas, *A sermon . . . St Anne's, Westminster . . . April 29, 1752* (London, 1752), p. 19; Glaister, *Smellie*, pp. 92, 97; W. Douglas, *A letter to Dr Smelle, shewing the impropriety of his new-invented wooden forceps* (London, 1748, reprinted in Glaister, *Smellie*, pp. 74–84).
21. Glaister, *Smellie*, p. 79.
22. W. Douglas, *A second letter to Dr Smellie and an answer to his pupil* (London, 1748, summarized in Glaister, *Smellie*, pp. 89–97), at p. 92. This was produced in response to a defence of Smellie published by an anonymous pupil. It named these men as "Dr S—ds, Sir R—d M–n–g–m, and Dr H—y". Here (p. 90) Douglas also swiped at La Motte, translated at Smellie's behest two years earlier (see Ch. 9 above).
23. Douglas's method was clearly an instrument of some sort, and not the forceps. The circumstantial evidence surrounding the vectis would suggest that Douglas had no knowledge of that device; the only qualification concerns Sandys's instrument (see n.15 to Ch. 10). The only other known possible instrument apart from the fillet was a device used once by Smellie in 1744, and described by him as "the common method at that time", yet not mentioned in any other source: "a blunt hook, that had a round button on the end", applied "above the chin". See McClintock, *Smellie's midwifery*, vol. II, Case 257, and n.24 to Ch. 9 above.
24. Douglas had an appointment to the household of Frederick, Prince of Wales; given the melange of interests which clustered around that household, this could imply any of a number of political allegiances. But all his identifiable associations were Whig.
25. *Gentlemen's Magazine*, 1757, p. 7; B. Exton, *A new and general system of midwifery* (London, 1751), 1766 edn, pp. 2 (Chapman), 9–10 (Manningham), 5 (the forceps not the Chamberlen secret), 57 (obliquity of the womb), 102–3 (turning in all such cases), 58–105 (manual delivery), 106–117 (craniotomy permitted, occasioned chiefly by "the bad formation of the pelvis"), 118 (fillet).
26. *Account . . . of the Middlesex Hospital . . . 1761*, p. 2; McClintock, *Smellie's midwifery*, vol. II, note appended to Case 261.
27. Hunter disagreed with Deventer as to the frequency of the oblique uterus and the early use of turning which this legitimated, and he did not mention Deventer's manoeuvre with the hand on the coccyx; yet he described the oblique uterus and recommended Deventer to his students. On the other hand, he also praised La Motte. See Hunter, lectures, pp. 10, 45–6, 59, 105.
28. See Ch. 13 below.
29. From 1752 Layard apparently became physician to the hospital, a post from which he resigned in 1755: Brock, *William Hunter*, p. 9.
30. George Macaulay: of Poland Street in 1752; not the "Dr M—y" sued by Richard Maddocks in 1753 (this was Matthew Morley); at some date before 1754 sent Smellie a case-description; in 1756 carried out the first premature induction of labour as a prophylactic measure in a woman with contracted pelvis. See *Account of the . . . British Lying-in Hospital* (1752); Glaister, *Smellie*, p. 322; Ch. 10 above; McClintock, *Smellie's midwifery*,

vol. II, Case 9; Munk, *Roll*.

31. In 1767 they were its two "men-midwives extraordinary" (the "man-midwife in ordinary" at this date being Dr Herman Heineken). See *An account of the City of London Lying-in Hospital*, appended to John Nichols, *A Sermon* (London, 1767), p. 18.
32. T. Denman, *Introduction to the practice of midwifery* (first published 1782; 3rd edn, London, 1801), vol. II, p. 118. Moses Griffith: born *c*.1724, at Lapidon, Salop; sizar at St John's College, Cambridge, 1742; MD Leyden, 1744 (thesis on abortion); LRCP London, 1747; of Mincing Lane, 1752; physician and man-midwife extraordinary to the City of London Lying-in Hospital, and also a governor there, 1752, 1753, 1767; retired to Colchester, 1768; published a book on fevers and haemorrhages, 1775; died at Colchester, probably March 1785. See *DNB*; Munk, *Roll*; Wallis, *Medics*; Innes Smith, *Students at Leyden*; and lists of officers in the 1752, 1753, and 1767 *Accounts* of the City of London Lying-in Hospital.
33. Samuel Wathen: born before 1730; of Devonshire Square, 1752; man-midwife-in-ordinary to the City of London Lying-in Hospital, 1752 (when a Mrs Elizabeth Wathen was a governor there); MD Aberdeen 1752; voluntarily disfranchized from Company of Surgeons 6 December 1753; book-subscriptions 1755–58; translated Boerhaave's lectures, 1765; man-midwife extraordinary to the City of London Lying-in Hospital, 1767; died at Dorking, Surrey, 1787. See Munk, *Roll*; Wallis, *Medics*; Brock, *William Hunter*, p. 35; *Critical Review* (1765), vol. 19, p. 51, and vol. 20, p. 466; and lists of officers in the 1752, 1753, and 1767 *Accounts* of the City of London Lying-in Hospital.
34. Jonathan Wathen: born probably after 1724; book-subscription 1755; dedicatee of Thomas Cogan's Leyden thesis, 1767; of Bartholomew Lane, 1769; subscriber to the Lying-In Charity, 1769; surgical mastership in 1780. See Wallis, *Medics*; Denman, *Midwifery*, vol. II, pp. 118–19; *Account of the Lying-in Charity* (1769), p. 51; *DNB*, entry for Thomas Cogan (for whom see *n*.39 to Ch. 10).
35. Donnison, Note on . . . Queen Charlotte's Hospital, pp. 398–400, at p. 399; *Account of the rise, progress, and state of the General Lying-in Hospital* (1768); *n*.20 to Ch. 2 above.
36. Rhodes, *Doctor John Leake's Hospital*, p. 49.
37. *Ibid.*, pp. 30–31. On Cogan see *n*.39 to Ch. 10.
38. There is possibly a parallel, and perhaps there was even a connection, between Leake's three-bladed forceps and the earlier instrument of Middleton Walker. Walker contrived a forceps with some asymmetry; this was perhaps a lock, perhaps a difference between the blades (see *n*.32 to Ch. 5). If the latter was the case, then it is intriguing that Walker was based in Southwark, and that Leake a generation later created his hospital in adjacent Lambeth. However, Leake himself lived across the river: in 1770 in Craven Street, at his death in 1792 in Parliament Street. See J. B. de Mainaduc, *The lectures of J. B. de Mainaduc* (1798), preface (I thank Patricia Fara and Reeve Parker for this) and Rhodes, *Doctor John Leake's hospital*, p. 45.
39. Candidates and political identifications from Sedgwick, *History of Parliament*. Whig candidates: Middlesex (poll held 2 July): Sir Hugh Smithson and Sir William Beauchamp Proctor, two of the four vice-presidents of the Middlesex Hospital; when the Brownlow Street Lying-in Hospital split off in 1749, both remained with the Middlesex, Smithson (now Earl of Northumberland) becoming president (replacing the defecting Earl of Portland). Westminster (1 July): Viscount Trentham and Sir Peter Warren, the other two vice-presidents of the Middlesex Hospital, also remaining with the Middlesex after the 1749 split. City of London (10 July): Sir William Calvert and Sir John Barnard, both governors of the Brownlow Street Lying-in Hospital by 1756; Slingsby Bethell and Stephen T. Janssen, both founding governors of the City of London Lying-in Hospital (Bethell as

President).
40. Tory candidates: Middlesex: George Cooke (a governor of the Brownlow Street Lying-in Hospital by 1756); Sir Roger Newdigate (no association with any lying-in hospital in the 1750s; however by 1768 a governor of the General Lying-in Hospital, n.45 below). Westminster: Sir Thomas Clarges and Sir Thomas Dyke (neither had any association with any lying-in hospital). City of London (only two Tory candidates): Sir Robert Ladbroke (a governor of the Brownlow Street Lying-in Hospital by 1756); Sir Daniel Lambert (no association with any lying-in hospital).
41. The odds against this being a chance association are 65 to 1.
42. L. Sutherland, "The City of London in eighteenth-century politics", in *Essays presented to Sir Lewis Namier,* R. Pares & A. J. P. Taylor (eds) (London: Macmillan, 1956), pp. 49–74; D. Marshall, *Dr Johnson's London* (London: Wiley, 1968), pp. 77–99, esp. pp. 95–9; N. Rogers, "Resistance to oligarchy: the City opposition to Walpole and his successors, 1725–47", in *London in the age of reform,* J. Stevenson (ed.) (Oxford: Blackwell, 1977), pp. 1–29.
43. For Hodges see L. Colley, *In defiance of oligarchy: the Tory party 1714–60* (Cambridge: Cambridge University Press, 1982), p. 280. Doughty's sermon *Christian sympathy* (London, 1752) referred favourably to works by the Tory divines of an earlier generation Bishop Smalridge (p. 12) and Jeremy Collier (pp. 6 and *passim*). For Church see DNB.
44. For Tory views see R. K. McClure, *Coram's children: the London Foundling Hospital in the eighteenth century* (New Haven, Conn.: Yale University Press, 1981), pp. 106–9. The 1768 appeal was *Account of the rise, progress, and state of the General Lying-in Hospital* (1768); details which follow are taken from this.
45. Military Whigs included the Dukes of Kingston and Marlborough, the Earl of Northampton, Lord Clive, and Admiral Keppel. Known Tories included the Earl of Bute, Sir Watkin Williams Wynn, John Morton Esq., and Sir Roger Newdigate. For political identities see A. C. Valentine, *The British establishment 1760–84: an eighteenth-century biographical dictionary* (2 volumes, Norman, Oklahoma: University of Oklahoma Press, 1970).
46. Cobden, *The parable of the talents,* p. 16. For Cobden see DNB.
47. E. Cobden, *Poems on several occasions* (London, 1748), pp. 160–63; see my The politics of medical improvement, pp. 29–33.
48. Cobden, *Poems,* pp. 139–44 (quoted below from p. 143), 145–8.
49. The only other known men-midwives "W——" who would fit the metre are the Wathens, Samuel and Jonathan, both probably of a later generation (see n.33 & 34 above) and certainly not known names for allusion in 1735. "C——" might be Matthew Carter of Dublin, or the Mr Clayton referred to by James Houstoun as training at the Hôtel-Dieu in 1714 but otherwise unknown; but these are unlikely on grounds of location and obscurity respectively. For these see S. A. Brody, "The life and times of Sir Fielding Ould: man-midwife and master physician", *Bulletin of the History of Medicine* 52 (1978), pp. 228–50, at pp. 232, 238, and n.37 to Ch. 6.
50. M. C. Versluysen, "Midwives, medical men, and 'poor women labouring with child': lying-in hospitals in eighteenth century London", in *Women, health and reproduction,* H. Roberts (ed.) (London: Routledge, 1981), pp. 18–49.
51. The lying-in ward was opened in July, 1747; 16 women had been delivered by March 1749. In 1760–61 137 women were delivered. See *Account of the Middlesex-Hospital,* appended to Cobden, *The parable of the talents, passim,* and *Account of the Middlesex-Hospital . . . 1761,* pp. 2, 8.

Part IV
The man as midwife

Chapter Twelve
The varieties of man-midwifery

Recapitulation: new practices, old forms

By the mid-1740s, male medical involvement in childbirth had advanced a vast distance within a single generation – from surgery to man-midwifery, from extracting a dead child to delivering a living baby. Its techniques, its tasks and its knowledge had all been transformed. At the accession of George I, very few English practitioners could deliver a living child in obstructed births by the head – the commonest source of obstetric difficulty. By the 1740s the midwifery forceps had been published and hundreds of young men were learning how to use it; Deventer's methods and the fillet were well known; and the vectis, although still secret and probably in the hands of only John Bamber and Starkey Middleton, was on the eve of passing to a wider circle. Correspondingly, men were now called much more swiftly to difficult births. Emergency calls were being made after hours rather than days, and the man was now expected to save the lives of both mother and child; onset calls with a midwife had become increasingly common. Public knowledge in midwifery had also expanded to an unprecedented degree. Hitherto, practical techniques, together with understanding of the bodily processes of birth, had been enclosed within the private realm of craft skill. Now this practical and theoretical knowledge was rapidly moving into the public domain, through systematic, specialized teaching and a new wealth of publications.

Yet the new practices were contained within the old forms: man-midwifery had not begun to displace the female midwife. Normal delivery was still managed by midwives within the framework of the traditional childbirth ritual. The "paths" to childbirth of the men-midwives were no different from those of their predecessors the obstetric surgeons. Forceps practitioners received emergency calls, followers of Deventer received onset calls (or advance calls) with a midwife, vectis practitioners were apparently called in both these ways. Such men also received an occasional onset or advance call in lieu of a midwife, but so had their predecessors a century earlier.[1] For all their criticisms of female midwives, men-midwives had no ambition to replace them: the midwife's management of normal birth was still assumed both by forceps practitioners and by Deventerians, and was subsequently enshrined in the lying-in hospitals. Even John Douglas, so hostile to the encroachments of "midmen", did not suggest in his polemic of 1736 that men were taking over normal birth from midwives, nor did other commentators writing in the 1740s.[2] Moreover, the obstetric divisions of the late 1740s were much the same as those of the previous generation. Just as Manningham's short-lived Lying-in Infirmary of 1739 had been a Whig and anti-forceps initiative, so too this was largely true of the more successful lying-in hospitals created a decade later. Just as John Bamber had kept the vectis secret and avoided public controversy since the 1720s, so his numerous heirs in the City would maintain the same low profile until the 1780s. And just as Giffard, the Westminster forceps practitioner of the late 1720s, had used case-histories to embody his obstetric arguments, so too Smellie, his successor in the 1740s, published two volumes of such histories. The one major exception to this story of continuity is the fact that Smellie was a Whig, whereas the forceps practitioners of the previous generation had been Tories. Yet this very exception doubly confirmed the rule – both in that Smellie had gone through a phase of rejecting the forceps, and in that he was a "Country" Whig, not a Court Whig. And while Smellie's synthesis transcended the division between Deventer and the forceps, it also embodied these very resources of the previous generation.

The persistence of the old social forms until mid-century was manifested in practical obstetric doctrines over the management of the placenta, of twin births, and of malpresentations. Today the delivery of the *placenta* is regarded as a natural process, accomplished by the uterus and constituting the "third stage of labour". And some early-modern midwives (though not all) took the same view, leaving the delivery of the placenta to Nature.[3] But the *men*-midwives of the early eighteenth century saw matters quite otherwise: almost without exception, they believed that the placenta should be removed manually, either by pulling on the umbilical cord or by putting the hand all the way into the uterus and taking hold of the placenta itself.[4] The reason for their concern to remove the placenta was that from time to time, they found themselves called to do precisely this job: that is, they received emergency calls either because the placenta had not been delivered, or for bleeding after labour that turned out to result from the retention of part of the placenta. Manual removal of the placenta, they believed, would eliminate this potential problem. By implementing this policy they made it self-confirming: an experience that arose from emergencies was transferred, as prophylactic advice, to normal labour. This package of experiences and precepts had been characteristic of male surgeons since the sixteenth century.[5] And we find it unchanged among eighteenth-century male practitioners until about 1750.[6] In this respect the men-midwives had similar experiences to the earlier obstetric surgeons, and drew the same conclusion.

The management of *twin* births seems to have produced a similar, and sharper, disagreement between midwives and male practitioners. Most midwives believed that the delivery of the second twin should be left to nature; but male practitioners thought that as soon as the first twin was delivered, the second should be extracted at once by the feet. In fact, within their very different spheres of practice, both were correct.[7] If the first twin was delivered spontaneously, then the powers of the uterus would usually complete the delivery of the second twin; this was what midwives saw and knew. But if the delivery of the first twin had been difficult, it was likely that the second twin would also come slowly, if at all – not least because the protracted initial labour had exhausted the mother. And it was the difficult births that the male practitioners usually encountered.[8] Just as with the delivery of the placenta, this doctrine was self-confirming.

Malpresentations posed the choice between turning the child to the head (cephalic version) and turning to the feet (podalic version). As described in the surviving texts of the ancients (chiefly Soranus), both of these were passive practices: after turning, the delivery was left to Nature. But Ambroise Paré had introduced the technique of podalic version *with traction*, which brought about an asymmetry: turning to the *feet* now permitted active delivery, without depending on the natural powers, and this was how podalic version was practised throughout our period.[9] From the mid-seventeenth century onwards, most male practitioners strenuously advocated podalic version and dismissed cephalic version as impracticable. Men such as Mauriceau, Willughby, Cooke, Deventer, La Motte and Heister, who differed on many other matters, were of one mind over this issue.[10] Thus the historian is tempted to dismiss cephalic version as a useless technique, particularly when one of the two main contrary voices (Sir Richard Manningham) gave no illustrative case-histories, while the other (Henry Bracken) delivered only a few births each year.[11] Yet it is abundantly clear that cephalic version could work just as well as podalic version, *provided that it was carried out early in the labour.*[12] But in our period cephalic version was difficult to employ because, as Smellie explained with unusual candour, "the cases in which we are most commonly called are after the membranes have been broken, the waters discharged, and the uterus strongly contracted around the body of the child".[13]

That is, the preference of most male practitioners for podalic version resulted from the dominance of emergency calls in their practical experience. (The exception of Manningham confirms the rule, as he probably experienced onset calls with a midwife, giving him much earlier access to such cases.[14]) This doctrine, too, was self-confirming: the more podalic version was practised and seen to work, the greater the vehemence with which cephalic version was rejected.[15]

Thus despite its technical advances, the man-midwifery of the 1740s was contained within the same social forms – the "paths" to childbirth – that had obtained in the earlier era dominated by craniotomy. Even though male practitioners were now called much more quickly, their province was still the delivery of *difficult* births. And although the threshold of difficulty had fallen considerably, the threshold itself remained firmly in place.

Man-midwifery transformed

Yet within the next few years – starting in about 1748 and clearly visible from 1751 – there emerged a man-midwifery of a very different kind: booked onset calls (and among the very wealthy advance calls), *in lieu of a midwife*. Such calls had been experienced by male practitioners before this – for instance by Willughby in the 1660s, by Henry Bracken around 1730, by Smellie in the early 1740s – but they had been very rare, and there was no sign that they were increasing.[16] But in the late 1740s and the 1750s this form of practice suddenly became common in several different places: in London, where it particularly impinged on Smellie; at Chelmsford, Essex, in the practice of Benjamin Pugh; at Wells in Somerset, Pontefract in Yorkshire, and probably also in parts of Lancashire and Cheshire.[17] During the next two decades it became clear that this was a permanent and irreversible shift: the midwife's hegemony had been decisively fractured.[18]

Smellie was beginning to be called in this way in 1748. Even now, this form of practice was at first associated with expected difficulty: thus in 1748 he was "bespoke" eight times "to attend women in their first children by their friends, who were apprehensive that they would have difficult or dangerous labours, because they were distorted in their backs". But the threshold of difficulty had plummeted, for in the event six of these mothers "had easy natural labours".[19] And whereas previously Smellie had been called to such cases as an adjunct to the midwife, he was now being given sole responsibility for the delivery. As a result, he accumulated far more experience of normal birth than ever before. Hence the fact that most of the cases in his "Collection" of "Natural Labours" dated from 1748 and after.[20] Hence, too, his renewed ambivalence towards the forceps at this time, and his associated concern "to make them appear less terrible to women": the forceps were "terrible" in the new form of practice, centred on normal birth, whereas they had been life-saving in the context of emergency work.[21] And hence his concern when writing his *Treatise*, in 1751, "to inform young practitioners that difficult cases do not frequently occur", and his consequently conservative estimates of the incidence of difficult births.[22] Ironically, just when he was publishing his synthesis of the resources of the previous generation, Smellie was being caught up in the new form of practice.

But the change at mid-century was obscured by a continuity of terminology. Most observers used the same word, "man-midwife", to describe two very different kinds of practice: the old form that supplemented the midwife, and the new one displacing her. Thus practitioner labels are a poor guide to underlying actions. The major change in *terminology*, from "surgeon" to "man-midwife", took place around 1720. So too at that time some medical men coined new names for the male practitioner of midwifery, i.e. "midman" (Edward Baynard in 1715) and "andro-boethogynist" (John Maubray in 1724).[23] Although those terms were not taken up – save by John Douglas, who argued strongly for "midman" in his polemic of 1736 – their emergence was symptomatic: both "man-midwife" and its ephemeral alternatives reflected the new expectation that the male practitioner would deliver a living child. But that shift, momentous though it was, involved no change in "paths" to childbirth. In contrast the momentous change in *path* a generation later, when the man-midwife replaced the midwife, went almost unmarked at the level of terminology (with the singular and important exception of William Hunter, as we shall later see). This confusing state of affairs is summarized in Table 12.1.

Table 12.1 The varieties of man-midwifery: terminology and schematic periodization.

Period	Type of call	Task: to deliver the child	Practitioner-label
pre *c.*1720	emergency	...dead	surgeon
	advance/onset *with* midwife	...dead	surgeon
*c.*1720–50	emergency	...alive	man-midwife
	advance/onset *with* midwife	...alive	man-midwife
post *c.*1750	advance/onset *in lieu of* midwife	...alive	man-midwife

Notes: (1) Most onset calls were probably *booked* in all three phases. (2) The changes around 1720 and 1750 *supplemented* the previous patterns rather than replacing them completely: calls of the older types persisted for many decades thereafter. Both changes, but especially that around 1750, were most marked and occurred first among wealthier mothers.

If practitioner labels confuse the issue, so too do the three London lying-in hospitals created in a sudden rush between 1749 and 1752. For it just so happened that those hospitals were founded at the same moment that the new form of man-midwifery was emerging, yet this was merely coincidence. It is true that in the tiny lying-in ward at the Middlesex Hospital, normal births were delivered by the man-midwife from 1748 until about 1755, and moreover that this ward was the starting-point of the whole London lying-in hospital movement. Yet while this radical practice at the Middlesex doubtless reflected the wider change taking place at this time, the lying-in hospitals themselves neither promoted nor reflected that change. One signal of this is the fact that male practice in lieu of a midwife emerged around 1750 in many different places, whereas the lying-in hospitals were located solely in London. Another is that the new man-midwifery arose from the choices of women (as we shall see in the following chapters), whereas the lying-in hospitals were created by men. Moreover, in some respects those hospitals were backward-looking. Their procedures reproduced the old forms, since they all employed a midwife to deliver normal births; and as far as can be ascertained, most of their men-midwives used existing techniques.[24]

The mid-century shift to calls in lieu of a midwife, although masked by terminology and complicated in London by the lying-in hospitals, was manifested in several ways. Hitherto medical men had accepted without question the traditional childbirth ritual, taking for granted such practices as the hot and darkened room, the use of caudle, the presence of gossips, the swaddling of the child. But now they began to criticize these traditional practices of women – starting with William Cadogan's *Essay upon nursing* of 1748, and culminating with Charles White's *Treatise on the management of pregnant and lying-in women* (1772).[25] It was precisely because the midwife's hegemony had been fractured that such a critique of female practices had become thinkable. Simultaneously, the new form of man-midwifery was reflected in literature: by 1755 Christopher Smart could depict a man-midwife as sole deliverer, in a widely reprinted epilogue to a stage production at Covent Garden.[26] And from mid-century there appeared a new kind of obstetric controversy. In the previous generation, public contests over midwifery had been between practitioners of different allegiances, sometimes female (Sarah Stone), mostly male, each promoting their own practice and attacking their rivals: even the pro-midwife intervention of John Douglas in 1736 had conformed to this pattern.[27] But now, after 1750, came critiques of the social role of the man-midwife – beginning with the campaign waged by Frank Nicholls in 1751–52.

Nicholls attacked not only the new man-midwifery, but also a particular group of men-midwives headed by Dr Robert Nesbit; and he castigated the College of Physicians for its failure to take action against these men.[28] He conducted this struggle both within the College and in anonymous printed satires (of which his authorship was immediately recognized), such as *The petition of the unborn babes to the Censors of the College of Physicians of London*. His final blow (March 1752) was a long letter to the College, proposing that it should provide lecture courses for midwives to improve their knowledge and skill, in order to restore childbirth to women practitioners; remarkably, Nicholls offered £1000 to endow such lectures.[29] Although he had supporters both inside and outside the College, his proposal came to nothing: the College formally rejected it in June 1752, upon which his campaign lapsed.[30] At first sight Nicholls's hostility to man-midwifery in 1751–52 seems paradoxical and inexplicable. He had taught anatomy to two of the leading men-midwives, Hunter and Smellie.[31] The practical methods he criticized – craniotomy and turning to the feet – were entirely traditional, as he well knew: he had included them in his own medical teaching at Oxford almost 20 years earlier, and he had never objected to Deventerian man-midwifery, which used these very techniques.[32] Nor was his onslaught precipitated by the vectis, used by his adversary Nesbit, for he was unaware of that instrument. And unlike John Douglas 15 years earlier, Nicholls was not moved by professional rivalry, for he did not himself practise midwifery.[33] It seems that he had a personal grievance both against Nesbit and, since January 1749, against the College, but at most this explains part of his target, and cannot account for his wider argument.[34] Finally, while the new lying-in hospitals received passing criticism in one of his satires, making it clear that he associated them with man-midwifery, these institutions were not his main target.[35] In short, Nicholls's arguments against man-midwifery have to be approached on their own terms.

The offence of the men-midwives, in Nicholls's eyes, was twofold. They were displacing midwives, "to the manifest violation of modesty and the scandal of all good people". And in this usurped role, they were killing children:

> And whereas men-midwives in order to give themselves the credit of quickness and despatch in the execution of their office frequently force the delivery without any necessity, either by using instruments or by turning the child, by which sudden violence the child is frequently killed and the mother . . . damaged . . . and oftentimes upon the least apprehension of difficulty (however insufficiently founded) they avowedly and professedly kill the children either by cutting off their limbs or by opening their heads and squeezing out their brains . . .[36]

This charge was almost certainly unfair. No doubt there were *some* cases in which men-midwives were killing living children — but there was nothing new about that. Rather, what was new was the social role of the man-midwife: instead of complementing the midwife, the male practitioner was now acting in her stead. This was why the men-midwives of 1751 provoked Nicholls's hostility, whereas their predecessors of the 1730s and '40s had elicited no such response from him. *The technical art of killing unborn children had become heinous because it could now be practised in a new context.* Under the old social arrangements, the presence of the midwife had acted as a barrier against craniotomy. Under the new arrangements, no such barrier existed. Nicholls apparently believed that men-midwives were carrying into primary midwifery, and applying to normal births, the same suite of techniques they had previously used for difficult births (whether in emergency calls, or in onset calls with a midwife). Nicholls had no objection to male practitioners helping in cases of difficulty: hence his inclusion of obstetric themes in his own teaching to male students, his silence during the controversies of the 1730s, and his friendship with Smellie and Hunter in the 1740s. But for a male practitioner to displace the midwife was a double crime, for it violated "modesty", and he believed that it transposed methods appropriate for difficult births into the realm of normal deliveries.

Nicholls's campaign has been portrayed as eccentric;[37] in fact, it was precocious. He was the first observer to notice the new form of man-midwifery, and the accuracy of his perception was confirmed by the subsequent contrasting attacks of Elizabeth Nihell (1760) and Philip Thicknesse (1763–64).[38] But while these critics were correct in recognizing that man-midwifery had taken a new form, their polemical depictions of its methods were wide of the mark. For they all described man-midwifery as interventionist and dominated by instruments; yet in fact, as we shall see in the next chapter, the new form of practice was pulling men-midwives in the opposite direction — towards reliance on the natural powers — for delivering births by the head. And a corresponding shift is apparent in other aspects of practical obstetrics. Now, as they accumulated experience of normal birth, male practitioners began to see for themselves what midwives had long known — that both the placenta and the second twin would be delivered spontaneously – and they altered their practices accordingly. After about 1750 the delivery of the placenta was increasingly left to the natural powers; Smellie's views moved markedly in this direction between 1751 and 1754, and this was symptomatic of a wider shift.[39] The same is true of the delivery of twins.[40] And Smellie even began to experiment with cephalic version for malpresentations. Remarkably enough, he began to alter his methods in this way as early as 1751, at the very time when he was endorsing *podalic* version in the first volume of his *Treatise*.[41] Indeed, it was probably this very contradiction which led Smellie to be so frank at this time in his rationale for podalic version. As we saw above, he argued that turning to the feet was preferable because male practitioners were usually called "after the membranes have been broken [and] the waters discharged". Such insight was unusual: male practitioners usually justified their practical obstetric preferences without reference to the underlying social processes. But Smellie's recent increasing exposure to normal births, presenting a sharp contrast with his previous experience over almost 30 years, had doubtless made him peculiarly aware of the social contingency of his obstetric experiences.[42]

Although some places experienced the watershed around 1750, this was not true everywhere; and as a result we find at this time men-midwives of both the old type and the new. This diversity is nicely illustrated by two provincial men who published on midwifery in the early 1750s – John Burton of York, a prominent Tory later satirized as "Doctor Slop" in Sterne's *Tristram Shandy*, and Benjamin Pugh of Chelmsford.[43] They were near-contemporaries – Burton had started practice around 1733, Pugh around 1739 – and their careers showed several parallels.[44] Both began as emergency practitioners, initially performing craniotomies and then using the forceps.[45] Both were mechanically ingenious, inventing variant surgical and obstetric instruments of their own, and both had wider cultural interests: Burton was a noted antiquary, Pugh later published travel works.[46] In midwifery they both transcended the London division of obstetric allegiances (as had their provincial predecessors in the 1730s), for each combined the use of the forceps with some resort to Deventer: Burton largely supported Deventerian theory, while Pugh opposed that theory yet made some use of Deventer's manoeuvre.[47] Yet despite these various similarities between the two men, their midwifery practice in the early 1750s took very different forms. Burton resembled men of the previous generation: on his account, a "man-midwife" delivered *difficult* births, and it seems that he was still only practising as an adjunct to the midwife in 1753 (in contrast with his colleagues at nearby Pontefract).[48] But Pugh was already receiving many calls in lieu of a midwife, and by 1754 he had delivered over 2000 women.[49] Given that he had started around 1739 as an emergency practitioner, his practice must have been transformed in the interim. He may perhaps have experienced that transformation in the early 1740s, several years before any other known man-midwife in the kingdom. But the shift probably occurred around 1748, in line with the experience of other individuals – in which case, Pugh must have been delivering about 300 births a year between then and 1754. Whatever the precise chronology, by about 1750 Pugh must have been the practitioner of first resort for the whole population of Chelmsford and the surrounding area.[50]

It is hardly surprising that the timing of the change varied in this way, as we have repeatedly encountered local variation at earlier stages of our story. No doubt the process of transition had different inflections in each of the major towns such as Birmingham, Bristol, Exeter, Liverpool, Manchester, Newcastle and Norwich.[51-56] Yet the overall result is not in doubt: by the 1770s men had taken over the most lucrative sphere of practice – the deliveries of wealthy mothers – throughout the kingdom. To follow this process in its local manifestations is beyond my present scope; the remaining chapters will focus chiefly on the London manifestations of the new man-midwifery. I shall first examine the teachings of its chief exemplar, William Hunter, and then suggest an explanation for the emergence of "the man as midwife".

Notes

1. See Ch. 4.
2. Ch. 8 above (John Douglas); *The state of physic* (London, 1742); Thomas Dover, *The ancient physician's legacy to his country* (London, 1742), pp. 213–19.
3. Willughby, *Observations*, pp. 11, 66, 117–18; Giffard, *Cases*, Cases 84, 207, 151; E. Chapman, *A reply to Mr Douglas's short account of the state of midwifery in London and Westminster* (London, 1737), pp. 30–32, 40. But for midwives delivering the placenta, see Willughby, *Observations*, pp. 170–71, 178, 184–5; Giffard, *Cases*, Cases 176 and possibly 53.
4. The sole exception was Fielding Ould: see E. Shorter, "The management of normal deliveries and the generation of William Hunter", in *William Hunter*, Bynum & Porter (eds), pp. 371–83, at pp. 377–8.
5. See E. Jones, "The life and times of Gulielmus Fabricius Hildanus (1560–1634)", *Medical History* 4 (1960), pp. 112–34, 196–209, at p. 200; N. Culpeper, *A directory for midwives* (London, 1651), p. 176; Willughby, *Observations*, pp. 26–7, 115–19, 236–7; Cooke, *Mellificium chirurgiae* (1685 edn), p. 171; William Cowper, *The anatomy of humane bodies* (1698), Table 54.
6. Giffard, *Cases*, Cases 84, 87 (with discussion), 100, 111, 150, 163, 180 (with rationale); John Douglas, *A short account of the state of midwifery in London, Westminster, &c.* (London, 1736), pp. 49, 72; Chapman, *Reply to Mr Douglas's short account*, pp. 30–32, 40; Sir Richard Manningham, *An abstract of midwifery for use in the Lying-In Infirmary* (London, 1744), pp. 6, 10, 20, 26; B. Pugh, *A treatise of midwifery, chiefly with regard to the operation. With several improvements in that art* (London, 1754), pp. 29–30.
7. Willughby, *Observations*, p. 45. Sarah Stone resembled male practitioners in believing that the second twin should be fetched immediately: *Complete practice*, p. 65; cf. Ch. 4.
8. Chapman, *Reply to Mr Douglas's short account*, p. 40; Giffard, *Cases*, Cases 86, 147, 220–21; F. Ould, *A treatise of midwifery. In three parts* (Dublin, 1742), p. 55. Manningham mentioned twins as a possible cause of difficulty (*Abstract of midwifery*, p. 15), but did not give directions on the management of twin births.
9. See Ch. 2 and E. Ingerslev, Rösslin's *Rosegarten*: its relation to the past (the Muscio manu-

scripts and Soranos, particularly with regard to podalic version, *Journal of Obstetrics and Gynaecology of the British Empire* 15 (1909), pp. 1–25, 73–92.

10. An exception was Robert Barret, *A companion for midwives, childbearing women, and nurses* (London, 1699), who practised turning to the feet in some cases (pp. 26–7, 32), turning to the head in others (p. 30, 32). Neither he nor Henry Bracken (below) exerted any influence over subsequent male writers. See Willughby, *Observations*, p. 120; Cooke, *Mellificium chirurgiae*, 1685 edn, p. 166; Radcliffe, *Milestones*, p. 25 (Mauriceau); Ch. 6 above (Deventer); La Motte, *Midwifery, passim*; L. von Heister ("Laurence Heister"), *A general system of surgery in three parts* (trans. anon., London, 1743), pp. 211–12 (slightly qualified, p. 217).

11. See H. Bracken, *The midwife's companion, or, a treatise of midwifery; wherein the whole art is explained* (London, 1737), pp. 127, 151, 134, 150, 164–7, 170–72. For Manningham see below.

12. Galabin, *Manual of midwifery*, pp. 694–5.

13. McClintock, *Smellie's midwifery*, vol. I, p. 343 (and cf. p. 344). For other rationales, for and against turning to the feet, see Giffard, *Cases*, Case 73, p. 170; Bracken, *The midwife's companion*, pp. 171–2.

14. See Ch. 6. Manningham wrote that if "the infant is situated a-cross", then "just after the breaking of the waters, the head is to be sought for and brought into the passage, if easy to be done, otherwise the child must be drawn out by its feet" (*Abstract of midwifery*, p. 17). This implies an early call, since the foetus has not yet descended and the waters have only just broken.

15. However, support for cephalic version could be combined with traditional views over the placenta (Manningham, above), and support for podalic version could be combined with anti-interventionism for the placenta and twins (William Hunter, below and Ch. 13).

16. McClintock, *Smellie's midwifery*, vol. II, Case 236 (1743); Ch. 4 above.

17. For Chelmsford, see below; for Wells, I. Loudon, *Death in childbirth: an international study of maternal care and maternal mortality 1800–1950* (Oxford: Clarendon Press, 1992), p. 169 n.11; for Pontefract, A. J. Vickery, *Women of the local elite in Lancashire, 1750–1825* (PhD thesis, University of London, 1991), p. 147 (I thank Dr Vickery for a copy of this chapter of her thesis); for Lancashire and Cheshire, David Harley, "Provincial midwives in England: Lancashire and Cheshire, 1660–1760", in Marland, *Art of midwifery*, pp. 27–48, at pp. 39–41.

18. Donnison, *Midwives*, Ch. 2.

19. McClintock, *Smellie's midwifery*, vol. II, p. 10.

20. *Ibid.*, Collection No. XIV, Cases 100–112.

21. Ch. 9 above.

22. McClintock, *Smellie's midwifery*, vol. I, p. 197; Ch. 2 above.

23. See Ch. 8 above.

24. See Ch. 11 above.

25. See Ch. 15 below.

26. Admittedly, this was for the benefit of the Middlesex Hospital, which had, uniquely, been using male practitioners in lieu of a midwife (Ch. 11). See Charles Ryskamp, "Christopher Smart and the Earl of Northumberland", in *The Augustan milieu: essays presented to Louis A. Landa*, H. K. Miller et al. (eds) (Oxford: Clarendon, 1970), pp. 321–32, at pp. 324–5. I thank Simon Schaffer for this reference.

27. See Ch. 8 above.

28. For Frank Nicholls see *DNB*; Munk, *Roll*; G. C. Boase & W. P. Courtney, *Bibliotheca*

cornubiensis (3 volumes; London: Longman, 1874–82), vol. I, pp. 387–8, and references there cited.
29. Royal College of Physicians, Annals, 23 March 1752. For titles of his satires see *n.*9 to Ch. 10 above.
30. *Ibid.*, 13 April and 25 June 1752. Nicholls was allied in different ways with Richard Mead, Thomas Lawrence, Isaac Schomberg, the *Gentleman's Magazine*, and the Court midwife Mrs Kennon. See Clark, *College of Physicians*, vol. II, p. 503; T. Lawrence, *Franci Nicholsii vita* (London, 1780); Ch. 10 above; *Gentleman's Magazine*, March, 1752; P. Thicknesse, *Man-midwifery analyzed* (London, 1765), p. 33.
31. Brock, *William Hunter*, p. 3; McClintock, *Smellie's midwifery*, vol. III, p. 108.
32. Frank Nicholls, *Compendium anatomico-oeconomicum ea omnia complectens, quae ad cognitam humani corporis oeconomicum spectant* (London, 1733), 5th edn (1746), Appendix, pp. 15–16.
33. For John Douglas, see Ch. 8.
34. See Clark, *College of Physicians*, vol. II, p. 503. Curiously, Nicholls and his protégé Thomas Lawrence had attended together with Nesbit and his fellow vectis practitioner Starkey Middleton at a post-mortem conducted by Middleton in Guy's Hospital on 15 October 1747. The deceased women had been a patient of Bamber's whom he passed on to Middleton in 1735. See *Philosophical Transactions of the Royal Society*, No. 484 (1747), pp. 617–21, at p. 620, and cf. Ch. 10 above.
35. *Petition*, pp. 8–9.
36. Royal College of Physicians, Annals, 23 March 1752.
37. Clark, *College of Physicians*, vol. II, pp. 503–5.
38. See Ch. 15.
39. Compare McClintock, *Smellie's midwifery*, vol. I, pp. 230–36, esp. p. 235, with vol. II, pp. 285–9 (Case 218, from 1752, and autobiographical reflections); and see vol. II, p. 252, where Smellie recorded Hunter's assistance in this. See also Hunter, lectures, pp. 95, 99f, 139f, 151–5; Shorter, The management of normal deliveries. For a later example of the new, more conservative approach see W. Perfect, *Cases in midwifery, with references, quotations, and remarks* (2 volumes; Rochester, n.d. & 1783), vol. I, pp. 93–4.
40. See McClintock, *Smellie's midwifery*, vol. I, pp. 354–8; vol. III, pp. 202–13 (Cases 411–420); Hunter, lectures, pp. 136–40 (cf. *n.*18 to Ch. 13 below). In vol. I, written in 1751, Smellie's position was a compromise: he advocated leaving the second twin to Nature only "if the pelvis is narrow, the woman strong, and the head presents" (pp. 356–7) – that is, when turning would be both difficult (from the narrow pelvis) and unnecessary. When he came to compile vol. III, only completed around 1763, he included seven twin cases of his own; only one of these came from before 1748 (Case 415, vol. III, p. 207), probably because Smellie had been intervening more in the early and mid-1740s than he now believed was appropriate.
41. Compare *ibid.*, vol. I, pp. 341–5, esp. pp. 343–4, with vol. II, pp. 196–8 (Cases 138 & 139, from 1751 & 1752). In this respect William Hunter's views (as expressed in his lectures of the 1760s) were anomalous, in that he was dogmatically opposed to cephalic version. See Hunter, lectures, pp. 126, 130–35, and *n.*22 to Ch. 13.
42. It was perhaps also for this reason that in 1750 Smellie began to be critical of the practice of stretching the labiae (although he still used it sometimes). See McClintock, *Smellie's midwifery*, Cases 226, 265; cf. Cases 230, 231, 235, 236, 246, 257, 264, 266, 269, 270, 271, 273, and Ch. 3 above.
43. J. Burton, *An essay towards a complete new system of midwifery, theoretical and practical*

(London, 1751); *idem*, *A letter to William Smellie, MD, containing critical and practical remarks upon his treatise* (London, 1753); Pugh, *Treatise of midwifery*. On Burton, Sterne and Tristram Shandy, see A. H. Cash, "The birth of Tristram Shandy: Sterne and Dr Burton", in *Studies in the eighteenth century*, R. F. Brissenden (ed.) (Canberra: Australian National University Press, 1968), pp. 133–54.

44. Burton graduated MD in 1733, and invented his "terebra occulta" before 1734; Pugh in 1754 had been practising for over 14 years. See Innes Smith, *Students at Leyden*; Burton, *Essay*, p. 221; Pugh, *Treatise of midwifery*, p. iv.

45. Burton, *Essay*, p. 221; Pugh, *Treatise of midwifery*, p. 54.

46. For Pugh's innovations in the design of the forceps see Radcliffe, *Milestones* and *The secret instrument*; his instrument-maker was Mr Stanton of Lombard Street, London (*Treatise of midwifery*, p. 152). Pugh's travel works appeared *c*.1770; in 1785 he translated a French treatise on mineral waters, adding "remarks on the city of Montpellier" (WIHM, catalogue; BL Catalogue). For Burton's publications, see *DNB*.

47. Burton, *Essay*, pp. viii–ix, 21, 162, 172–84, 200, 225–6 (explicitly or implicitly pro-Deventer), 5–6 (anti-Deventer); *Letter to Smellie*, pp. 32–51 (pro-Deventer). Pugh, *Treatise of midwifery*, pp. 6, 69 (opposition to Deventer), 20 (use of Deventer's manoeuvre, without acknowledgement). On provincial publications of the 1730s see Ch. 8.

48. Burton, *Letter to Smellie*, passim; *Essay*, title-page ("the most dangerous cases"), pp. 162, 181, 194, 196–7 (man-midwife as emergency practitioner), 59, 185 (man-midwife as practising onset calls with a midwife). However, note his interest in the nutrition of the foetus (*Essay*, pp. 28–55, 64ff, 67–75). For Pontefract, see *n*.17 above.

49. Pugh, *Treatise of midwifery*, p. iv.

50. Pugh would amply repay closer study. Note that almost uniquely among British practitioners of midwifery, he used the forceps to dilate the maternal soft passages (*ibid.*, p. 85; cf. *n*.10 to Ch. 5).

51. It was perhaps in Birmingham that a Caesarean section was carried out in 1748 or earlier by "Dr Altree, now of Norfolk Street, late of Wolverhampton": see *Gentleman's Magazine*, 1748, p. 112. This was probably John Altree, apprenticed at Wolverhampton to John Kent in 1716 and a master surgeon there in 1741: see Wallis, *Medics*.

52. Bristol medical practice in general is discussed in M. E. Fissell, *Patients, power and the poor in eighteenth-century Bristol* (Cambridge, 1991). Some earlier Bristol cases are included in Stone, *Complete practice*, pp. 145ff. William Cadogan was practising in Bristol when he wrote his *Essay upon nursing* of 1748, which began the medical critique of women's traditional practices. Bristol is given in Wallis, *Medics* as one of the two addresses (the other being Fareham, Hants.) of George Counsell, whose *The art of midwifery* (London, 1752) was yet another work bridging the forceps/Deventerian divide. Its overall frame was clearly Deventerian, with illustrations of normal and contracted female pelves, support for Deventer's manoeuvre, and insistence that craniotomy is unavoidable in some cases (pp. 57, 73). But there were several casual references to the forceps as one of the instruments of the male practitioner (pp. 79, 95, 142, 147, 150). The book, dedicated to Edward Hody, instructed midwives to summon male practitioners early in difficult cases; in London, this would have been a rather dated injunction by mid-century.

53. In Liverpool in 1757 two men-midwives, Ralph Holt (a former pupil of Henry Bracken) and John Wareing, were conducting a dispute in the local press, while a third, Matthew Turner (a former Smellie pupil) was offering training to midwives; see Harley, "Provincial midwives", pp. 27–48, at p. 41, and *idem*, "Honour and property: the structure of professional disputes in eighteenth-century English medicine", in *The medical enlightenment of*

the eighteenth century, A. Cunningham & R. French (eds) (Cambridge: Cambridge University Press, 1990), pp. 138–64, at p. 148.

54. In Manchester, note Thomas White, who performed a Caesarean section "before 1740" (Young, *Caesarean section,* p. 37) and his more famous son Charles White (cf. Ch. 15).
55. In Newcastle-upon-Tyne, a lying-in charity was established in 1760; and midwifery was being taught to both male and female practitioners by Mr Smith, surgeon, in 1765, and by Mr Francis Humble, surgeon and man-midwife, in 1785. See M. C. Versluysen, "Midwives, medical men, and 'poor women labouring with child': lying-in hospitals in eighteenth century London", in *Women, health and reproduction,* H. Roberts (ed.) (1981), pp. 18–49, at p. 44; *Newcastle Courant,* 6 February 1765; *Newcastle Chronicle,* 19 February 1785. For the latter two references I thank Tom Peck.
56. Thomas Jones of Norwich had published a translation of Mauriceau's *Aphorisms* in 1739; Mrs Phoebe Crewe, a notable midwife, began practice there in the late 1770s (she delivered 9730 children in 40 years, dying in 1817); a Mr Martineau was a man-midwife there in 1780. See Ch. 8 above; Donnison, *Midwives,* p. 60 and p. 212 *n.*82; J. Beresford (ed.), *The diary of a country parson 1758–1802 by James Woodford: passages selected* (Oxford: Oxford University Press, 1978), p. 164.

Chapter Thirteen
William Hunter: the man as midwife

The man as midwife

When William Hunter lectured on midwifery in London in the 1760s, to his own vast profit from the fees of his male students, he gave the male practitioner a new name – neither "surgeon" nor "man-midwife", but *midwife*. This curious terminological twist was not to survive: other practitioners preferred Hunter's alternative designation, the French *"accoucheur"*, which was succeeded in the nineteenth century by the British "obstetrician". But although it was idiosyncratic and ephemeral, Hunter's use of the word "midwife" for the male practitioner was precise. Below is an example of Hunter's usage, taken from notes of his lectures (my emphases):

> A lady was prejudiced from the manner of her *midwife's* entering the room only, that she would not suffer *him* to come near her, and ordered another operator to be sent for. Hence the necessity of being particularly cautious of *our* behaviour as *midwives,* as it not only gains esteem and practice but retains it.[1]

Clearly "midwife" here refers to the male practitioner. (Female midwives Hunter referred to variously as "women practitioners", "woman operators" and, inconsistently, "midwives".[2]) Hunter's unusual terminology reflected the fact that he was receiving *booked onset calls in lieu of a midwife* – the new form of practice that supervened around 1750. Hunter was the most famous and influential of the male practitioners concerned; it was entirely appropriate that it was he who embarked, from around 1750, on the systematic anatomical researches that were to culminate in 1773 with his *Anatomy of the gravid uterus*.[3] The man who entered the womb and resolved the anatomy of the placenta was the same man who had most successfully entered the lying-in chamber. So too Hunter cultivated and gained the reputation of relying on the powers of Nature to effect the delivery of both child and placenta.

Hunter's lectures make it abundantly clear that the male practitioner had to *work* to gain such practice. A new niche of practice was already available, but to enter it required a politic deportment that had to be cultivated and learnt. The passage already quoted illustrates this; another among many further examples recommends that:

> In all degrees of midwifery the accoucheur's behaviour should be conducted in such a manner as not to merit the calumnious censure of the family through precipitation [i.e. precipitate action] or temerity. A proper degree of seeming tenderness and sympathy can never do a man any disservice but often the contrary.[4]

And this was the theme of the final lecture – "Advice to young accoucheurs" on "the dress and address" of the aspiring practitioner. This little sermon on manners concluded:

> It is not the mere safe delivery of the woman will recommend an accoucheur, but a sagacious, well-conducted behaviour of tenderness, assiduity, and delicacy.[5]

Strikingly, those who have to be impressed are exclusively women; Hunter makes no reference to husbands as significant agents in calling the male practitioner. Correspondingly, while the main appeal to be cultivated is to the mother herself, the collectivity of women is still important – just as Smellie's rush of "bespoke" calls in 1748 came from the "friends" of the various mothers.[6] Thus the young male practitioner "should never . . . proceed to anything of consequence relating to the obstetrical operations without the approbation of the gossips after having stated the case".[7]

While the gossips are to be placated, Hunter has a different and more complex attitude towards the lying-in nurse. Managing such nurses, he tells his students, is a particularly difficult and vexatious task.

> We see every day proofs of the nurses' obstinacy in not watching their women. A lady of quality whom I delivered and left extremely well I found the day after delivery sitting up in bed and she very cheerfully asked me if she might change her linen. I cautioned her against it and candidly stated the danger: I ordered the nurses not to suffer her to do anything of that kind. Notwithstanding which I had not been long gone but the nurse hearkened to her importunities . . . [The mother] dressed and powdered her hair, but was soon taken ill and died before night. I knew two other cases where they died very soon. These are circum-

stances which might with propriety be imputed to the nurse's negligence, and ought to awaken our vigilance in overlooking [i.e. overseeing] and superintending nurses in general.[8]

(Notice that Hunter is insisting on traditional lying-in – a point to which we will return.) Yet while the nurse is a target of criticism, she is also an important figure who can give useful information and even advice: the young accoucheur should be "particularly obliging and ready to reap advice from old experienced nurses who may be of great service to him". This is a further testimony to the continuing importance of women as managers of childbirth; at the same time, it is only "old experienced" nurses who merit such respect.[9]

Hunter's practice was concentrated in an elevated social sphere – the wives of the aristocracy and presumably the upper merchant classes in London. (We have seen his patients described as "a lady" and as "a lady of quality"; when his practice enlarged, apparently in the 1760s, he kept it within manageable bounds by charging new patients 10 guineas.[10]) And this had implications for obstetric practice, as his lectures repeatedly demonstrate. The clearest example – concerning the diagnosis of pregnancy – illustrates the distance between Hunter and his erstwhile teacher William Smellie:

> Smellie advises introducing a finger *in ano*, which will more likely ascertain the pressure, but the indelicacy of this operation has exploded its practice in private [i.e. as distinct from in lying-in hospitals, where the patients were poor]. Such practice is improper when you are called to satisfy a lady. Here you should for your own reputation's sake endeavour to use some ambiguous answer, and by prescribing some inoffensive medicine . . . to amuse her a month longer.[11]

This and other aspects of his practice led naturally to Hunter's famous anti-interventionism.[12] Onset calls in lieu of a midwife marginalized difficult births, and the need for intervention plummeted to around 2% of deliveries. Wealthy mothers paid him for hanging around, so that patience and expectancy were rewarded in guineas. And "delicacy" dictated minimal use of even the hands, let alone of instruments.

Like the forceps practitioners, Hunter illustrated his approach by means of case-histories; but he used these as arguments *against* surgical intervention. For instance:

> A lady whose pubis was not well formed, [nor] yet could it be called narrow, after her first labour had always two eminent men of the profession to attend her, who without loss of time always proceeded to open the head [i.e. to deliver by craniotomy]. Because the labour was tardy they concluded the pelvis was narrow.[13]

These "two eminent men of the profession" were presumably followers of Deventer, as they justified craniotomy on the grounds of pelvic deformity. Perhaps they were acting as a physician–surgeon team, as I have suggested for John Douglas's practice.[14] Hunter's account does not mention a midwife, but this does not mean that no midwife was present. Hunter continued:

> At last [i.e. for a further delivery] I was employed and instead of falling into these erroneous practices suffered the labour to go on four days (no bad symptoms occurring), at the expiration of which she was delivered of a living child by the natural pains. She has been delivered four or five times since of living children but her labours were all laborious.

This is one example among many of Hunter's well-known reliance on the natural powers to effect delivery. That reliance was far from new: a century earlier Willughby had similarly extolled "Dame Nature, Eve's midwife" and "friendly nature, the best of midwives".[15] But Hunter put this idea to new use, appropriating it on behalf of the man as midwife, and using it to distance himself from earlier generations of male practitioners, who used the forceps or, as in the above example, the crotchet. Those practitioners had not experienced the luxury of primary responsibility for the delivery. The natural powers predominated for Hunter precisely because normal birth was his routine experience of childbirth. Thus Hunter initiated the new movement towards leaving the delivery of the placenta to Nature, and cautioned patience before proceeding to deliver the second child if there should be twins.[16]

Hunter, Smellie and the forceps

Yet Hunter's lectures reveal that his anti-interventionism was less extreme than has usually been thought, for he devoted nearly a tenth of the lecture course (15 pages in the manuscript notes) to instructions on the use of the forceps. It is true that he criticized their injudicious or over-hasty use, and repeatedly advised patience and caution, yet at this time, probably the 1760s, his approach to the instrument was not hostile but measured or even ambivalent. Indeed, on the use of the forceps for face-presentation Hunter actually contradicted himself. When introducing such cases, he began: "I inculcate it as a rule always to submit face cases to nature". But in the next lecture, discussing those face-presentations where the chin was to the sacrum, he directed that these should be delivered with the forceps, concluding that "the mechanic delivery [i.e. using forceps] should be observed in all face cases, but particularly in this".[17] This remarkable inconsistency suggests that each course of lectures was a palimpsest, subject to partial revision from year to year in the light of Hunter's changing experiences and views.[18]

The lectures reveal a similar ambivalence towards Smellie, who emerged not only as the foil for Hunter's own anti-interventionism, but also as the great man, towering over all other authors combined in Hunter's citations. As we would expect, many of these allusions depicted Smellie as too ready to intervene. But Hunter also praised Smellie – indeed, almost as often as he criticized him – and he followed him in depicting Deventer and La Motte as the leading earlier theorists.[19] All this suggests that Hunter saw Smellie as a father-figure. For this there was good reason: he had spent his first year in London (1740–41) as Smellie's living-in pupil, and had had repeated dealings with him thereafter. This almost certainly included instruction with the forceps in the later 1740s, after Smellie had made his pivotal discovery of forceps rotation.[20] Subsequently the former pupil had become both colleague and rival, rapidly outpacing Smellie in the arts of social mobility and self-presentation, and relations between them had duly fluctuated, with ambivalence on both sides. In 1750 Smollett was trying to smooth over some quarrel between them; this apparently succeeded, for they had dealings together again in 1752, and in 1754 Smellie acknowledged in print that Hunter had helped him "in reforming the wrong practice of delivering the placenta". But a few years later, on the eve of Smellie's retirement in 1759, they had fallen out again, never to be reconciled.[21] Hunter's lectures reflected this complex legacy: whatever his criticisms, he took Smellie's approach as the starting-point for his own midwifery.[22]

Hunter's ambivalent stance in the 1760s towards Smellie and the forceps indicates a process of transition. Already he had abandoned the very manoeuvre that had convinced Smellie of the utility of the forceps, i.e. its use to rotate the child's head.

> Pushing up the head is attended with too great an inconvenience to be eligible as it is more than ten to one against the blades keeping their hold. . . . If the head (as it will in well-formed women) advances pretty quickly by the natural pains, the mechanical turn would not only be needless, but dangerous.[23]

Subsequently Hunter was to retreat still further from the instrument. By 1778 he could state in print:

> A new practice, salutary and useful perhaps in a few rare cases, may, very naturally, by an indiscriminate and frequent use, do much more harm than good. This sentiment will not surprise those of the profession who know my opinion of the *Forceps*, for example, in midwifery. I admit that it may sometimes be of service, and may save either the mother or the child. I have sometimes used it with advantage; and, I believe, never materially hurt a mother or child with it, because I always used it with fear and circumspection. Yet, I am clearly of opinion, from all the information which I have been able to procure, that the *Forceps* (midwifery instruments in general, I fear) upon the whole, has done more harm than good.[24]

And in his lectures at around this time he was more trenchant, exclaiming that "where they save one, they murder twenty ... 'tis a thousand pities that they were ever invented".[25]

In short, Hunter's development had a consistent direction: away from the use of the forceps, and towards reliance on the natural powers. Clearly this pull towards anti-interventionism arose from the new form of practice — that of the man-as-midwife — in which normal births predominated. But it also reflects Hunter's exquisite sense of what mothers themselves required and expected of those who were to deliver them. Midwives had traditionally used manual methods; male practitioners had used instruments, and this was true even of Deventer and his followers.[26] *To turn away from the forceps was to be more like a midwife.* Smellie, in the late 1740s, had tried to make the forceps more acceptable to mothers by making the blades non-metallic — first by constructing them of wood, then by applying a leather covering to the traditional metal blades. But these devices only showed Smellie's attachment to his earlier roots in the role of obstetric surgeon.[27] Over the years Hunter gradually took one vital step further, pressing to the limit the practical implications of being a midwife.

"Their counsellor and adviser"

These implications extended far beyond the technical management of childbirth. For Hunter was drawn into the very role of wide-ranging support for women already played by the traditional, female midwife. Hence his collusion with "a lady of fortune whose husband was unhappy on account of her not breeding": Hunter diagnosed her faked miscarriage as a piece of boiled liver, but did not give her away to her husband, "who was very sorry for her and sent her to Bath to recuperate". Hence also his running errands for women, his participation in women's sociable activities, and perhaps also his reputation for gossip.[28] And it was probably this new social role that led Hunter to develop a particular sympathy for unmarried mothers. In the 1770s, when "the daughter of a peer ... confessed herself pregnant, and requested his assistance", Hunter arranged that the Foundling Hospital would take in her child for a payment of £100. He delivered her clandestinely, as it chanced of twins, and took the twins to the Hospital himself, together with £200.[29] Nor was his sympathy directed only towards wealthy women in such a plight. A few years later, towards the end of his life, he wrote a paper (published posthumously) in support of women accused of infanticide. Under existing law, an unmarried mother who gave birth to a stillborn child was presumed to have murdered the child and was subject to capital punishment.[30] Hunter argued that the traditional signs of infanticide were inconclusive; that the fear and distress occasioned by bearing a bastard child made such births difficult, and thus liable to end in a stillbirth; and that the presumption in such cases should therefore shift from the mother's guilt to her innocence.[31] Central to this argument was

Hunter's claim to understand the passions and motives of women. Accordingly, he began his paper with an eloquent justification of that claim.

> The world will give me credit, surely, for having had sufficient opportunities of knowing a good deal of female characters. I have seen the private as well as the public virtues, the private as well as the more public frailties of women in all ranks of life. I have been in their secrets, their counsellor and adviser in the moments of their greatest distress in body and mind. I have been a witness to their private conduct, when they were preparing themselves to meet danger, and have heard their last and most serious reflections, when they were certain they had but few hours to live.

Just as Hunter's words alluded to the profound intimacy of his role as midwife, so too the wider argument of his paper attested to *the effects of that role upon him*. He took the side of unmarried mothers because the experience of being a midwife had drawn him into sympathy towards women "in the moments of their greatest distress in body and mind".

In his midwifery practice and teaching, just as in his other medical activities, William Hunter was a supremely successful opportunist: although he did not create the new social niche of the man-as-midwife, he exploited it with conspicuous and probably unique skill.[32] Hunter therefore reveals to us something of the nature of that niche itself, and the striking feature is that childbirth was still under the collective control of women. It was to women, not to their husbands, that the male practitioner had to appeal; childbirth was still a collective female affair; and many aspects of the traditional ceremony remained intact. Hunter's attitude to the ritual procedures of women was complex, falling somewhere between the passive acceptance of previous generations and the wide-ranging attack of his own pupil Charles White in 1772. For example, he proposed that caudle should be drunk during lying-in but strongly opposed its use to assist delivery. The passage devoted to this latter point is highly revealing.

> It is very wrong . . . to suffer the gossips to give her hot stimulating liquors when the labour proceeds slow and painful, such as crude or burnt wine, saffron, castor, drams or any spirituous liquors, and you should take care they do not make too free with spices etc., as they may produce the most terrible consequences, and not withstanding the notion imbibed by them of its promoting delivery.[33]

Thus the very circles of women who had already welcomed the male practitioner in lieu of the midwife were still following traditional methods (caudle) and retained great confidence not only in those methods but also in their own understanding of what was best for the mother. And this poses still more sharply our fundamental question: how had Hunter's niche become possible? What had happened by about 1750 to drive out the midwife and replace her with a man?

Notes

1. Hunter, lectures, pp. 70–71; see also pp. 52, 79. For "accoucheur" see pp. 99, 115, 119, 172–6. These lectures appear to date after Smellie's retirement in 1759, as references to Smellie as a practitioner are in the past tense; they were surely pre-1772, for they make no mention of Charles White's *Treatise on the management of pregnant and lying-in women*, published in that year; and they were probably pre-1769, as they do not refer to Wallace Johnson's *New system of midwifery* (1769).
2. Hunter, lectures, pp. 49–50, 133–4.
3. W. Hunter, *Anatomy of the gravid uterus* (Birmingham, 1774). See L. J. Jordanova, "Gender, generation and science: William Hunter's obstetrical atlas", in *William Hunter*, Bynum & Porter (eds), pp. 385–412.
4. Hunter, lectures, p. 150.
5. *Ibid.*, pp. 172–6, quoted from p. 176.
6. Ch. 12.
7. Hunter, lectures, p. 173.
8. *Ibid.*, pp. 162–3.
9. The fact that the male practitioner is enjoined to control the nurse suggests that the traditional, female midwife had managed the lying-in nurse; if so, this would confirm that midwives' activities extended into post-partum care (cf. Ch. 3).
10. Brock, *William Hunter*, p. 8.
11. Hunter, lectures, p. 39; cf. also p. 70.
12. See Ch. 1, at *n*.5.
13. Hunter, lectures, pp. 146–7. Other cases, all undated, appear on pp. 40, 45, 48–9, 50, 53–4, 57, 62, 64, 66–8, 70, 72–3, 76, 80–81, 101, 118–19, 127, 130, 132–4, 149–50, 162–3, 174–5.
14. Ch. 6.
15. Willughby, *Observations*, pp. 42–3 (see also pp. 233–4, 274–5), 32.
16. Placenta: Hunter, lectures, pp. 95, 99f, 139–40, 151–5, and Ch. 12 above. Twins: Hunter, lectures, pp. 40, 136–40, and *n*.18 below.
17. *Ibid.*, pp. 117, 120.
18. Such a reading is also consistent with the passage on twins (*ibid.*, pp. 136–40), which combines interventionist and expectant advice, with the latter dominant.
19. In the lectures proper Hunter mentioned Smellie 27 times, as against 18 for all other authors combined. With three further references in the introductory historical lecture, Smellie had 30 citations in all; of these, 14 were critical, 10 were favourable, and the remaining 6 were ambiguous or neutral. *Ibid.*, pp. 7, 8, 10, 25, 28, 32, 34, 35, 39 (twice), 47, 51, 59, 73–4, 90, 92, 97, 101, 102, 104 (twice), 111, 115, 119, 122, 131, 134, 139, 147, 173. For Deventer and La Motte see p. 10.
20. Brock, *William Hunter*, pp. 2–3; Chs 9 & 11 above.
21. Brock, *William Hunter*, pp. 48–9; McClintock, *Smellie's midwifery*, vol. III, p. 199 (Case 408); vol. II, p. 252.
22. One interesting anomaly is that Hunter dogmatically preferred podalic over cephalic version: he stated his choice briefly with respect to breech births, and did not even discuss the issue when subsequently considering arm presentation (Hunter, lectures, pp. 126, 130–35). This is surprising, given that Manningham and Bracken had supported cephalic version a generation earlier, and given also the promptness with which Smellie had re-experimented with the technique once his own practice changed in the direction of normal birth, around 1750 (see Ch. 12 above).

NOTES

23. Hunter, lectures, pp. 115–16. On Smellie and forceps rotation see Ch. 9 above.
24. See J. Vaughan, *Cases . . . hydrophobia . . . Caesarean section* (London, 1778), pp. 74–98, at p. 81, quoted in Glaister, *Smellie*, p. 123.
25. Spencer, *British midwifery*, pp. 72–3, quoting from MS notes of Hunter's lectures; Ch. 1 above.
26. There were of course exceptions on both sides, such as the midwife of Ticknall, Derbs., whom Willughby criticized for performing craniotomies (*Observations*, pp. 153–6), and on the male side, in France, Cosme Viardel, who used his fingers and hand as a crotchet: *Observations sur la pratique des accouchemens* (Paris, 1671, reprinted 1673, 1674), *passim.*, e.g. pp. 186, 223–5.
27. Ch. 9.
28. Brock, *William Hunter*, pp. 65 (faked miscarriage; words in quotes are Hunter's, others partly quoted and partly paraphrased from Brock), 56 (errands, sociability), 59 (gossip, which Brock construes rather differently).
29. *Ibid.*, pp. 59–60.
30. 21 James I, *c*.27. See K. Wrightson, "Infanticide in European history", *Criminal Justice History* 3 (1982), pp. 1–20, and R. W. Malcolmson, "Infanticide in the eighteenth century", in *Crime in England, 1550–1800,* J. S. Cockburn (ed.) (London: Methuen, 1977), pp. 187–209.
31. On the uncertainty of the signs of murder, in the case of bastard children. By the late William Hunter . . . Read July 14, 1783, *Medical Observations and Inquiries* 6 (1784), pp. 266–90, quoted below from p. 269. The paper was read to the London Medical Society four months after Hunter's death in March 1783.
32. Hunter's opportunism is brought out well by R. Porter, "William Hunter: a surgeon and a gentleman", in *William Hunter*, Bynum & Porter (eds), pp. 7–34.
33. Hunter, lectures, p. 91.

Chapter Fourteen
Two female cultures

Our exploration has now posed with renewed force the very question with which we began: how did men come to play the role of midwives? The answer to that question, I shall now suggest, lies in the wider sphere to which childbirth was closely tied: the lives of women.[1] What we must remember is that the traditional role of the midwife was embedded in the collective culture of women. It was the ceremony of childbirth that conferred authority on the midwife; the mother's personal choice extended only to the selection of *which* midwife, of those locally available, would deliver her. What gave the ritual itself its immense power was collective female authority, which transcended the whims and wishes of the individual mother: hence the importance of the gossips in the management of childbirth. Mothers, midwives and gossips were bound together by the same web of social bonds that constituted the collective culture of women in general. That culture was made possible by the range of experiences and activities shared by mothers of all social ranks. The basis of this sharing was the patriarchal order, that is, the laws and customs that conferred upon husbands property in the sexuality, the goods and the labour of their wives.[2] Even the aristocratic wife was subsumed within this order; all women found themselves bound by it. Hence the fact that the relatively humble midwife could assert power over a mother who belonged to the ruling class.[3]

A new female culture

Surely the midwife can only have been displaced from this role if the collective culture of women fragmented. And in fact there are grounds for believing that the old culture did indeed break up during the first half of the eighteenth century.

Wealthy mothers began to detach themselves from their humbler sisters and to construct a new cultural space – most conspicuously in London but also elsewhere. After about 1750 there were two distinct cultures of women: the old, traditional, *oral* culture, characteristic of the lower orders, and a new, fashionable, *literate* culture, the culture of 'the ladies', visible among the aristocracy and the wealthy middle classes.

The two hallmarks of this new female culture were literacy and leisure – of which literacy is far easier to document. In the period 1680 to 1730, women in London acquired writing literacy (visible to the historian as the ability to sign their names) to a degree that probably had no historical precedent, and certainly had none in England. Over 50% of London women were able to sign by 1730; the rate had more than doubled in 50 years.[4] Moreover, the absolute numbers of literate women had grown still faster, since the base population of London was increasing rapidly at this time; thus the number of London women able to write probably increased about threefold in a generation or so. Still more widespread – although by how much more is difficult to assess – was the ability to read.[5] Not surprisingly, this transformation was reflected in the creation of a new literature, written both *for* women and increasingly *by* women. Almanacs for women appeared as early as the 1680s; in the 1690s the *Athenian Mercury* popularized Newton's new natural philosophy, with women among its audience; and a host of similar initiatives followed in the early eighteenth century.[6] The high point of these developments was of course the novel – a new literary form that emerged in this period and was intimately bound up with women, as readers, as subject-matter, and increasingly as authors.[7] In the 60 years from 1690, an impressive roll of at least 13 new women novelists appeared on the literary scene, producing some dozens of works between them. But the pace of female recruitment into novel writing accelerated dramatically from 1750, for a further 13 new women novelists appeared in print between 1750 and 1765.[8] That is, the rate at which women novelists emerged multiplied almost fourfold from mid-century (it was to increase again with similar sharpness in the 1780s).[9]

Many of these women writers were, like their male counterparts, writing for a living. But if writing was work, reading was leisure; what called forth the novel was a new female reading public, and this much wider circle of women, numbered in tens of thousands, was enjoying a new measure of freedom from domestic labour. Habits of domestic life were changing among a large group of London married women. By the early eighteenth century, in the words of Dorothy George, "London and its neighbourhood had reached a stage of industrial development where spinning, weaving, baking, brewing and candle-making were no longer done by housewives".[10] For poorer women this was no emancipation – indeed, it probably helped to propel them into low-paid semi-casual labour – but for the wives of the upper artisan stratum and above, it must have made available a significant expansion of leisure time. (One cannot imagine the wife of an eighteenth-century Admiralty official physically doing the washing with her maid, as Elizabeth Pepys had done in the 1660s.) This development gradually but inexorably separated wealthier women from their less affluent peers. Its cultural corollary was literacy, which at first set such women apart from the old oral culture but then brought some of them together in a new culture based on the written and printed word.

I suggest that together, literacy and leisure began to break the bonds that had united women in a common culture. As long as the middle-class wife was engaged in manual labour, she shared a certain set of experiences with her fellow women far down the social scale. And so long as female literacy was relatively low, the literate/literary woman was individualized and uncommon – whence the tendency for midwives, who were local leaders of women, to be endowed with literacy.[11] But as female literacy expanded, accompanied by an increased degree of leisure, there became possible a new collective culture of women: the culture of "the ladies", that is, a culture distinct both from that of their husbands and from that of humbler women.[12] In the Restoration period we see the solitary virago (Aphra Behn), the isolated literary lady deriving her main support from her husband (Margaret Cavendish), the educated woman driven to despair by "the retiredness of her life and how unpleasant it was" (Elizabeth Pepys), or, at the end of the century, the individual campaigner proposing semi-monastic institutions for female education and mutual support (Mary Astell).[13] By the mid-eighteenth century the educated woman is a far commoner phenomenon, and although she remains constrained by the patriarchal order, isolation is not her main problem. She now belongs to active circles of collective literary involvement, and even the men (Samuel Richardson, Henry Fielding, Samuel Johnson) recognize something of her worth.[14] And as the literary lady made new companions, so she detached herself from the traditional, oral, collective culture – once the collective culture of all women, now that of the lower orders of women. This finds symbolic expression, as early as 1709, in Delariviere Manley's *The New Atalantis,* in which a midwife (Mrs Nightwork) is made into a comic character – not quite an object of ridicule or satire, but certainly given a voice far removed from that of the genteel authoress.[15]

The new female culture was complex, both internally and in its relations with men. We might suppose that reading and writing were simple acquisitions that at last made it possible for the authentic voice of women to be heard directly and unambiguously. But this was far from being the case. For the new literary culture of women was saturated with the presence of men, as models, as publishers, as critics, as readers, and as opponents or supporters of the very enterprise of women's writing. Some individual men gave notable support to particular women writers: for instance, Sarah Fielding was helped both by her brother Henry – just as she helped him – and by his political and literary opponent Richardson.[16] But such instances of male support derived their meaning from a wider context of male condescension, criticism and disapproval.[17] Literary culture offered the woman writer not the chance of independence, but rather the opportunity for a new form of dependence upon men; the gender order placed her between the literary equivalent of the hard man and soft man of the interrogation cell. The female writer ran the risk of a specific kind of character assassination: her writing and her life were both scrutinized for their moral qualities, and if she was found to fail in either sphere, she would be condemned in both through the medium of male-dominated literary criticism.[18] Even after women novelists were well established, this risk was almost sufficient to paralyse the efforts of one of the most gifted of them, Fanny Burney, who assured her chief personal supporter, Samuel Crisp, "I would a thousand times rather forfeit my character as a writer, than risk ridicule or censure as a female". Crisp had already explained to her, quite unblushingly it seems, what was required of a female writer:

> Do you remember, about a dozen years ago, how you used to dance . . . on the grass plot . . . like a mad thing? Now you are to dance . . . with fetters on; there is the difference.

The nature of the "fetters" was plain enough. Burney was required, despite her already proven comic gifts, to maintain every "grain" of her "female delicacy". That "delicacy" amounted to a genteel, polite subordination, and the careful avoidance of the bedroom in literary productions.[19]

Nevertheless, the new female culture retained, or constructed, a certain degree of independence from men and, as we shall see below, it preserved some aspects of the older oral culture. The dilemma facing the eighteenth-century "lady" was precisely that of maintaining simultaneously a female identity and an identity of gentility. There were many different responses to this challenge; those that are best known and most accessible are of course those of the women writers who now emerged as a major cultural force. It would require a vast research enterprise to reconstruct the corresponding responses among the much wider circle of their readers. Even more interesting would be a study of the complex interplay between the changing reality of women's lives and the equally changing content and form of literature itself, above all, of the novel. Literature simultaneously reflected, deflected and informed the lives of its readers.[20] One indication of this is the highly popular epistolary form. There seems to be a continuum between the epistolary novel (Delariviere Manley, Eliza Haywood, Samuel Richardson), the published correspondence (Mary Delaney), the "private" letter written with an eye to later publication (as one suspects of many of Mrs Delaney's letters), the personal letter that circulated extensively in manuscript (as happened with some of the letters of Lady Mary Montagu) and, finally, the genuinely private letter, written only for the eyes of a single reader, yet in all probability powerfully influenced in style and in content by published epistolary models.[21] It was precisely this complex connection between life and art that was displayed in the novel, with its conventions of verisimilitude, character, plot, and intimate involvement of the reader.[22] More generally, it was the new female reading public that actually called forth the novel; and the leading male novelists (Richardson, Fielding) were keenly aware of both their female readers and their female authorial colleagues.[23]

The new female readership (as well as authorship) was responsible for the –

literally – intimate concerns of the new "domestic novel" of the eighteenth century.[24] Rosemary Bechler's compelling analysis of Richardson's purposes strongly suggests that the new leisure and literacy of women gave particular urgency and shape to Richardson's driving moral and religious aims. For Richardson, Bechler argues, *time* was sacred: following Jacob Boehme, he saw time as a battleground for life's unremitting contest or dialectic between good and evil, "light" and "fire", sin and redemption: "Human nature, good and evil, coexist and suffer in human time in order that we should come to know God's truth. *Hence the horror at 'kill-time' amusements*".[25] And such "amusements" (notably card-playing) were exactly the worldly eighteenth-century response to the new leisure enjoyed, or suffered, by genteel women. Richardson's writing was designed to restore to women's lives a moral seriousness, an ability to experience time as the Creator intended, a capacity to find in even the most mundane occupations the opportunity for fulfilment and for grasping both practically and contemplatively the spiritual destiny of humanity. This Richardson attempted both through such examples as his heroine Pamela, and through making available to his female readers texts that would enable them to spend long hours in serious reading. His twofold exhortation had a dazzling success, specifically among women readers, in the late eighteenth century.[26] Mass female leisure, then, was one of the fundamental new conditions that evoked Richardson's deeply serious project, and the central weapon he deployed was a particular use of the corresponding phenomenon of mass female literacy.[27]

The new kind of woman who thus emerged during the first half of the eighteenth century of course posed a threat to men – as the women themselves were well aware. Educated girls, wrote Mary Astell, were "stared upon as monsters"; or as Lady Mary Wortley Montagu put it, it was "looked upon as in a degree criminal to improve our reason, or fancy we have any".[28] In response women learnt to conceal their learning, to wear it lightly, and, if they chose to become writers, to make a positive display of their reluctance to be published. By mid-century, men had apparently evolved a way of coming to terms with the new phenomenon of the literary lady: they held up as examples those women who *combined* accomplishments in literature with traditional domestic activities, with, as Richardson put it, "those more necessary, and therefore not meaner, employments which will qualify her to be a good mistress of a family, a good wife and a good mother". Dr Johnson made the point more pithily, praising Elizabeth Carter because she "could make a pudding, as well as translate Epictetus".[29] By such delicate accommodations on both sides, the new literary lady was absorbed into a patriarchal gender order that was left largely undisturbed.[30] Marriage still conferred conjugal property on the husband; a woman like Charlotte Lennox might be one of England's foremost writers in the 1750s, yet in law she did not exist, while in daily life she was wracked by the perpetual debts of her spendthrift husband. All the patronage that Dr Johnson could exercise on her behalf could not alleviate her material situation – a situation forced upon her by the prevailing relations of marital property.[31] Thus, while the cultural transformation we have been considering was indeed profound, what it offered for educated women was not an escape from subordination but new ways of living that subordination.

The new female culture had both male and female roots. In its literary manifestations it was male-influenced, both in its self-separation from the traditional collective culture of women, and through the pervasive impact of men – as patrons, publishers, readers, critics – on what was acceptable in a woman writer and her works. Yet at the same time it was in many ways distinctively female. Most obviously, the woman writer was never allowed to forget that she was female; this was as true of Fanny Burney in the 1780s as it had been of Aphra Behn over a century earlier. Necessarily, therefore, whether she liked it or not, her writing was gendered, and in response to this, women novelists gradually developed a well-modulated, distinctive voice.[32] Moreover, the new women's culture as a whole preserved, or perhaps one should say it re-created, the *collective* character that had been such a marked feature of the traditional female culture from which it was separating itself. The new collectivity was bounded by class, in sharp contrast to its predecessor, but it was a collectivity nonetheless. Ladies took many of their recreations together, and in separation or semi-separation from men. One of the oblique indications of this is the acceptability to ladies of the solitary *bachelor* male as part-serious, part-trivial companion both in their gatherings and in their correspondence. This role was accepted and enjoyed by many literary men – and, significantly, by the lifelong bachelor, William Hunter.[33]

There can be little doubt about the phenomena we have been considering: the expansion of women's literacy, the commercialization of domestic activities, the growth of female readership and the emergence of women writers are all well-documented. Yet before returning to our own theme, we must observe that these wider cultural changes raise many unresolved questions. What, for instance, was the role within these developments of women's aspirations for education? Did such aspirations – best known through the initiatives of Bathsua Makin in 1673 and Mary Astell in the 1690s – simply reflect the wider changes, or did they significantly help to bring those changes about?[34] Furthermore, and here Mary Astell is again an exemplar, why was it that down to perhaps 1720 or so, literary women were overwhelmingly of Cavalier and then Tory allegiance?[35] How did the processes we have been considering impinge on the debate over women's "nature" in the learned literature on "generation" around 1700?[36] Can we say that by about 1750 there emerged, among the middle and upper classes, a new conjugal ideology?[37] And in general, what set in motion this train of developments? One could certainly wish for a more precise chronology of the relevant changes. The growth of women's literacy in London was most marked between perhaps 1690 and 1720, yet the process of commercialization, while undoubtedly already at work then, became much more apparent around 1750.[38] I hope that any study undertaken to explore these questions will take into consideration the emergence of man-midwifery as one facet of this cultural transformation.[39]

Ladies as mothers

Hitherto, childbirth had been the great leveller – in several interlocking ways. It had physically brought together women of different social ranks. It had exposed the aristocratic lady and the cottager's wife to the same risks of illness and even death. With its inevitable blood and pain, it vividly contradicted the phrase "gentle birth" used to describe the origins of members of the landed classes. And in subordinating the lady to the midwife, it had ceaselessly reminded that lady that she was, for all her pretensions to rank and breeding, a woman like other women; manual labour she might eschew, delegating this to servants, but labour in its other sense, that of childbirth, remained her inescapable lot. As long as women's traditional collective culture remained intact across all social classes, childbirth retained this levelling quality. And surely this was why the man-midwife was so attractive to those wealthy and literate women who by about 1750 had collectively constructed a new female culture. The male practitioner was a midwife who was not a midwife, a childbirth practitioner who stepped into the midwife's shoes and yet differed in all other respects from the traditional female midwife. The midwife, by her very presence – whatever her actual deportment – served as a tangible reminder that ladies were mere women. But the man-midwife offered proof of their superior social status: who but ladies could afford the 10 guineas that William Hunter charged for deliveries? The putative skills of the male practitioner, we may venture, went to support this: whatever the real distribution of skill between male and female practitioners, the ladies doubtless assured themselves that exclusive fees meant exclusive technical abilities. Mentally, therefore, they detached themselves from the dangers of childbirth – a further separation from their less fortunate sisters.

In these terms we can begin to understand the role of "fashion" in giving momentum to man-midwifery. It has always been alleged that fashion played a crucial part in the making of the man-midwife, but, as we saw at the outset, such explanations beg the question as to how this process got started.[40] Set in the context of the new split in women's culture, this ceases to be mysterious. Fashion was in general the symbolic reflection of the new culture of class; in the world of women, for which childbirth was so crucial, fashion dictated the need for the man-midwife. In the same moment as it effected a separation between social ranks, fashion offered a bridge by which those of intermediate or ambiguous status could symbolically climb the ranks and "ape the quality". The artisan's wife might not be able to afford a carriage, but every couple of years she could afford a man-midwife. Man-midwifery thus became an area of conspicuous consumption; the new men-midwives cashed in, and the loser was of course the traditional midwife, who saw draining away her most lucrative sphere of practice.

In the management of childbirth, the new culture actually preserved significant aspects of the traditional collectivity. The swaddling of the newborn child was attacked by William Cadogan in 1748 – but, according to James Nelson, "the ladies" thought Cadogan quite mistaken. With regard to swaddling, then, the new culture preserved traditional methods.[41] By the 1770s it was seen as "old-fashioned" to drink the mother's caudle when visiting her – but it was still being done.[42] Most significant of all is that William Hunter, in delineating the route to male practice as a midwife, laid great stress on pleasing and appeasing the "gossips" and never mentioned husbands in this connection at all.[43] In this matter, as in technical obstetrics, Hunter was the supreme expert. His account thus offers powerful evidence that even in distancing themselves from their humbler fellow women, in abandoning the female midwife, and in resorting instead to male practitioners, the ladies of mid-eighteenth-century London nevertheless preserved for childbirth a collective female ritual of management.

Viewed with hindsight, the man-midwifery of the previous generation – from the 1720s to the 1740s – had served as a *precondition* for the new form of practice of the man-as-midwife. As mothers became aware that male practitioners could deliver a living child, whether by Deventer's methods or by one of the Chamberlen instruments, they summoned them more frequently as an adjunct to the midwife, and more quickly in cases of emergency. But although this was a necessary condition for the mid-century shift, it was not a sufficient condition; nor was this further step inevitable. In their "paths" to childbirth, in their practical methods, and in their obstetric doctrines, the men of the previous generation had still been concerned specifically with difficult births. Nor had these male practitioners wanted to act in the role of midwife: on the contrary, their ambitions were confined within the bounds of their own experiences. Forceps practitioners, who received early emergency calls, merely wanted these to come still earlier; the followers of Deventer, who experienced onset calls with a midwife, merely wanted these to be more frequent. Male practitioners were turned into midwives not by their own desire but through the choices of women. Only *after* mothers summoned into being the man-as-midwife was this form of practice rationalized as natural by Smellie and taught as deportment by Hunter.[44] The making of man-midwifery was the work of women.

Notes

1. The argument developed here was prompted by reading M. Benjamin, *Women and natural philosophy in eighteenth century England* (MPhil thesis, University of Cambridge, 1986). I thank Timothy Ashplant, Ludmilla Jordanova, Neil McKendrick, Valerie Rumbold, Simon Schaffer, Richard Smith and Margaret Spufford for advice, and Lois Chabor, Peter Clark, Sandy Cunningham, Elizabeth Nathaniels and Janet Todd for helpful comments on earlier drafts. The main works cited below are I. Watt, *The rise of the novel: studies in Defoe, Richardson and Fielding* (London: Chatto & Windus, 1957; reprinted Hogarth Press, 1987); Todd, *Women writers*; J. Spencer, *The rise of the woman novelist: from Aphra Behn to Jane Austen* (Oxford: Blackwell, 1986); D. Spender, *Mothers of the novel: 100 good women writers before Jane Austen* (London: Routledge, 1986); N. Armstrong, *Desire and domestic fiction: a political history of the novel* (Oxford: Oxford Uni-

NOTES

versity Press, 1987).
2. Ch. 3.
3. Willughby, *Observations*, pp. 142–5, 226.
4. D. Cressy, *Literacy and the social order* (Cambridge: Cambridge University Press, 1980), p. 147. For some qualifications see P. Earle, "The female labour market in London in the late seventeenth and early eighteenth centuries", *Economic History Review*, 2nd series, **42** (1989), pp. 328–53, at pp. 333–6.
5. M. Spufford, *Small books and pleasant histories: popular fiction and its readership in seventeenth-century England* (Cambridge: Cambridge University Press, 1981), pp. 19–44.
6. Benjamin, Women and natural philosophy, *passim*.
7. For women as readers see Watt, *Rise of the novel*. For women as writers see Spencer, *Rise of the woman novelist*; Spender, *Mothers of the novel*; Todd, *Women writers*; F. Morgan, *The female wits: women playwrights on the London stage 1660–1720* (London: Virago, 1981).
8. Spender, *Mothers of the novel*, pp. 119–37.
9. There is now a rapidly growing body of work on the social origins and significance of the novel. In addition to other works cited, see R. Perry, *Women, letters and the novel* (New York, 1980); T. Eagleton, *The rape of Clarissa* (Minneapolis: University of Minnesota Press, 1982); J. Barrell, *English literature in history 1730–80: an equal, wide survey* (London: Hutchinson, 1983); M. McKeon, *The origins of the English novel 1600–1740* (Baltimore: John Hopkins University Press, 1987); L. B. Faller, *Turned to account: the forms and functions of criminal biography in late seventeenth- and early eighteenth-century England* (Cambridge, 1987); A. D. Harvey, *Literature into history* (Macmillan 1988); J. P. Hunter, *Before novels: the cultural context of eighteenth century fiction* (New York & London: W. W. Norton, 1990); R. Kroll, *The material word: literate culture in the Restoration and early eighteenth century* (Baltimore & London: Johns Hopkins University Press, 1991); R. Ballaster, *Seductive forms: women's amatory fiction from 1684 to 1740* (Oxford: Clarendon, 1992).
10. D. George, *London life in the eighteenth century* (first published 1925; Harmondsworth: Penguin, 1966), p. 172. Cf. D. Davis, *A history of shopping* (London: Routledge, 1966).
11. Ch. 3.
12. A. Calder-Marshall, *The grand century of the lady* (London: Gordon & Cremonesi, 1976).
13. For Aphra Behn and Margaret Cavendish, see Spencer, *Rise of the woman novelist*, pp. 24–5, 27–30, 42–52; Spender, *Mothers of the novel*, pp. 35–46, 64–6. For Elizabeth Pepys, see S. H. Mendelson, "Stuart women's diaries and occasional memoirs", in *Women in English society 1500–1800,* M. Prior (ed.) (London, 1985), pp. 181–210, at p. 184. For Mary Astell, see *DNB*; J. Kinnaird, "Mary Astell and the conservative contribution to English feminism", *Journal of British Studies* **19** (1979), pp. 53–75; B. Hill (ed.), *The first English feminist: "Reflections upon marriage" and other writings by Mary Astell* (Aldershot: Gower/Temple Smith, 1986).
14. Spencer, *Rise of the woman novelist*, p. 91.
15. M. D. Manley, *Secret memoirs and manners of several persons of quality, of both sexes. From the New Atalantis, an island in the Mediterranean* (London, 1709).
16. Spencer, *Rise of the woman novelist*, pp. 91–4. On Sarah Fielding's career see Spender, *Mothers of the novel*, pp. 180–93.
17. There were also women critics: see Armstrong, *Desire and domestic fiction*, p. 265 n.2.
18. Spencer, *Rise of the woman novelist*, Ch. 3.
19. *Ibid.*, p. 97.
20. Watt, *Rise of the novel,* depicted the novel as a reflection of social forces; Armstrong, *Desire and domestic fiction,* stresses the social effects of writing. For an interesting discussion of

the issues, see N. Tadmor, "'Family' and 'friend' in *Pamela*: a case-study in the history of the family in eighteenth-century England", *Social History* 14 (1989), pp. 289–306, at pp. 290–91.
21. R. A. Day, *Told in letters: epistolary fiction before Richardson* (Ann Arbor, Michigan: University of Michigan Press, 1970); cf. Watt, *Rise of the novel*, pp. 189–96.
22. J. Preston, *The created self: the reader's role in the eighteenth century* (London: Heinemann, 1970); cf. Watt, *Rise of the novel*, pp. 200–201.
23. On the female reading public see Watt, *Rise of the novel, passim*. For male novelists' awareness of women see *ibid.*, pp. 152–3; Spencer, *Rise of the woman novelist*, p. 91; T. C. Duncan Eaves & B. D. Kimpel, *Samuel Richardson: a biography* (Oxford: Clarendon Press, 1971), p. 557.
24. This phrase is Armstrong's: see *Desire and domestic fiction*.
25. R. Bechler, "Triall by what is Contrary": Samuel Richardson and Christian Dialectic, in *Samuel Richardson: passion and prudence,* V. G. Myer (ed.) (London: Vision, 1986), pp. 93–113 (quoted from p. 99, my emphasis).
26. On the popularity of *Pamela* – and of Pamela – see Watt, *Rise of the novel*, pp. 55, 148, 151–4.
27. For a different interpretation, although also stressing the gendered quality of the novel, see Armstrong, *Desire and domestic fiction*.
28. Todd, *Women writers*, Introduction, p. 4.
29. Spencer, *Rise of the woman novelist*, p. 86.
30. Susan Moller Okin, "Patriarchy and married women's property in England: questions on some current views", *Eighteenth-Century Studies* 17 (1983), pp. 121–38.
31. Todd, *Women writers*, p. 196.
32. Spencer, *Rise of the woman novelist, passim*; Todd, *Women writers*, Introduction.
33. Brock, *William Hunter*, pp. 53–4; Watt, *Rise of the novel*, pp. 146–7. Richardson, although married, played a similar role (*ibid.*, pp. 152–3).
34. Bathsua Makin, *An essay to revive the antient education of gentlewomen* (London, 1673); reprinted, P. L. Barbour (ed.), Augustan Reprint Society Publication No. 202 (William Andrews Clark Memorial Library, 1980). On Makin and Astell, see Todd, *Women writers*, and *n.*14 above.
35. Todd, *Women writers*, Introduction, p. 4; Kinnaird, Mary Astell.
36. E. Cohen, "Medical debates on women's 'Nature' in England around 1700", *Bulletin of the Society for the Social History of Medicine*, No. 39 (1985), pp. 7–11.
37. Susan Moller Okin, "Women and the making of the sentimental family", *Philosophy and Public Affairs* 11 (1982), pp. 65–88; cf. Armstrong, *Desire and domestic fiction*.
38. See N. McKendrick et al., *The birth of a consumer society* (Bloomington, Indiana: Indiana University Press, 1982).
39. An intriguing sub-plot is the place of childbirth in the novel itself: it was present in *Pamela*, was more or less expunged as the novel developed towards a focus on courtship in the late eighteenth century, and yet remained present off-stage as a site of pain and suffering; finally it returned in realistic mode in 1954. See M. Riley, *Brought to bed* (London: Dent, 1968). The issue has a wider significance, for as Riley comments (p. 69) G. D. Read regarded "the screams and moans issuing from the pages of novels" as among "the chief promoters of fear in his women patients". See G. D. Read, *Revelation of childbirth* (London: Heinemann, 1942), reissued as *Childbirth without fear* in 1954.
40. Ch. 1.
41. See Ch. 15 below.

NOTES

42. R. Trumbach, *The aristocratic family in England, 1690–1780. Studies in childhood and kinship* (Johns Hopkins PhD thesis, 1972), p. 38.
43. Ch. 13. A. Vickery (personal communication) has found confirming evidence from family letters in London and Lancashire.
44. For Smellie's rationale, see Ch. 15.

Chapter Fifteen
Conclusion

Counterattacks

The main lines of resistance against the new form of man-midwifery were laid down by Frank Nicholls as early as 1751 – "modesty", opposition to instruments and the defence of the midwife. Between 1757 and 1764 such resistance led to further public initiatives from three different quarters, and although these failed to stem the advance of the man-as-midwife, they left some enduring effects and are of interest in their own right.

In 1757 a small group of women and men set up a new London charity to increase "the number of skilful and honest midwives" by giving them free instruction "in their art", and also to provide "midwives and medicines" for poor mothers "in their time of travail". This, the "Lying-in Charity for delivering poor married women at their own habitations", was initially based in Southwark, the one major region of London that lacked a lying-in hospital; but around 1760 it expanded into the City of London (particularly around Bishopsgate and Cheapside), and thereafter it competed for funds with the lying-in hospitals.[1] In this it increasingly succeeded during the 1760s: by 1768 it had 467 subscribers and was delivering almost 3000 mothers in a single year – over 10% of all births in London, an unprecedented scale of philanthropic achievement. Through a combination of free training and pledged service, the Charity's midwives gained vast experience: in 1769 the 19 midwives had an average case-load of over 150 births per year. In the delivery of difficult births they were now helped by a salaried "physician and man-midwife", Dr John Ford of Old Jewry. Subsequently Ford acquired two male helpers, Thomas Cogan and William Cooper, duly succeeded by Drs Douglas, Sims, Dennison, Squire and Croft.[2] All these men, on Denman's testimony, were users of the vectis – yet another connection between the vectis and the City.[3] But the Charity's most notable feature was that it produced a cadre of trained midwives. Thus, although it did not present itself as opposed to man-midwifery, it was certainly a pro-midwife initiative: hence its male practitioners only delivered difficult births.

During the Lying-in Charity's early years, man-midwifery came under contrasting polemical attacks from two authors who were unaware of the Charity's existence. In 1760 Elizabeth Nihell's *Treatise on the art of midwifery* mounted a sustained polemic against male practice, seeking to undermine its practical premises.[4] Herself a midwife who had been trained at the Paris Hôtel-Dieu and now practised from the Haymarket, Mrs Nihell had watched with horror the recent displacement of the midwife by the "he-midwife", "monsieur l'Accoucheur", the "gentleman-midwife", the "man-pretender to a purely female office".[5] Her aim was to reverse this by persuading "all fathers and mothers" that even the worst of midwives was preferable to the best of men. To cast doubt on male skill she extracted stories of difficult births from the books of men such as Smellie. (Contrast Sarah Stone a generation earlier, promoting her own practice by means of case-histories and reflections against other midwives.) To advance the midwives' cause, Nihell argued that the essential obstetric instrument was *the female hand*. Being soft, delicate and sensitive, the midwife's hand could both receive and impart the subtle impressions required to facilitate delivery. In particular, if the birth came by the head but the natural powers could not effect the delivery, the midwife's fingers could work directly on the cervix – for the feminine hand was naturally attuned to the uterus. Nihell's rationale for this used Deventer's theory of obliquity; but her method differed radically from Deventer's. Correcting the obliquity required enormous patience, working gently and gradually, in harmony with the progress of the labour itself. The midwife's hand thus became a part of the very mechanism of delivery, transcending the dichotomy between Nature and Art.[6] (Again it is instructive to compare Mrs Stone, who *combined* Nihell's method with the vectis-like use of the finger.[7]) Although Nihell's treatise did not achieve its intended effect, her attack on male practice struck home, for she provoked a lengthy response from Smellie's ally Tobias Smollett, leading to some further critical exchanges.[8]

In contrast, Philip Thicknesse, writing four years later, criticized the new "male imposters" from a male viewpoint.[9] Although he shared Nihell's hostility to instruments and her use of selective quotations from Smellie, his *Letter to a young lady* and *Man-midwifery analyzed* proceeded from very different premises from hers, and he did not mention her recent treatise. Instead he cited Frank Nicholls's earlier *Petition of the unborn babes*; and in fact his main arguments – that man-midwifery offended against "decency" and destroyed children – were simply lurid expansions of Nicholls's criticisms. Nevertheless, Thicknesse wrote in a style of his own. For him, "decency" meant the husband's conjugal property in the wife's sexuality: portraying the man-midwife as a dangerous seducer, Thicknesse combined censoriousness and prurience, sexualizing his text while deploring the need for this and blaming it on the men-midwives. And unlike both Nicholls and Nihell, Thicknesse showed no concern for the midwife. Indeed, he turned the realm of skill into a void: delivery had been achieved through the millenia "by the help *only*" (his emphasis) "of that excellent and scarce ever failing female midwife, Goody Nature".[10] Thus, despite his assertion that "I would have women properly instructed", Thicknesse had left them with nothing to be instructed in, and his proposed "fund for the instruction of women in the practice of midwifery" was a purely rhetorical device. Difficult labours were not only rare, but arose from man-midwifery itself: remove man-midwifery and the very need for skill would disappear.[11] The state of Nature was a happy condition in which labours were natural and easy, men-midwives unknown, and the midwife only had to "wait the course of nature, receive her hints, and gently assist her efforts".[12] Nihell had explained *how* the midwife was to "receive" Nature's "hints" and "assist her efforts" – that is, by working on the cervix – and had argued that the midwife could in this way turn a difficult birth into a natural one. Thicknesse elided this concrete activity on the part of the midwife, and dismissed difficult births as a mere by-product of man-midwifery.

Thicknesse's attacks had a slight and unfavourable reception, and evoked few echoes in either male or female readers.[13] A few years earlier (1757), John Brown's *Estimate of the manners and principles of the times*, although bemoaning the "effeminacy" of male manners and alleging that "the sexes have now little apparent distinction", had not mentioned man-midwifery.[14] And a decade after Thicknesse's polemics, Jonas Hanway dropped a brief criticism of man-midwifery into his *The defects of police* (1775), but devoted no serious attention to this theme.[15] Nor did Thicknesse's writings have any apparent practical effect. Man-midwifery continued to flourish, and neither Hunter's lectures nor treatises such as those of Wallace Johnson and Denman suggest that men-midwives had to assuage any fears on the part of husbands. Further critiques of man-midwifery appeared sporadically from 1779[16] until the mid-nineteenth century, particularly in the 1790s[17] and the 1820s.[18] Most of these rehearsed the arguments already developed by Nicholls, Nihell and Thicknesse, although *Man-midwifery dissected* (1793) also attacked the newly publicized vectis.[19] These polemics, too, had little effect; their very vehemence, like that of Nicholls, Nihell and Thicknesse, testifies to their impotence in the face of the massive cultural shift that had occurred in the mid-eighteenth century.[20]

Prospect

By the 1750s the man-as-midwife had been summoned into being, and the female midwife had lost her former monopoly, yet the rivalry between them was only beginning. Much practice remained in the hands of midwives, and although male practitioners were already getting some of the lucrative work among the "ladies", they did not attain instant hegemony even in this social sphere. Old forms of practice continued alongside the new: thus in the 1753 case that came to court over the malpractice of Matthew Morley, the call had been an emergency – an entirely traditional summons – and Morley's failing was that he had refused to come when called.[21] In subsequent decades male practice expanded dramatically, yet very unevenly. Among the aristocracy it appears that the female midwife had been abandoned by 1780.[22] Lower down the social scale, the pattern varied by locality. In some places, male practice in lieu of a midwife appeared with astonishingly speed: at Donington, Lincolnshire, Matthew Flinders was delivering about half the births in the mid-1770s.[23] Yet elsewhere, change was much slower, as at Bridgwater, Somerset, where the forceps was not introduced until around 1800.[24] And at Henley-in-Arden in the 1790s, Thomas Jones was receiving the full spectrum of possible types of call, from traditional emergency calls to deliver a dead child to booked onset calls in lieu of a midwife.[25] Moreover, local variation in the balance between midwives and medical men continued throughout the nineteenth century.[26]

Nevertheless, a profound revolution had already taken place by the early 1750s; and like other revolutions, this generated its own mythical history. The new men-midwives wanted to depict their own involvement in childbirth as natural, but this entailed explaining why they had been excluded for so long. The explanation was supplied by women's "modesty": male practice had been held back by – in Smellie's words – "the false modesty of the women, who were shy of male practitioners", by the "ridiculous prejudices which the fair sex had been used to entertain".[27] The rise of man-midwifery thus reflected the rational breaking down of this mistaken "modesty". This view provided a polemical tool that male practitioners would value well into the nineteenth century. Since we tend to be charmed by such notions – nothing so bewitches the social historian as a supposed prevailing "attitude" in the past – it is important to notice the mythical status of this "modesty". The surviving materials on the management of childbirth in early-modern England yield no evidence that it was female modesty that had previously barred the male practitioner. On the contrary, the concept of "modesty" was a construct, not an embedded attitude; it was not of ancient lineage but was produced in our period; and it emanated not from women but from men.[28] What had actually excluded men from the lying-in chamber was women's collective culture. The myth of "modesty" concealed this fact, even though it rendered a delicately oblique tribute to women's power.

The new man-midwifery did not fit into the formal tripartite structure of the London medical corporations. This problem had not arisen before: individual men-midwives had variously begun as apothecaries (Smellie), surgeons (Bamber), and physicians (Manningham); midwifery had affinities with each of these professions, just as they overlapped with each other. But male practice as a midwife posed a new problem of professional identity, producing two contrasting responses.[29] (1) Some saw midwifery as separate: this view was manifested from one side by Smellie, and from the other by the Surgeons' Company. In Smellie's eyes, midwifery was a further and distinct sphere of practice. Hence his pronouncements about "the honour of the profession" and the fact that when a consultation was required, he would seek the men "most eminent in my own way", that is, the most eminent men-midwives – not the most eminent physicians or surgeons.[30] In a complementary move the Company of Surgeons, which separated from the Barbers in 1745, soon afterwards declared that midwifery was not part of "pure" surgery – an oblique yet eloquent testimony to the gap between traditional obstetric surgery and the new man-midwifery. Half a century later, when the surgeons acquired Collegiate aspirations and status, this exclusionist view was to harden.[31] (2) The alternative response was to assimilate man-midwifery to one of the traditional medical professions. Surgery would have been the logical association, since midwifery was a manual practice, but physic was more prestigious and lucrative; men-midwives probably wanted to distance themselves from traditional obstetric surgery; and in any case the surgeons had proclaimed that midwifery was distinct from surgery. Thus most of the specialist men-midwives of the late eighteenth century – men such as William Hunter, Thomas Denman, William Osborne, John Ford – sought to join the London College of Physicians.[32] Their subordinate status was one of the issues at stake in the Licentiates' struggle of the late 1760s, in which Hunter played a prominent part.[33] In 1783 the College offered the grudging recognition of a "licence in midwifery" – a move that acknowledged the men-midwives' skills but assigned these to the second rank, below the attainments of the learned physicians. Even this licence was discontinued in 1800, leaving man-midwifery professionally adrift.[34] At a humbler level, midwifery training, skills and practice meanwhile came to be routine for the "surgeon-apothecaries" of the late eighteenth century.[35] In consequence the lower ranks of both the surgeons and the apothecaries, who began to press for corporate medical reform from the 1790s, wanted midwifery to be included in the formal requirements of a medical education.[36] But their hopes were dashed, precisely because midwifery lay outside the framework of the corporations; indeed its formal status remained problematical well into the nineteenth century.[37]

Despite its professional limbo, male practice in midwifery became the essential entrée into "general practice" – as the work of the surgeon-apothecary came to be called. Correspondingly, as Jean Donnison has shown, the century from around 1750 to 1850 witnessed "the decline of the midwife". Male practitioners delivered more and more births, especially among the wealthier classes, and many midwives became restricted to delivering working-class mothers.[38] Yet simultaneously another transformation was taking place: the very meaning of "midwife" was changing, perhaps specifically in middle-class circles. Formerly the midwife's standing had derived from her position as the central figure in a unified women's culture. As that culture broke up, so there developed a new demand that it should be technical expertise that qualified the midwife to practise; and this demand began to be met, at least in London, by a new cadre of trained midwives. Those midwives who were taught in the lying-in hospitals and by private male teachers probably acquired a restricted set of skills, just enough to "know" what male practitioners prescribed to be their limits. But other midwives developed greater autonomy and a wider range of skills. In the 1790s both Martha

Mears and Margaret Stephen were teaching midwifery in the capital, and Mrs Stephen actually taught midwives the use of forceps – an indication that a new female tradition could absorb the methods of its male rivals.[39] Moreover, it seems that some of their pupils went out to practice in the country, just as Smellie's male pupils had done half a century earlier: three London-trained midwives had settled in Suffolk by 1805.[40] And the Lying-in Charity, subsequently renamed the Royal Maternity Charity, continued to produce skilled midwives throughout the nineteenth century. Their practical attainments led to "consistently low maternal mortality rates" among the Charity's deliveries; and it was probably these midwives who pressed most strongly for the midwife's cause in the inter-professional struggles of the nineteenth century. Perhaps this was why British midwives survived so much more successfully than their American counterparts. In America, too, male practitioners began to deliver normal births in the late eighteenth century – responding, like William Hunter, to the needs of their patients. But from this similar starting-point, customs on the two sides of the Atlantic diverged in the course of the nineteenth century. In America, the "decline of the midwife" was seemingly inexorable, and medical men became the normal childbirth practitioners. In Britain, after a protracted struggle, midwives in 1902 were accorded professional status, with the effect that normal births largely returned into their hands.[41]

In technical male obstetrics, our period appears to end with the dominance of Smellie, with the triumph of the forceps (despite Hunter's strictures and Nihell's criticisms), and with publication replacing the former practice of secrecy. But in fact this image is a retrospective projection of later practices, including a focus on textbooks. What shatters this picture is the remarkable history of the vectis, which was being used and taught in secrecy long after the forceps had been published.[42] That secrecy was only broken in the early 1780s, when Thomas Denman announced his sudden conversion from forceps to vectis – a change of attitude bitterly attacked by his erstwhile partner in forceps teaching, William Osborne. This began a public contest that was to continue for something like a century. Only in the late nineteenth century did the forceps finally displace the vectis from practice, and as late as 1904 Galabin could still write that the vectis was preferable to the forceps for delivering the commonest type of obstruction.[43] Thus the apparent hegemony of Smellie's methods in the mid-eighteenth century actually reflects the views of one party, over a century later.

It has recently been established that maternal mortality fell considerably during the eighteenth century – probably from about 13.5 to 7 deaths per 1000 births in rural areas, and from about 17 to 10.5 in London.[44] Were men-midwives responsible for this change? In London they may well have played a part, but so also did the midwives trained by the Lying-in Charity. Elsewhere the issue is unclear, since nothing is yet known of the local history of childbirth management in the handful of communities on which we still rely for charting early-modern maternal mortality outside the metropolis. If male practitioners did have such an effect, this was not necessarily in the role of midwife, for it could have arisen through a changed emergency practice. To a large extent, albeit unevenly, the forceps probably displaced the crotchet in rural general practice between about 1750 and 1800. This doubtless saved significant numbers of infant lives, reduced the incidence of prolonged obstructed labour, and thus cut down one source of serious risk to mothers. But other influences such as diet (affecting the size and shape of the mother's pelvis) and general hygiene (influencing women's exposure to puerperal infection) will have been at work. To assess the relative contributions of these different possible causes is a delicate task, requiring large numbers (since it concerns low-frequency events) and yet a local focus. It would equally be worth investigating the historical origins of the very idea of measuring maternal mortality; and the same applies to the parallel practice of estimating and counting the incidence of different kinds of births. The first rough estimates of rates of presentation-types were produced by Smellie in 1751; the first empirical count came from Felix MacDonough in 1768; and it was not until 1781 that Robert Bland published detailed figures.[45] No doubt this was part of a wider conceptual transformation, in which the domain of the social and medical was brought within a more or less mathematical net; but the application of a mathematical approach to midwifery must have had its own distinctive timing and reasons.

Since the traditional ceremony of childbirth was exclusively female, we would expect that the arrival of the man-as-midwife profoundly disrupted that ritual. Certainly the new form of man-midwifery led some medical men to criticize various components of the ritual. In 1748 William Cadogan launched a blistering attack on swaddling as an irrational female practice, explicitly connecting this with "the suffocating atmosphere of the lying-in chamber".[46] Two decades later William Buchan criticized caudle and poured particular scorn upon the use of gossips, or as he put it,

> that ridiculous custom which still prevails in some country-places, of collecting a number of women together upon such occasions. These, instead of being useful, serve only to crowd the house, and obstruct the necessary attendants. Besides, they hurt the patient with their noise; and often by their untimely and impertinent advice, do much mischief.

Buchan's wording was rhetorical, not descriptive: the customs he was describing "still prevailed" in 1769 not just "in some country-places" but everywhere, and he wanted to overthrow them. And in 1772, in his *Treatise on the management of pregnant and lying-in women*, Charles White condemned the enclosure and heating of the lying-in room – along with caudle, nurses, prolonged bed-rest and gossips – as the causes of puerperal fever.[47] Moreover, these new views had some echoes among mothers and their husbands. In the 1770s caudle was becoming "old-fashioned", while Mrs Delaney's term for lying-in became "confinement", suggesting a new perception of the process as imprisoning – and initiating the modern usage of "confinement" for birth. And in the 1790s the radical artisan Francis Place was satisfied to find that the male practitioner employed for his wife's second delivery dispensed with the caudle ("stimulating messes") and candles that the midwife had arranged at the birth of their first child.[48]

However, it is as hazardous in this sphere as in the realm of obstetric technique to build direct bridges between the eighteenth and twentieth centuries. Several considerations suggest that the new male criticisms of the ritual represent only one aspect of a more complex story. Cadogan's advice was resisted by "the ladies", and in 1769 Wallace Johnson observed that swaddling was still being practised; caudle may have been "old-fashioned", but ladies were still drinking it.[49] We recall that William Hunter – the very man who most clearly embodied the new role of the man-as-midwife, and the dedicatee of White's *Treatise* attacking the practices of women – endorsed many aspects of the traditional ceremony of childbirth.[50] In 1786 *Chambers's cyclopaedia* was still advising warmth, sweating, a darkened room and nine days' bed-rest after labour, and moreover that the mother should not leave the *room* "until a month, or until five or six weeks are over" – even though "the person who assists" at labour was assumed to be male.[51]

Among the poor the traditional ritual was observed throughout the eighteenth century and beyond. This is especially apparent in the bitter conditions of the 1790s, which brought to the attention of middle-class commentators the plight of the poor, their own response to that plight in the form of Friendly Societies, and the local welfare arrangements made under the Poor Law. The resulting documentation makes it clear that childbirth and lying-in had a high priority. Sir Frederick Morton Eden, the most systematic observer, stated that the central purpose of "Female Benefit Clubs" (women's friendly societies) was "to ensure a decent subsistence during the lying-in month". Eden also found that workhouses in the larger towns made provision for childbirth.[52] Especially revealing are the agricultural labourers' budgets collected by Eden's contemporary, the Anglican minister David Davies. Davies reckoned the expenses of lying-in at 20 shillings, assumed that this happened once in two years, and so concluded that 10 shillings per year was required. Out of an annual family budget of £7 this was a very large sum.[53] The lying-in expenses included the midwife's fee, "attendance of a nurse for a few days", "a bottle of gin or brandy always had upon this occasion" and "half a bushel of malt brewed, and hops". The fact that these expenses were standard among the poorest families in a time of extreme hardship vividly attests to the popularity of the lying-in ritual. Indeed, some features of that ritual persisted well into the nineteenth century, such as the "monthly" nurse (so named from the 1830s) and the popularity of the churching service; and medical men of the late nineteenth and early twentieth centuries endorsed the need for prolonged rest after childbirth.[54] Relatedly, the personal recollections of working women – published in the striking *Maternity letters* of the Women's Co-operative Guild (1915) – suggest that in this respect, there was no difference between having a doctor and having a midwife.[55] Thus it seems that nineteenth-century medical men supported at least some aspects of the traditional ritual.

Yet in one vital respect that ritual had disappeared by about 1900: childbirth was no longer a collective event. There is nothing in the *Maternity letters*, nor in the interview material collected by Elizabeth Roberts, to suggest the presence of friends and neighbours at working-class deliveries – where, if anywhere, the traditional ritual might have lasted longest.[56] On the contrary, these accounts suggest that birth and lying-in was now a solitary, lonely affair. The mother might have one or two female relatives present, particularly her own mother, but the gossips had now gone, and with them the caudle: childbirth had lost its convivial aspect.[57] (Perhaps it was this that led to the shift in terminology from *lying-in* to *maternity*.) Although women's collective culture and resistance to men still flourished, childbirth was now marginal in this domain.[58] What had happened to remove the gossips from the lying-in room? Arguably this was one of the effects of the new work-rhythms imposed by industrial capitalism. In the early-modern order, the separation between work and leisure was unknown: these very categories, as mutually exclusive divisions of time, are products of the age of the machine. The new work-rhythms imposed by factory and clock completely reconstructed the experience of the working day, and this had a double impact upon women: many working-class wives were themselves employed in wage-labour, and all of them had to structure their domestic labour around the routine of the husband's work. In this situation, women did not enjoy that elasticity of time required to attend labours in the capacity of gossips. A birth could last for one hour, or for two days; in the new industrial and commercial order of Victorian Britain, time was simply not available in such large and expansible chunks. For women this was especially so after 1870, since compulsory education removed the help of older children and added to wifely duties.[59] If this interpretation is correct, then it should prove possible to chart the process of transformation, between about 1800 and 1900, by which the lying-in chamber was emptied of the attending women. We should expect that this displayed very different timings in different localities, depending for instance upon social groupings, work-rhythms, relations between workplace and residence, and the involvement of women in wage-labour.

In fact, the moment at which the future of the childbirth ritual becomes most clearly visible – around 1900, through the retrospective *Maternity letters* of 1915 – was probably itself a point of transition. On closer inspection, these "letters from working women" suggest that the traditional ceremony was also declining in the domain of rest and recovery after childbirth. Several mothers wrote that they had been "lucky", able to have a good week or 10 days' rest after the birth, and not be subjected to sexual demands – "lucky", that is, to have a considerate husband.[60] And other letters attest to the opposite experience, that of being "unlucky" – forced to work, or to have sex, far too soon after the delivery.[61] Thus what had been a *right* now became a matter of *fortune* – subject to the vagaries of conjugal relations. It would seem that as the gossips disappeared from the delivery room and from lying-in, so the mother began to lose what the traditional ceremony had given her. Faced with the demands of her husband – himself under the relentless pressures of wage-labour and insecure employment – the working-class wife had to rely upon his consideration and kindness to get the period of rest and recovery that had earlier been policed by her female friends. We may suspect that the position worsened still further after 1900, and that this helped to fuel the very publication of the *Maternity letters* in 1915.

Thus it is not surprising that when hospital delivery began to be offered to working-class women on a large scale – starting in the 1930s and accelerating in the 1950s after the creation of the National Health Service – they jumped at the chance.[62] For the concomitant of birth in the hospital was a week or more of hospital rest after the delivery. Ironically, therefore, this moment of supreme medicalization probably restored to mothers something they had enjoyed for countless generations, and were only recently losing. And the medical profession, by decreeing that bed-rest after childbirth was essential, acted as the material allies of working women. What the women wanted, I am suggesting, was *lying-in*; the hospital was the only available place for this, and birth in the hospital was a means to this end. Thus the hospitalization of childbirth was an ambiguous event: while it medicalized childbirth, it also offered mothers a massive donation of human labour. To be fed, to be washed, to be removed from the demands of husband and children, to recline in bed – these were highly attractive luxuries.

What is more, the hospital maternity ward immersed the mother once more in a collective female space. Admittedly this was a different collectivity from that of the traditional ritual: the mother was now surrounded not by relatives, friends and neighbours she had invited to attend, but instead by uninvited strangers. Yet on the other hand, the little *ad hoc* society of the maternity ward was tightly focused upon childbirth: fellow-mothers were sharing the experience of giving birth, midwives and nurses were highly familiar with the needs of lying-in mothers. What bonds were forged between the women thus thrown together? What was the collective subculture of the hospital ward? How did the maternity hospital appear from the various viewpoints of the mother, the nurse and the midwife? It may be ventured that alongside the white coats, the technical apparatus, the rigid routine, the antiseptic odours of the hospital – the whole massive visibility of its medical paraphernalia – there flourished an earthy, collective, social world of shared experiences, largely forgotten after the return home, inaccessible to the outside observer, yet vital to mothers themselves in humanizing – or rather feminizing – the experience of hospital childbirth.

Notes

1. In Southwark it was led by Mrs Elizabeth Alldist, Mrs Calverley, James Burt and William Collinson (identified as founders from the numbers of their recommendations by 1769). This and other details from *An account of the Lying-in Charity for Delivering Poor Married Women at their Own Habitations. Instituted 1757.* (London, 1769). See also S. A. Seligman, "The Royal Maternity Charity", *Medical History* 24 (1980), pp. 403–18.
2. John Ford (*c.*1736–1806): see Munk, *Roll*, vol. II, p. 272. To be distinguished from his namesake, *c.*1731–1807, of Bristol and London (below).

NOTES

3. Denman, *Midwifery* (1801 edition), vol. II, p. 118; cf. Chs 10 & 11 above. In addition, Jonathan Wathen of Bartholomew Lane, another vectis practitioner, was a subscriber to the Charity in 1769: *Account of the Lying-in Charity*, p. 51.
4. Elizabeth Nihell: Born 1723; married (n.d.) James Nihell, (below); trained two years at Hôtel-Dieu, Paris, through dispensation of Duc d'Orléans; then practised, with husband, from the Haymarket; published *Traité des eaux Minerales de la Ville de Rouen* (1759); widowed 1759; date of death unknown: see Todd, *Women writers*. James Nihell: born c.1708, prob. Limerick, Ireland; medical student at Leyden 1731; MD Rheims 1733; practised at Cadiz then London; published *Observations concerning the prediction of crises by the pulse* (London, 1741), as from "the Grecian Coffee House, Devereux Court, London"; FRS 1742; died 1759: see Innes Smith, *Students at Leyden*; Wallis, *Medics*.
5. E. Nihell, *A treatise on the art of midwifery* (London, 1760), pp. 314, 320, 325, 352, 355.
6. *Ibid.*, pp. 347–8, 332.
7. Ch. 4.
8. *Critical Review*, March, 1760, pp. 187–97; E. Nihell, *An answer to the author of the Critical Review, for March, 1760, upon the article of Mrs Nihell's treatise on the art of midwifery* (London: Morley, 1760); *Critical Review*, May, 1760, p. 412; *Monthly Review*, 22 (1760), June, pp. 525–6.
9. *A letter to a young lady* (London, 1764); *Man-midwifery analyzed* (London, 1764), both published anonymously; *Man-midwifery analyzed* (2nd edn, London, 1765). On Thicknesse, see *DNB* and Philip Gosse, *Dr Viper: the querulous life of Philip Thicknesse* (London: Cassell, 1952). His anti-man-midwifery writings were perhaps directed against Dr John Ford, uncle of Thicknesse's third wife Ann Ford (who married him 1762); certainly Ford was the target of his 1790 edition. John Ford (c.1731–1807): moved from Bristol to London c.1790; taught Edward Ford, surgeon (apparently no relation); to be distinguished from his namesake, of the Lying-in Charity (above). See Munk, *Roll*, vol. II. p. 413; *DNB*, entry for Edward Ford (1746–1809); *A Letter from Miss Fo–d, addressed to a person of distinction* (London, 1761), pp. 17, 19, 23; *DNB*, entry for Ann Thicknesse (1737–1824); Philip Thicknesse, *Man-midwifery analyzed* (third edition, London, 1790), dedication.
10. *Man-midwifery analyzed* (1765 edn), p. 3.
11. *Ibid.*, pp. 21, 31–2, 13.
12. *Ibid.*, p. 13.
13. *Critical Review*, January, 1764; *ibid.*, December, 1764, p. 478, 479; *Monthly Review*, May, 1764, p. 410; *ibid.*, January 1765, pp. 71–3; *Gentlemen's Magazine*, booklists, 1764, 1765; *A letter to the author of a letter to a young lady* (London, 1764); RCSL, Tr.B.77, item 7 (a set of newspaper cuttings of anti-man-midwifery letters).
14. J. Brown, *An estimate of the manners and principles of the times* (London, 1757), pp. 29 and *passim*, 51 (quoted).
15. J. Hanway, *The defects of police* (London, 1775), pp. xx–xxi.
16. *Thoughts for the times but chiefly on the profligacy of our women* (1779); see Donnison, *Midwives*, p. 30.
17. P. Thicknesse, *Man-midwifery analyzed* (3rd edn, London, 1790); John Blunt (pseud.) *Man-midwifery dissected: or, the obstetric family instructor* (London: S. W. Fores, 1793).
18. Donnison, *Midwives*, pp. 47–8; I. Loudon, "Deaths in childbed from the eighteenth century to 1945", *Medical History* 30 (1986), pp. 1–41, p. 8, n.20; *Observations on the impropriety of men being employed in the business of midwifery* (1827); W. Cobbett, *Advice to young men and (incidentally) to young women in the middle and higher ranks of life* (1829–30). On

such literature generally see R. Porter, "A touch of danger: the man-midwife as sexual predator", in *Sexual underworlds of the Enlightenment,* G. S. Rousseau & R. Porter (eds) (Manchester, 1987), pp. 206–32.

19. Blunt (pseud.) *Man-midwifery dissected*, p. 17.
20. *The good nurse* (London, 1825), discussing lying-in, made no mention of man-midwifery, either for or against.
21. *The trial of a cause between R. Maddox, plaintiff, and Dr M—y, defendant* (London, 1754), p. 19 (cf. Glaister, *Smellie*, p. 322).
22. J. S. Lewis, *In the family way: childbearing in the British aristocracy, 1760–1860* (New Brunswick, NJ: Rutgers University Press, 1986).
23. LAO, Diary and account book of Matthew Flinders, surgeon, 1775–1784, *passim*. This assessment from a comparison of Flinders's deliveries with the population of Donington in *1801 Census*. See also I. Loudon, *Medical care and the general practitioner 1750–1850* (Oxford: Clarendon, 1986), pp. 103–5.
24. Loudon, *Medical care*, p. 90.
25. J. Lane, "A provincial surgeon and his obstetric practice: Thomas W. Jones of Henley-in-Arden, 1764–1846", *Medical History* 31 (1987), pp. 333–48, at pp. 339–40, 345.
26. I. Loudon, *Death in childbirth: an international study of maternal care and maternal mortality 1800-1950* (Oxford: Clarendon Press, 1992), pp. 177–8, and Loudon, Deaths in childbed, pp. 9–10.
27. McClintock, *Smellie's midwifery,* vol. I, pp. 58, 62. For some slightly earlier uses of women's "modesty" see John Douglas, *A short account of the state of midwifery in London and Westminster* (London, 1736), p. 36; Sarah Stone, quoted by Donnison, *Midwives*, p. 23.
28. The structure of this myth resembles the myth of the taboo on dissection. See M. Foucault, *The birth of the clinic: an archaeology of medical perception* (trans. A. M. Sheridan, London: Tavistock, 1973). An exception was Sarah Stone (see previous note); but her stance had something in common with that of male practitioners (see Ch. 4 above).
29. Loudon, *Death in childbirth*, pp. 172–3; Loudon, *Deaths in childbed*, pp. 10–11. In Dublin this problem arose slightly earlier, and took a different form, because its College of Physicians issued licences in midwifery; see S. A. Brody, "The life and times of Sir Fielding Ould: man-midwife and master physician", *Bulletin of the History of Medicine* 52 (1978), pp. 228–50, at pp. 236–7.
30. McClintock, *Smellie's midwifery,* vol. I, p. 78; vol. III, p. 222, Case 431.
31. Donnison, *Midwives*, p. 43; B. Hamilton, "The medical professions in the eighteenth century", *Economic History Review*, 2nd series, 4 (1951), pp. 141–69, at pp. 150–51; I. Waddington, "The struggle to reform the Royal College of Physicians, 1767–1771: a sociological analysis", *Medical History* 17 (1973), pp. 107–26, at p. 121. William Douglas alluded to the problem in 1748: see Glaister, *Smellie*, p. 75.
32. A notable exception was Felix Macdonough of the General Lying-in Hospital, who was a member of the Company of Surgeons and in 1772–73 became one of its two "wardens of anatomy". See C. Wall, *The history of the Surgeons' Company, 1745–1800* (London, 1937), p. 231.
33. L. G. Stevenson, "The siege of Warwick Lane: together with a brief history of the Society of Collegiate Physicians (1767–1798)", *Journal of the History of Medicine and Allied Sciences* 7 (1952), pp. 105–21; I. Waddington, "The struggle to reform the Royal College of Physicians"; Clark, *College of Physicians*, vol. II, pp. 562–4; *Medico-Mastix* (London, 1774). This gives us another way of looking at Frank Nicholls (Ch. 12); also relevant in this connection is the midwifery-licensing initiative of George Counsell, in his *The art of mid-*

wifery (London, 1752).
34. Denman and Osborne acquired this licence on 22 December 1783, Michael Underwood on 5 April 1784; Hunter and Ford were already "licentiates" in the general sense. See Munk, *Roll*, and Loudon, *Medical care*, pp. 92–3.
35. Loudon, *Medical care*, Ch. 4.
36. Donnison, *Midwives*, p. 45; Hamilton, The medical professions, p. 158.
37. See Loudon, *Death in childbirth*, p. 173, and O. Moscucci, *The science of woman: gynaecology and gender in England, 1800–1929* (Cambridge: Cambridge University Press, 1990).
38. Donnison, *Midwives*, Chs 2 & 3.
39. *Ibid.*, pp. 37–40, 61.
40. Loudon, *Death in childbirth*, p. 175.
41. *Ibid.*, p. 18 (quoted); Donnison, *Midwives*, Chs 4–8; J. B. Donegan, *Women and men midwives: medicine, morality and misogyny in early America* (Westport, Conn.: Greenwood Press, 1978); C. M. Scholten, *Childbearing in American society: 1650–1850* (New York: New York University Press, 1985), pp. 109–10; J. W. Leavitt, *Brought to bed: childbearing in America, 1750–1950* (New York & Oxford: Oxford University Press, 1986).
42. Ch. 10.
43. Galabin, *Manual of midwifery*, pp. 651–2.
44. Estimating the 1700 level as the mean of 1650–1700 and 1700–1750, and correspondingly for 1800. See R. Schofield, "Did the mothers really die? Three centuries of maternal mortality in 'the world we have lost'", in *The world we have gained*, L. Bonfield et al. (eds) (London, 1986), pp. 230–60. See also Loudon, *Death in childbirth*, pp. 158-62, and B. M. Willmott Dobbie, "An attempt to estimate the true rate of maternal mortality, sixteenth to eighteenth centuries", *Medical History* 26 (1982), pp. 79–90.
45. Ch. 2.
46. J. Rendle-Short, "Infant management in the eighteenth century with special reference to the work of William Cadogan", *Bulletin of the History of Medicine* 34 (1960), pp. 97–122; A. Wilson, "The Enlightenment and infant care", *Bulletin of the Society for the Social History of Medicine,* No. 25 (1979), pp. 44–7.
47. W. Buchan, *Domestic medicine, or, the family physician* (Edinburgh: Balfour et al., 1769), p. 571 (labelled 569); C. White, *A treatise on the management of pregnant and lying-in women* (London, 1772), *passim.*
48. R. Trumbach, *The aristocratic family in England 1690–1780: studies in childhood and kinship* (PhD thesis, John Hopkins University, 1972), p. 38; *OED*, "confine" and "confinement"; M. Thale (ed.), *The autobiography of Francis Place* (Cambridge: Cambridge University Press, 1972), p. 184.
49. J. Nelson, *An essay on the government of children under three general heads, viz. Health, Manners, and Education* (London, 1753); R. W. Johnson, *A new system of midwifery, in four parts* (London, 1769), pp. 213–14.
50. Ch. 13.
51. *Chambers's cyclopaedia* (Abraham Rees (ed.), 4 volumes; London, 1783–6), under "lying-in women", "delivery".
52. F. M. Eden, *The state of the poor* (3 volumes; London, 1797), vol. I, p. 630 (quoted on Female Benefit Clubs); vol. II, pp. 56, 239 (lying-in rooms), 189 (Bristol), 327 (Liverpool); vol. III, p. 744 (Birmingham).
53. D. Davies, *The case of the labourers in husbandry stated and considered* (London, 1795), p. 16.
54. Ch. 3 above; Galabin, *Manual of midwifery*, pp. 298, 305; T. W. Eden & E. Holland, *A*

manual of obstetrics (first published 1906; 8th edn, London: Churchill, 1940), p. 533; E. Roberts, *A woman's place: an oral history of working-class women 1890–1940* (Oxford: Blackwell, 1984), pp. 108–9.
55. *Maternity. Letters from working-women collected by the Women's Co-Operative Guild* (London: Bell, 1915): Letters 18, 37, 72, 100, 114, 134, 140, 160. See A. Davin, "Imperialism and motherhood", *History Workshop Journal* 5 (1978), pp. 9–65.
56. On the middle classes at the mid-nineteenth century, see C. A. Huff, "Chronicles of confinement: reactions to childbirth in British women's diaries", *Women's Studies International Forum* 10 (1987), pp. 63–8.
57. Roberts, *A woman's place*, p. 109; *Maternity letters*, Letters 13, 71, 99, 138, 158, 160.
58. E. Ross, "Survival networks: women's neighbourhood sharing in London before World War I", *History Workshop Journal* 15 (1983), pp. 6–27 (childbirth, pp. 10–11); *idem*, "Fierce questions and taunts: married life in working-class London, 1870–1914", *Feminist Studies* 8 (1982), pp. 575–602 (childbirth, p. 587).
59. Ross, Fierce questions and taunts, p. 578.
60. *Maternity letters*, Letters 15, 71, 82, 88, 95, 101, 123.
61. *Ibid.*, Letters 21, 73, 89, 107; also Letters 37, 41, 63, 93, 104, 111, 142, 156. Most eloquent was Letter 8, pp. 27–8: "no amount of State help can help the sufferings of mothers until men are taught . . . that the wife's body belongs to herself. . . .Very much injury and suffering comes to the mother and child through the father's ignorance and interference. . . . No animals will suffer this: why should the woman? Why, simply because of the Marriage Laws of the woman belonging to the man, to have and to own, etc.".
62. Loudon, *Deaths in childbed*, p. 22.

Bibliography

Abbreviated names and titles used in the notes are listed in alphabetic order of abbreviation.

Repositories of manuscript sources

BL: British Library
CUL: Cambridge University Library
Cumbria Record Office
Henry E. Huntingdon Library, San Marino, California
Hunterian Library, University of Glasgow
LAO: Lincolnshire Archives Office
NNRO: Norfolk and Norwich Record Office
RCPL: Royal College of Physicians, London
RCSL: Royal College of Surgeons, London
Royal Society Library
WIHM: Wellcome Institute for the History of Medicine Library, London

Manuscript sources are cited in full in the notes, except:
Hunter, lectures: RCSL, MS 42.d.25, Lecture notes on midwifery taken from William Hunter's lectures, n.d. (?1760s)

Printed primary sources

1801 Census: *Parliamentary Papers* (1802), vols VI and VII: *Abstract of the answers and returns.*
An account of the City of London Lying-in Hospital for Married Women at Shaftesbury-House in Aldersgate-Street, instituted March 30, 1750 (London, 1752).
An account of the City of London Lying-in Hospital, appended to J. Nichols, *A sermon* (London,

1767).
An account of the Lying-in Charity for Delivering Poor Married Women at their own Habitations. Instituted 1757. (London, 1769).
An account of the Lying-in Charity (London, 1776).
An account of the Middlesex-Hospital, appended to E. Cobden, *The parable of the talents. A sermon* (London, 1749).
An account of the Middlesex-Hospital, appended to J. Dalton, *A sermon . . . St Anne's, Westminster . . . April 25, 1751* (London, 1751).
An account of the Middlesex-Hospital, appended to John Thomas, *A sermon . . . St Anne's, Westminster . . . April 29, 1752* (London, 1752).
An account of the Middlesex-Hospital . . . to 24 June 1761, appended to C. Dodgson, *A sermon . . . St James Westminster . . . April 28, 1761* (London, 1761).
An account of the rise, progress, and state of the British Lying-in Hospital for Married Women . . . Brownlow-Street (London, 1756).
An account of the rise, progress, and state of the General Lying-in Hospital, the corner of Quebec-Street, Oxford-Road (London, 1768).
Allen, J., *Synopsis medicinae* (2 volumes; London, 1749 edn).
Ballard, G., *Memoirs of several ladies of Great Britain* (Oxford, 1752).
Barret, R., *A companion for midwives, childbearing women, and nurses* (London, 1699).
The Battiad (London, 1750).
Baynard, E., Appendix to Sir John Floyer, *The history of cold bathing both ancient and modern* (4th edn, London, 1715).
Bland, R., Some calculations . . . taken from the midwifery reports of the Westminster General Dispensary, *Philosophical Transactions of the Royal Society*, 71, Part I, No. 22 (1781), pp. 35–72.
Bland, R., *Some account of the invention and use of the lever of Roonhuysen* (London, 1790).
Blunt, John (pseud.), *Man-midwifery dissected: or, the obstetric family instructor* (London: S. W. Fores, 1793).
Bracken, H., *The midwife's companion, or, a treatise of midwifery; wherein the whole art is explained* (London, 1737).
Braithwaite, T., *Remarks on a short narrative . . . as published by Mr St André, Anatomist to His Majesty. With a proper regard to his intended recantation* (London, 1726).
Brown, J. *An estimate of the manners and principles of the times* (London, 1757).
Brugis, T., *The marrow of physic. Or a learned discourse of the several parts of mans body* (London, 1648).
Buchan, W., *Domestic medicine, or, the family physician* (Edinburgh: Balfour et al., 1769).
Burton, J., *An essay towards a complete new system of midwifery, theoretical and practical* (London, 1751).
Burton, J., *A letter to William Smellie, MD, containing critical and practical remarks upon his treatise* (London, 1753).
Butter, A., Description of a forceps, etc., *Medical Essays and Observations from a Society in Edinburgh* 3 (1733), p. 254.
Chambers's cyclopaedia, A. Rees (ed.) (4 volumes; London, 1783–86).
Chapman, E., *An essay on the improvement of midwifery, chiefly with regard to the operation* (London, 1733).
Chapman, E., *A treatise on the improvement of midwifery, chiefly with regard to the operation* (London, 1735).
Chapman, E., *A reply to Mr Douglas's short account of the state of midwifery in London and Westminster* (London, 1737).

Clark, W., *The province of midwives in the practice of their art* (London, 1751).
Cobbett, W., *Advice to young men and (incidentally) to young women in the middle and higher ranks of life* (London, 1829–30).
Cobden, E., *Poems on several occasions* (London, 1748).
Cockburn, W., *Symptoms . . . of gonorrhoea* (London, 1713; 2nd edn, London, 1715).
Cooke, J., *Mellificium chirurgiae; or, the marrow of chirurgery* (1648, 1662, 1676, 1685, 1693, 1717).
Counsell, G., *The art of midwifery* (London, 1752).
Cowper, W., *The anatomy of humane bodies* (London, 1698).
Crooke, H., *Microscosmographica* (2nd edn, 1631).
Culpeper, N., *A directory for midwives* (London, 1651).
Davies, D., *The case of the labourers in husbandry stated and considered* (London, 1795).
Dawkes, T., *The midwife rightly instructed* (London, 1736).
Dawkes, T., *Prodigium Willinghamense* (London, 1747).
de Mainaduc, J. B., *The lectures of J. B. de Mainaduc* (London, 1798).
de Visscher J., & H. van de Poll, *Het Roonhysiaansch geheim, in de vroedkunde ontdekt* (Leyden, 1754).
A defence of Dr Pocus and Dr Malus against the petition of the unborn babes to the Censors of the College of Physicians of London (London, 1751).
Denman, T., *Introduction to the practice of midwifery* (first published 1782; 3rd edn, London, 1801).
Diderot, D. & J-R. D'Alembert (eds), *Encyclopédie ou dictionnaire raisonnée des sciences, des arts et des métiers, par une société des gens de lettres* (Paris: Briasson, David, Le Breton & Durand, 17 volumes; 1751–57, 1765).
Dionis, P., *Traité général des accouchemens* (Paris, 1718), p. 303; trans. anon. as *A general treatise of midwifery* (London, 1719).
Doughty, S., *Christian sympathy* (London, 1752).
Douglas, James, *An advertisement occasion'd by some passages in Sir R. Manningham's diary lately publish'd* (London, 1727).
Douglas, James, *The history of the lateral operation* (London, 1726).
Douglas, John, *A dissertation on the venereal disease* (London, 1737).
Douglas, John, *A dissertation on the venereal disease. Part II* (London, 1737).
Douglas, John, *A dissertation on the venereal disease. Part III* (London, n.d.).
Douglas, John, *A short account of the state of midwifery in London, Westminster, &c.* (London, 1736).
Douglas, W., *A letter to Dr Smelle, shewing the impropriety of his new-invented wooden forceps* (London, 1748, reprinted in Glaister, *Smellie*, pp. 74–84).
Douglas, W., *A second letter to Dr Smellie and an answer to his pupil* (London, 1748, summarized in Glaister, *Smellie*, pp. 89–97).
Dover, T., *The ancient physician's legacy to his country* (London, 1742).
Drake, J., *Anthropologia nova* (1707).
Eden, Sir Frederick Morton, *The state of the poor* (3 volumes; London, 1797).
Exton, B., *A new and general system of midwifery* (London, 1751; 2nd edn, 1766).
Flamingo (pseud.), *A shorter and truer advertisement by way of supplement, to what was published the 7th instant: or, Dr D–g–l–s in an extasy, at Lacey's Bagio, December the 4th, 1726* (London, 1727).
Ford, A., *A letter from Miss Fo–d, addressed to a person of distinction* (London, 1761).
Gibson, E., *Codex Juris Ecclesiae Anglicani* (2nd edn, 2 volumes; Oxford, 1761).

Giffard, W., *Cases in midwifery, revis'd and edited by Edward Hody, MD* (London, 1734).
The good nurse (London, 1825).
Goodall, C. *The College of Physicians . . . established by law* (London, 1684).
Groeneveldt, John (Johannes), *Tutus cantharidum in medicina usus internus* (1679).
Gulliver, Lemuel (pseud.), *The anatomist dissected* (London, 1726).
Hanway, J., *The defects of police* (London, 1775).
Harrison, E., *Remarks on the ineffective state of the practice of physic in Great Britain; with proposals . . . and the resolutions of the members of the Medical Benevolent Society in Lincolnshire* (London, 1806).
Herbinieaux, M. G., *Traité sur divers accouchemens laborieux* (Brussels, 1782).
Houstoun, J., *Memoirs of the life and travels of James Houstoun, MD, collected and written by his own hand* (London, 1747).
Hunter, W., *Anatomy of the gravid uterus* (Birmingham, 1774).
Hunter, W., On the uncertainty of the signs of murder, in the case of bastard children. By the late William Hunter . . . Read July 14, 1783, *Medical Observations and Inquiries* 6 (1784).
Iatro-Rapsodica: or, a physical rhapsody (London, 1751).
Johnston, R. W., *A new system of midwifery, in four parts* (London, 1769).
The lady's decoy: or, the man-midwife's defence (London, 1738).
La Motte, G. M., *A general treatise of midwifery: illustrated with upwards of four hundred curious observations and reflexions concerning that art* (French original 1722; trans. Thomas Tomkyns, London, 1746).
Lawrence, T., *Franci Nicholsii vita* (London, 1780).
A letter to the author of a letter to a young lady (London, 1764).
Manley, M. D., *Secret memoirs and manners of several persons of quality, of both sexes. From the New Atalantis, an island in the Mediterranean* (London, 1709).
Manningham, Sir Richard, *Artis obstetricariae compendium tam theoriam quam praxin spectans* (London, 1739); trans. anon. as *An abstract of midwifery for use in the Lying-In Infirmary* (London, 1744).
Manningham, Sir Richard, *An exact diary of what was observed during a close attendance upon Mary Toft* (London, n.d.).
Maternity. Letters from working-women collected by the Women's Co-Operative Guild (London: Bell, 1915).
Maubray, J., *The female physician* (London, 1724).
Maubray, J., *Midwifery brought to perfection by manual operation* (London, 1725).
Mauriceau, F., *Traité des maladies des femmes grosses* (Paris, 1668); trans. Hugh Chamberlen as *The accomplisht midwife* (London, 1673), reissued as *The diseases of women with child* (1683, 1697, 1710, 1716, 1718, 1727, 1736, 1752).
Mauriceau, F., *Aphorisms . . . Translated by Thomas Jones* (London & Norwich, 1739).
Medico-Mastix (London, 1774).
Milward, E., *Trallianus reviviscens* (London, 1734).
Milward, E., *A circular invitatory letter . . . concerning . . . an history . . . of the most celebrated British physical and chirurgical authors* (London, 1740).
Mulder, J. *Historia litteraria et critica forcipium et vectium obstetriciorum* (Leyden, 1794).
Nelson, J., *An essay on the government of children under three general heads, viz. Health, Manners, and Education* (London, 1753).
Nicholls, F., *Compendium anatomico-oeconomicum ea omnia complectens, quae ad cognitam humani corporis oeconomicum spectant* (London, 1733; 5th edn, 1746).
Nihell, E. *Traité des eaux minerales de la Ville de Rouen* (1759).

Nihell, E. *A treatise on the art of midwifery* (London, 1760).
Nihell, E. *An answer to the author of the Critical Review, for March, 1760, upon the article of Mrs Nihell's treatise on the art of midwifery* (London: Morley, 1760).
Nihell, J. *Observations concerning the prediction of crises by the pulse* (London, 1741).
Observations on the impropriety of men being employed in the business of midwifery (1827).
Osborn, W., *Essays on the practice of midwifery in natural and difficult labours* (London, 1792).
Ould, F., *A treatise of midwifery* (Dublin, 1742).
Parsons, J., *Praelecturi Jacobi Parsons, MD, elenchus gynaico pathologicus et obstetricarius* (London, 1741).
Perfect, W., *Cases in midwifery, with references, quotations, and remarks* (2 volumes; Rochester, n.d. & 1783).
The petition of the unborn babes to the Censors of the College of Physicians (1751).
Philalethes (pseud.), *The sooterkin dissected. In a letter to John Maubray, MD, alias Dr Giovanni. By a lover of truth and learning* (London, 1726, reprinted 1727).
Pilkington, L., *Memoirs of Mrs Laetitia Pilkington* (first published 1748; reprinted, 3 volumes in 1; London: Routledge, 1928).
Portal, P., *The complete practice of men and women midwives ... illustrated with a considerable number of observations* (French original 1685; trans. anon., London, 1705).
Pugh, B., *A treatise of midwifery, chiefly with regard to the operation. With several improvements in that art* (London, 1754).
Read, A., *Chirurgorum comes, or the whole practice of chirurgery* (London, 1687).
Rueff, J., *De conceptu et generatione hominis* (Zurich, 1554).
Scultetus, J., *The chyrurgeon's store-house* (trans. J. Ruding; London, 1674).
Sharp, J., *The midwives book* (London, 1671).
Southwell, T., *Remarks on some of the errors both in anatomy and practice, contained in a late treatise of midwifry, published by Fielding Ould, man-midwife* (Dublin: Thomas Bacon, 1742).
Southwell, T., *A continuation of remarks on Mr Ould's midwifry* (London: Thomas Meigham, 1744).
The state of physic (London, 1742).
Stone, S., *A complete practice of midwifery* (London, 1737).
Stuart, A., *New discoveries in surgery* (London, 1738).
Thicknesse, P., *A letter to a young lady* (London, 1764; published anonymously).
Thicknesse, P., *Man-midwifery analyzed* (London, 1764; published anonymously).
Thicknesse, P., *Man-midwifery analyzed* (2nd edn, London, 1765).
Thoughts for the times but chiefly on the profligacy of our women (1779).
Torriano, N., *Compendium obstetricii: or, a small tract on the formation of the foetus, and the practice of midwifery* (London, 1753; in his English translation of J. B. L. Chomel, *An historical dissertation on ... sore throat*, French original Paris, 1749).
The trial of a cause between R. Maddox, plaintiff, and Dr M—y, defendant (London, 1754).
Turner, D., *The art of surgery* (2nd edn, London, 1725).
van Deventer, H., *Operationes chirurgicae, novum lumen exhibentes obstetricantibus* (Leyden, 1701).
van Deventer, H., *The art of midwifery improv'd* (trans. Robert Samber, London, 1716).
van Deventer, H., *New improvements in the art of midwifery* (London, 1724), translated from *Operationes chirurgicae* (Leyden, 1724), Part II. James Vaughan, *Cases ... hydrophobia ... Caesarean section* (London, 1778).
Viardel, C., *Observations sur la pratique des accouchemens* (Paris, 1671, reprinted 1673, 1674).
A vindication of man-midwifery, being the answer of Dr Pocus, Dr Malus, and Dr Barebones, and

others, their brethren, who, like Legion, are many, to the petition of the unborn babes, &c. In a letter to the President and Censors, and The Elect, of the College of Physicians, London (London, 1752).

von Heister, L., ("Laurence Heister"), *A general system of surgery in three parts* (German original 1718; trans. anon., London, 1743).

Wheatley, C., *A rational illustration of the Book of Common Prayer of The Church of England* (1st edn 1710; 4th edn, London, 1722).

White, C., *A treatise on the management of pregnant and lying-in women* (London, 1772).

Newspapers and periodicals

Adams's Weekly Courant
Commons Journals
Critical Review
Gentleman's Magazine
Historical Register
Medical Essays and Observations from a Society in Edinburgh
Monthly Review
Newcastle Chronicle
Newcastle Courant
Philosophical Transactions of the Royal Society

Editions and compilations of original sources

Barbour, P. L. (ed.), *An essay to revive the antient education of gentlewomen* by Bathsua Makin (London, 1673); Augustan Reprint Society Publication No. 202 (William Andrews Clark Memorial Library, 1980).

Beresford, J. (ed.), *The diary of a country parson: the Reverend James Woodforde. Vol. I, 1758–1781* (Oxford: Clarendon, 1924).

Beresford, J. (ed.), *The diary of a country parson 1758–1802 by James Woodford: passages selected* (Oxford: Oxford University Press, 1978).

Bloom, J. H. & R. R. James, *Medical practitioners in the diocese of London, licensed under the Act of 3 Henry VIII, c. 11: an annotated list 1529–1725* (Cambridge, 1935).

Brock, *William Hunter*: Brock, C. H. (ed.), *William Hunter 1718–1783: a Memoir by Samuel Foart Simmons and John Hunter* (Glasgow: University of Glasgow Press, 1983).

Campion, W. M. & W. J. Beaumont (eds), *The Prayer Book interleaved with historical illustrations* (10th edn, London, 1880).

Cartwright, J. J. (ed.), *Wentworth papers 1705–39* (London, 1883).

Clark, A. (ed.), *The life and times of Anthony Wood, antiquary, of Oxford, 1632–1695, described by himself* (5 volumes; Oxford, 1891–1900).

Cohen, R. A., Documents concerning James Cooke, surgeon, of Warwick, *Medical History* 1 (1957), pp. 168–73.

CSPD: Calendar of State Papers, Domestic Series (London: HMSO, various dates).

Hearne, *Remarks*: C. E. Doble et al. (eds), *Remarks and collections of Thomas Hearne*, (11 volumes; Oxford, 1885–1921),.

Hey, D. (ed.), *The history of Myddle* by Richard Gough (Harmondsworth: Penguin, 1981).
Hill, B. (ed.), *The first English feminist: "Reflections upon marriage" and other writings by Mary Astell* (Aldershot: Gower/Temple Smith, 1986).
Hitchcock, J., A sixteenth-century midwife's license, *Bulletin of the History of Medicine* 41 (1967), pp. 75–6.
HMC *Egmont*: Historical Manuscripts Commission: *Manuscripts of the Earl of Egmont: Diary of Viscount Percival, afterwards First Earl of Egmont* (3 volumes; London: HMSO, 1920–23).
Hobhouse, E. (ed.), *The diary of a West Country physician AD 1684–1726* (London: Simpkin Marshall, 1934).
Holmberg, B., *James Douglas on English pronunciation c.1740* (Lund: C. W. K. Gleerup, 1956).
Innes Smith, *Students at Leyden*: R. W. Innes Smith, *English-speaking students of medicine at the University of Leyden* (Edinburgh: Oliver & Boyd, 1932).
Jackson, C. (ed.), *The autobiography of Mrs. Alice Thornton, of East Newton, Co. York* (Surtees Society Publications, vol. LXII), 1873.
James, G. P. R. (ed.), *Letters illustrative of the reign of King William III* (3 volumes; London: Colburn, 1841).
Johnson, H. C. & J. H. Hodson (eds), *Warwick County Records Volume VIII: Quarter Sessions records Trinity, 1682, to Epiphany, 1690* (Warwick, 1953).
Johnson, H. C. & N. J. Williams (eds), *Warwick County Records Volume IX: Quarter Sessions records Easter, 1690, to Michaelmas, 1696* (Warwick, 1964).
Josselin, *Diary*: A. Macfarlane (ed.), *The diary of Ralph Josselin 1616–1683* (British Academy Records of Social and Economic History, New Series, III), 1976.
Kennedy, W. P. M., *Elizabethan episcopal administration* (3 volumes; London, 1924).
Linnell, C. D. (ed.), The diary of Benjamin Rogers, Rector of Carlton, 1720–71, *Publications of the Bedfordshire Historical Records Society,* 30 (1950).
Linnell, C. L. S. (ed.), *The diaries of Thomas Wilson, DD, 1731–37 and 1750, son of Bishop Wilson of Sodor and Man* (London: SPCK, 1964).
Lady Llanover (ed.), *The autobiography and correspondence of Mary Granville, Mrs Delany* (3 volumes; London, 1861).
Magrath, J. R. (ed.), *The Flemings in Oxford; being documents selected from the Rydal papers in illustration of the lives and ways of Oxford men 1650–1700* (3 volumes; Oxford Historical Society, 1904–24).
Matthews, R. C. & W. Latham (eds), *The diary of Samuel Pepys* (11 volumes; London, 1970–83).
McClintock, *Smellie's midwifery*: McClintock, A. H. (ed.), *Smellie's treatise on the theory and practice of midwifery* (3 volumes; New Sydenham Society, London, 1876–8).
Moody, H. M. The Monnington letters 1720–25, *Worcestershire Recusant* 3, No. 21 (1973), pp. 8–19.
Moore, N., *The history of St Bartholomew's Hospital* (2 volumes; London: C. Pearson, 1918).
Morsley, C. *News from the English countryside 1750–1850* (London: Harrap, 1979).
Nankivell, P. H., Certificate of attendance at William Smellie's lectures, 1757, *Medical History* 1 (1957), pp. 279–80.
Nichols, J., *Literary anecdotes of the eighteenth century* (9 volumes; London, 1812–16; facsimile reprint New York, 1986).
Pady, D. S., A London medical satire of 1607, *Journal of the History of Medicine and Allied Sciences* 33 (1978), pp. 409–16.
Parkinson, R. (ed.), *The autobiography of Henry Newcome, MA, vol. I* (Chetham Society, *Remains Historical and Literary*, 26, 1852).
Pollock L. (ed.), *A lasting relationship: parents and children over three centuries* (London, 1987).

Roberts, P. (ed.), *The diary of Sir David Hamilton 1709–1714* (Oxford: Clarendon, 1975).
Second report of the Commissioners appointed to inquire into the Rubrics, Orders, and directions for regulating the course and conduct of public worship, &c. (London: HMSO, 1868).
Smith, D. N. (ed.), *The letters of Thomas Burnet to George Duckett, 1712–1722* (London, Roxburgh Club, 1914).
Spalding, R. (ed.), *The diary of Bulstrode Whitelocke 1605–1675* (British Academy: Records of Social and Economic History, New Series, XIII; Oxford University Press, 1990).
Thale, M. (ed.), *The autobiography of Francis Place* (Cambridge: Cambridge University Press, 1972).
Vaisey, D. (ed.), *The diary of Thomas Turner 1754–1765* (Oxford: Oxford University Press, 1985).
Venn, J & J. A. Venn, *Alumni cantabrigiensis: a biographical list of all known students, graduates and holders of office at the University of Cambridge . . . Part I, from the earliest times to 1751* (4 volumes; Cambridge, 1922–27).
Verney, M. M. (ed.), *Memoirs of the Verney family* (4 volumes; London: Longmans, 1892–9).
Wigfield, W. McD., *The Monmouth rebels, 1685* (Gloucester: Alan Sutton, 1985).
Williams, H. (ed.), *Journal to Stella* by Jonathan Swift (2 volumes; Oxford, 1948).
Willughby, *Observations*: H. Blenkinsop (ed.), *Observations in midwifery. As also the country midwife's opusculum or vade mecum*, by Percival Willughby (Warwick, 1863; facsimile reprint John L. Thornton (ed.), Wakefield, 1972); *ibid.*, London version: BL, Sloane MS 529, fols. 1–19 (transcript in Wilson, Childbirth, Appendix B).
Young, S., *The annals of the Barber-Surgeons of London, compiled from their records and other sources* (London: Blades, East & Blades, 1890).

Secondary works

Amussen, S. D., Gender, family and the social order, 1560–1725, in *Order and disorder in early modern England*, J. Stevenson & A. Fletcher (eds) (Cambridge, Cambridge University Press 1985), pp. 196–217.
Andrew, D., *Philanthropy and police: London charity in the eighteenth century* (Princeton, NJ, 1989).
Armstrong, N., *Desire and domestic fiction: a political history of the novel* (Oxford: Oxford University Press, 1987).
Aveling, J. H., *The Chamberlens and the midwifery forceps: memorials of the family and an essay on the invention of the instrument* (London: Churchill, 1882).
Aveling, J. H., *English midwives: their history and prospects* (London: Churchill, 1872).
Aveling, J. H., Biographical sketches of British obstetricians: James Cooke, *Obstetrical Journal of Great Britain and Ireland* 1 (1873–74), pp. 449–52.
Baker, J. H., *An introduction to English legal history* (2nd edn; London, 1979).
Ballantyne, J. W., The "Byrth of Mankynde", *Journal of Obstetrics and Gynaecology of the British Empire*, 10 (1906), pp. 297–325; 12 (1907), pp. 175–94, 255–74; 17 (1910), pp. 329–32.
Ballaster, R., *Seductive forms: women's amatory fiction from 1684 to 1740* (Oxford, Clarendon, 1992).
Barrell, J., *English literature in History 1730–80: an equal, wide survey* (London: Hutchinson, 1983).
Bechler, R., "Triall by what is Contrary": Samuel Richardson and Christian dialectic, in *Samuel Richardson: passion and prudence*, V. G. Myer (ed.), (London: Vision, 1986), pp. 93–113.

Benedek, T. G., The changing relationship between midwives and physicians during the Renaissance, *Bulletin of the History of Medicine* 51 (1977), pp. 550–64.

Benjamin, M, Women and natural philosophy in eighteenth century England (MPhil thesis, University of Cambridge, 1986).

Berry, B. M. & R. S. Schofield, Age at baptism in pre-industrial England, *Population Studies* 25 (1971), pp. 453–63.

W. Berry, *County pedigrees: Essex* (London: Sherwood, Gilbert & Piper, 1840).

BL Catalogue: The British Library Catalogue of Printed Books to 1975 (360 volumes; London: K. G. Saw, 1979–87).

Boase, G. C. & W. P. Courtney, *Bibliotheca cornubiensis*, vol. I (3 volumes; London: Longman, 1874–82).

Boulton, J., *Neighbourhood and society: a London suburb in the seventeenth century* (Cambridge, 1987).

Brock, H., James Douglas of the pouch, *Medical History* 18 (1974), pp. 162–72.

Brock, H., James Douglas (1675–1742), botanist, *Journal for the Society for Bibliography of Natural History* 9 (1979), pp. 137–45.

Brock, H., The happiness of riches, in *William Hunter*, Bynum & Porter (eds), pp. 35–54.

Brody, S. A., The life and times of Sir Fielding Ould: man-midwife and master physician, *Bulletin of the History of Medicine* 52 (1978), pp. 228–50.

Butterton, J., The education, naval service and early career of William Smellie, *Bulletin of the History of Medicine* 60 (1986), pp. 1–18.

Bynum, W. F. & Roy Porter (eds), *William Hunter and the eighteenth century medical world* (Cambridge: Cambridge University Press, 1985).

Calder-Marshall, A., *The grand century of the lady* (London: Gordon & Cremonesi, 1976).

Capp, B., *Astrology and the popular press* (London: Faber, 1979).

Carwardine, H. H. (mis-spelt "Cansardine"), Brief notice presented to the medico-chirurgical society with the original obstetric instruments of the Chamberlens, *Medico-Chirurgical Transactions* 9 (1818), pp. 181–4.

Cash, A. H., The birth of Tristram Shandy: Sterne and Dr Burton, in *Studies in the eighteenth century*, R. F. Brissenden (ed.) (Canberra: Australian National University Press, 1968), pp. 133–54.

Cavallo, S., The motivations of benefactors: an overview of approaches to the study of charity, in *Medicine and charity before the Welfare State*, J. Barry & C. Jones (eds) (London: Routledge, 1991), pp. 46–62.

Clark, *College of Physicians*: Sir George Clark, *A history of the Royal College of Physicians of London* (2 volumes; Oxford, 1964–66).

Clark, H. E., *A rare medical book and its author* (Glasgow: Macdougall, 1899).

Clark-Kennedy, A. E., *London Pride: the story of a voluntary hospital* (London: Hutchinson, 1979).

Clay, C. G., *Economic expansion and social change: England, 1500–1700* (2 volumes; Cambridge, 1984).

Cohen, E., Medical debates on women's "Nature" in England around 1700, *Bulletin of the Society for the Social History of Medicine*, No. 39 (1985), pp. 7–11.

Colley, L., *In defiance of oligarchy: the Tory party 1714–60* (Cambridge: Cambridge University Press, 1982).

Collins, H., *Changing order: Replication and induction in scientific practice* (London: Sage, 1985).

Cook, H. J., *The decline of the old medical regime in Stuart London* (London: Cornell University

Press, 1986).

Cook, H. J., Practical medicine and the British armed forces after the "Glorious Revolution", *Medical History* 34 (1990), pp. 1–26.

Coster, W., Purity, profanity and Puritanism: the churching of women, 1500–1700, in *Women in the church,* W. J. Sheils & D. Wood (eds), (Oxford: Blackwell, for the Ecclesiastical History Society, 1990), pp. 377–87.

Cox, J., *The English churches in a secular society: Lambeth, 1870–1930* (Oxford, Oxford University Press, 1982).

Crawford, P., From the woman's view: pre-industrial England, 1500–1750, in *Exploring women's past,* Crawford (ed.) (2nd edn; Sydney, 1984), pp. 49–85.

Cressy, D., *Literacy and the social order* (Cambridge: Cambridge University Press, 1980).

Cressy, D., Purification, thanksgiving, and the churching of women in post-Reformation England, *Past & Present*, No. 141 (1993), pp. 106–46.

Cunningham, A., Medicine to calm the mind: Boerhaave's medical system, and why it was adopted in Edinburgh, in *The medical enlightenment of the eighteenth century,* A. Cunningham & R. French (eds) (Cambridge: Cambridge University Press, 1990), pp. 40–66.

Cunnington, P. & C. Lucas, *Costume for births, marriages and deaths* (London, 1972).

Das, K., *Obstetric forceps: its history and evolution* (Calcutta: The Art Press, 1929; reprinted by Medical Museum Publishing, Leeds, 1993).

Davin, A., Imperialism and motherhood, *History Workshop Journal* 5 (1978), pp. 9–65.

Davis, D., *A history of shopping* (London: Routledge, 1966).

Day, R. A., *Told in letters: epistolary fiction before Richardson* (Ann Arbor, Michigan: University of Michigan Press, 1970).

Dobbie, B. M. W., An attempt to estimate the true rate of maternal mortality, sixteenth to eighteenth centuries, *Medical History* 26 (1982), pp. 79–90.

DNB: *The Dictionary of National Biography,* L. Stephen & S. Lee (eds) (63 volumes; London, 1885–1900).

Donegan, J. B., *Women and men midwives: medicine, morality and misogyny in early America* (Westport, Conn.: Greenwood Press, 1978).

Donnison, J., *Midwives and medical men: a history of inter-professional rivalries and women's rights* (London: Heinemann, 1977).

Donnison, J., Note on the foundation of Queen Charlotte's Hospital, *Medical History* 15 (1971), pp. 398–400.

DSB: *Dictionary of Scientific Biography,* C. C. Gillespie (ed.) (16 volumes; New York, 1970).

Eagleton, T., *The rape of Clarissa* (Minneapolis: University of Minnesota Press, 1982).

Peter Earle, The female labour market in London in the late seventeenth and early eighteenth centuries, *Economic History Review*, 2nd series, 42 (1989), pp. 328–53.

Eaves, T. C. D. & B. D. Kimpel, *Samuel Richardson: a biography* (Oxford: Clarendon Press, 1971).

Eccles, A., *Obstetrics and gynaecology in Tudor and Stuart England* (London: Croom Helm, 1982).

Eden, T. W. & E. Holland, *A manual of obstetrics* (first published 1906; 8th edn, London: Churchill, 1940).

Ehrenreich, B. & D. English, *Witches, midwives and nurses: a history of women healers* (New York: Feminist Press, 1973).

Evenden, D., Mothers and their midwives in seventeenth-century London, in *Art of midwifery,* Marland (ed.), pp. 9–26.

Faller, L. B., *Turned to account: the forms and functions of criminal biography in late seventeenth-*

and early eighteenth-century England (Cambridge, 1987).

Filippini, N. M., The Church, the State and childbirth: the midwife in Italy during the eighteenth century, in *Art of midwifery,* Marland (ed.), pp. 152–75.

Finlay, R., *Population and metropolis* (Cambridge, 1981).

Fissell, M. E., *Patients, power and the poor in eighteenth-century Bristol* (Cambridge: Cambridge University Press, 1991).

Forbes, T. R., The regulation of English midwives in the sixteenth and seventeenth centuries, *Medical History* 8 (1964), pp. 235–44.

Forbes, T. R., *The midwife and the witch* (New Haven, Conn.: Yale University Press, 1966).

Forbes, T. R., *Chronicle from Aldgate: life and death in Shakespeare's London* (New Haven & London: Yale University Press, 1971).

Forbes, T. R., A jury of matrons, *Medical History* 32 (1988), pp. 23–33.

Foucault, M., *The birth of the clinic: an archaeology of medical perception* (trans. A. M. Sheridan; London: Tavistock, 1973).

Fraser, A., *The weaker vessel: woman's lot in seventeenth century England* (2nd edn; London, 1985).

Galabin, A. L., *A manual of midwifery* (6th edn; London: Churchill, 1904).

Garrison, *History of medicine*: F. H. Garrison, *An introduction to the history of medicine: with medical chronology, suggestions for study and bibliographic data* (Philadelphia: Saunders, 1929).

Gelbart, N., Midwife to a nation: Mme du Coudray serves France, in *Art of midwifery,* Marland (ed.), pp. 131–51.

George, D., *London life in the eighteenth century* (first published 1925; Harmondsworth: Penguin, 1966).

Glaister, *Smellie*: J. Glaister, *Dr William Smellie and his contemporaries: a contribution to the history of midwifery in the eighteenth century* (Glasgow: Maclehose, 1894).

Gosse, P., *Dr Viper: the querulous life of Philip Thicknesse* (London: Cassell, 1952).

Grundy, I., Sarah Stone: Enlightenment midwife, in *Medicine and the Enlightenment*, R. Porter (ed.) (Amsterdam: Rodopi, 1994).

Guy, J. R., Archbishop Secker as a physician, in *The church and healing,* W. J. Sheils (ed.) (Oxford: Blackwell, for the Ecclesiastical History Society, 1982), pp. 127–35.

Hamilton, B., The medical professions in the eighteenth century, *Economic History Review*, 2nd series, 4 (1951), pp. 141–69.

Harley, D. N., Ignorant midwives – a persistent stereotype, *Bulletin of the Society for the Social History of Medicine*, No. 28 (1981), pp. 6–9.

Harley, D., Historians as demonologists: the myth of the midwife-witch, *Social History of Medicine* 3 (1990), pp. 1–26.

Harley, D., Honour and property: the structure of professional disputes in eighteenth-century medicine, in *The medical enlightenment of the eighteenth century,* A. Cunningham & R. French (eds) (Cambridge: Cambridge University Press, 1990), pp. 138–64.

Harley, D., Ethics and dispute behaviour in the career of Henry Bracken of Lancaster, surgeon, physician and manmidwife, in *The codification of medical morality in the eighteenth and nineteenth centuries,* R. Baker et al. (eds), (Dordrecht, 1993), pp. 47–71.

Harley, D., Provincial midwives in England: Lancashire and Cheshire, 1660–1760, in *Art of midwifery*, Marland (ed.) pp. 27–48.

Harvey, A. D., *Literature into history* (London: Macmillan 1988).

Hess, A. G., Midwifery practice amongst the Quakers in southern rural England in the late seventeenth century, in *Art of midwifery*, Marland (ed.), pp. 49–76.

Higgins, P., The reactions of women, with special reference to the women petitioners, in *Poli-*

tics, religion and the English civil war, B. Manning (ed.) (London, 1973), pp. 179–222.

Horsfield, J. K., *British monetary experiments 1650–1710* (London: Bell, 1960).

Houtzager, H. L., Hendrik van Deventer, *European Journal of Obstetrics, Gynaecology and Reproductive Biology* 21 (1986), pp. 263–70.

Hudson, G., The politics of credulity: the Mary Toft case (MPhil dissertation, Cambridge, 1987).

Huff, C. A., Chronicles of confinement: reactions to childbirth in British women's diaries, *Women's Studies International Forum,* 10 (1987), pp. 63–8.

Hunter, J. P., *Before novels: the cultural context of eighteenth century fiction* (New York & London: W. W. Norton, 1990).

Ingerslev, E., Rösslin's "Rosegarten": its relation to the past (the Muscio manuscripts and Soranos), particularly with regard to podalic version, *Journal of Obstetrics and Gynaecology of the British Empire,* 15 (1909), pp. 1–25, 73–92.

Johnstone, R. W., *William Smellie, the master of British midwifery* (Edinburgh: Livingstone, 1952).

Jones, E., The life and times of Gulielmus Fabricius Hildanus (1560–1634), *Medical History* 4 (1960), pp. 112–34, 196–209.

Jordanova, L. J., Gender, generation and science: William Hunter's obstetrical atlas, in *William Hunter,* Bynum & Porter (eds), pp. 385–412.

Kenyon, J. P., The birth of the Old Pretender, *History Today* 13 (1965), pp. 418–26.

Keynes, G., *The life of William Harvey* (Oxford: Clarendon, 1966).

King, H., The politick midwife: models of midwifery in the work of Elizabeth Cellier, in *Art of midwifery,* Marland (ed.), pp. 115–30.

Kinnaird, J., Mary Astell and the conservative contribution to English feminism, *Journal of British Studies* 19 (1979), pp. 53–75.

Kitzinger, S., *Birth at Home* (Oxford: Oxford University Press, 1979).

Kitzinger, S., & J. Davis (eds), *The place of birth* (Oxford: Oxford University Press, 1978).

Kroll, R., *The material word: literate culture in the Restoration and early eighteenth century* (Baltimore & London: Johns Hopkins University Press, 1991).

Lane, J., The administration of an eighteenth century Warwickshire parish: Butlers Marston, *Dugdale Society Occasional Papers,* No. 21 (1973).

Lane, J., A provincial surgeon and his obstetric practice: Thomas W. Jones of Henley-in-Arden, 1764–1846, *Medical History* 31 (1987), pp. 333–48.

Lawson, J. B. & D. B. Stewart (eds), *Obstetrics and gynaecology in the tropics and developing countries* (London: Edward Arnold, 1967).

Leap, N. & B. Hunter, *The midwife's tale: an oral history of childbirth in the twentieth century* (London: Scarlet Press, 1993).

Leavitt, J. W., *Brought to bed: childbearing in America, 1750-1950* (New York & Oxford: Oxford University Press, 1986).

Lewis, J. S., *In the family way: childbearing in the British aristocracy, 1760–1860* (New Brunswick, NJ: Rutgers University Press, 1986).

Lindeman, M., Professionals? Sisters? Rivals? Midwives in Braunschweig, 1750–1800, in *Art of midwifery,* Marland (ed.), pp. 176–91.

Lipton, E. L. et al., Swaddling, a child care practice: historical, cultural and experimental observations, *Paediatrics,* Supplement, 35 (1965), pp. 519–67.

Loudon, I., *Medical care and the general practitioner 1750–1850* (Oxford: Clarendon, 1986).

Loudon, I., *Death in childbirth: an international study of maternal care and maternal mortality 1800-1950* (Oxford: Clarendon Press, 1992).

Loudon, I., Deaths in childbed from the eighteenth century to 1945, *Medical History* 30 (1986), pp. 1–41.
McClure, R. K., *Coram's children: the London Foundling Hospital in the eighteenth century* (New Haven, Conn.: Yale University Press, 1981).
Macdonald, M., *Mystical bedlam: madness, anxiety and healing in seventeenth-century England* (Cambridge: Cambridge University Press, 1981).
McKendrick, N. et al., *The birth of a consumer society* (Bloomington, Indiana: Indiana University Press, 1982).
McKeon, M., *The origins of the English novel 1600–1740* (Baltimore: John Hopkins University Press, 1987).
McLachlan, G. & T. McKeown (eds), *Medical history and medical care* (London, 1971).
Malcolmson, R. W., Infanticide in the eighteenth century, in *Crime in England, 1550–1800,* J. S. Cockburn (ed.) (London: Methuen, 1977), pp. 187–209.
Marland, *Art of midwifery*: Marland, H. (ed.), *The art of midwifery: early modern midwives in Europe* (London: Routledge, 1993).
Marland, H., *Medicine and society in Wakefield and Huddersfield 1780–1870* (Cambridge: Cambridge University Press, 1987).
Marland, H., The "burgerlijke" midwife: the stadsvroedvrouw of eighteenth-century Holland, in *Art of midwifery*, Marland (ed.), pp. 192–213.
Marshall, D., *The English poor in the eighteenth century: a study in social and administrative history* (London: Routledge, 1926).
Marshall, D., *Dr Johnson's London* (London: Wiley, 1968).
Mendelson, S. H. Stuart women's diaries and occasional memoirs, in *Women in English society,* M. Prior (ed.), *1500–1800* (London, 1985), pp. 181–210.
Morgan, F., *The female wits: women playwrights on the London stage 1660–1720* (London: Virago, 1981).
Moscucci, O., *The science of woman: gynaecology and gender in England, 1800–1929* (Cambridge: Cambridge University Press, 1990).
Munk, *Roll*: W. Munk, *Roll of the Royal College of Physicians of London* (3 volumes; 2nd edn, London, 1878).
Nichols, R. H. & F. H. Wray, *The history of the Foundling Hospital*, London, 1935.
OED: *The Oxford English Dictionary* (12 volumes; Oxford, 1933).
Okin, S. M., Women and the making of the sentimental family, *Philosophy and Public Affairs* 11 (1982), pp. 65–88.
Okin, S. M., Patriarchy and married women's property in England: questions on some current views, *Eighteenth-Century Studies* 17 (1983), pp. 121–38.
Ortiz, T., From hegemony to subordination: midwives in early modern Spain, in *Art of midwifery*, Marland (ed.), pp. 95–114.
Owen, D. E., *English philanthropy 1660–1960* (Cambridge, Mass.: Belknap, 1965).
Oxley, G. W., *Poor relief in England and Wales 1601–1834* (London: David & Charles, 1974).
Paulson, R., *The art of Hogarth* (London: Phaidon, 1975).
Perry, R., *Women, letters and the novel* (New York, 1980).
Pickstone, J. V. & S. V. F. Butler, The politics of medicine in Manchester 1788–1792: hospital reform and health services in the early industrial city, *Medical History* 28 (1984), pp. 227–49.
Pollock, L., Embarking on a rough passage: the experience of pregnancy in early-modern society, in *Women as mothers in pre-industrial England: essays in memory of Dorothy McLaren,* V. Fildes (ed.), (London: Routledge, 1990), pp. 39–67.
Porter, R., *English society in the eighteenth century* (Harmondsworth: Penguin, 1982).

Porter, R., William Hunter: a surgeon and a gentleman, in *William Hunter*, Bynum & Porter (eds), pp. 7–34.

Porter, R., A touch of danger: the man-midwife as sexual predator, in *Sexual underworlds of the Enlightenment,* G. S. Rousseau & R. Porter (eds) (Manchester, 1987), pp. 206–32.

Porter, R., The gift relation: philanthropy and provincial hospitals in eighteenth-century England, in *The hospital in history,* L. Granshaw & R. Porter (eds) (London: Routledge, 1990), pp. 149–78.

Pressey, W. J., Some seating experiences in Essex churches, *Essex Review* 35 (1926).

Preston, J., *The created self: the reader's role in the eighteenth century* (London: Heinemann, 1970).

Proctor F. & W. Frere, *A new history of the Book of Common Prayer, with a rationale of its offices* (London, 1905).

Quaife, G. R., *Wanton wenches and wayward wives: peasants and illicit sex in early seventeenth century England* (London: Croom Helm, 1979).

Radcliffe, W., *Milestones in midwifery* (Bristol: Wright, 1967).

Radcliffe, W., *The secret instrument (the birth of the midwifery forceps)* (London: Heinemann, 1947).

RCOG Catalogue: *Short-title catalogue of books printed before 1851 in the Library of the Royal College of Obstetricians and Gynaecologists* (2nd edn; London: Royal College of Obstetricians and Gynaecologists, 1968).

Read, G. D., *Revelation of childbirth* (London: Heinemann, 1942; reissued as *Childbirth without fear,* 1954).

Rendle-Short, J., Infant management in the eighteenth century with special reference to the work of William Cadogan, *Bulletin of the History of Medicine* 34 (1960), pp. 97–122.

Rhodes, P., *Doctor John Leake's hospital: a history of the General Lying-In Hospital, York Road, Lambeth, 1765–1971* (London: Davis-Poynter, 1977).

Riley, M., *Brought to bed* (London: Dent, 1968).

Rich, A., *Of woman born: motherhood as experience and as institution* (London: Virago, 1977).

Ringland, J., *Annals of midwifery in Ireland* (Dublin: Falconer, 1870).

Roberts, E., *A woman's place: an oral history of working-class women 1890–1940* (Oxford: Blackwell, 1984).

Roberts, M. "Words they are women, and deeds they are men": images of work and gender in early modern England, in *Women and work in pre-industrial England,* L. Charles & L. Duffin (eds) (London: Croom Helm, 1985), pp. 122–80.

Rogers, N., Resistance to oligarchy: the City opposition to Walpole and his successors, 1725–47, in *London in the age of reform,* J. Stevenson (ed.) (Oxford: Blackwell, 1977), pp. 1–29.

Rook, A., Medicine at Cambridge 1660–1760, *Medical History* 13 (1969), pp. 118–19, 252.

Rose, C., Politics and the London Royal Hospitals, 1683–92, in *The hospital in history,* L. Granshaw & R. Porter (eds) (London: Routledge, 1990).

Ross, E., Fierce questions and taunts: married life in working-class London, 1870–1914, *Feminist Studies* 8 (1982), pp. 575–602.

Ross, E., Survival networks: women's neighbourhood sharing in London before World War I, *History Workshop Journal,* No. 15 (1983), pp. 6–27.

Rubini, D., Politics and the battle for the Banks, 1688–1697, *English Historical Review* 85 (1970).

Ryskamp, C., et al., in *The Augustan milieu: essays presented to Louis A. Landa,* H. K. Miller et al. (eds) (Oxford: Clarendon, 1970), pp. 321–32.

Sarton, G., review of A. J. M. Lamers, *Hendrik van Deventer, medicinae doctor, 1651–1724*

(Assen, 1946), *Isis* **39** (1948), pp. 182–4.

Savage, W., *A Savage enquiry: who controls childbirth?* (London: Virago, 1986).

Saxby, T. J., *The quest for the New Jerusalem: Jean de Labadie and the Labadists, 1610–1744* (Dordrecht: Nijhoff, 1987).

Schaffer, S., Glass works: Newton's prisms and the uses of experiment, in *The uses of experiment*, D. Gooding et al. (eds) (Cambridge: Cambridge University Press, 1989), pp. 67–104.

Schaffer, S., The consuming flame: Tory mystics and electrical showmen in the world of goods, in *Consumption and the world of goods*, J. Brewer & R. Porter (eds) (Routledge, 1993).

Schofield, R. S., Perinatal mortality in Hawkshead, Lancashire, 1581–1710, *Local Population Studies*, No. 4 (1970), pp. 11–16.

Schofield, R. S., Did the mothers really die? Three centuries of maternal mortality in "the world we have lost", in *The world we have gained*, L. Bonfield et al. (eds), (London, 1986), pp. 230–60.

Scholten, C. M., *Childbearing in American society: 1650–1850* (New York: New York University Press, 1985).

Sedgwick, R., *History of Parliament: the House of Commons 1715–1754* (2 volumes; London: HMSO, for the History of Parliament Trust, 1970).

Seligman, S. A., The Royal Maternity Charity, *Medical History* **24** (1980), pp. 403–18.

Shorter, E., *Women's bodies: a social history of women's encounter with health, ill-health and medicine* (New Brunswick, NJ: Transaction Publications, 1990; first published 1982 as *A history of women's bodies*).

Shorter, E., The management of normal deliveries and the generation of William Hunter, in *William Hunter*, Bynum & Porter (eds), pp. 371–83.

Sloane index: Index to the Sloane Manuscripts in the British Museum (London: British Museum, 19xx).

Spencer, *British midwifery*: H. R. Spencer, *The history of British midwifery from 1650 to 1800* (London, 1927).

Spencer, J., *The rise of the woman novelist: from Aphra Behn to Jane Austen* (Oxford: Blackwell, 1986).

Spender, D., *Mothers of the novel: 100 good women writers before Jane Austen* (London: Routledge, 1986).

Sperling, C. F. D., An Essex pensioner in the days of Queen Anne, *Essex Review* **32** (1923), pp. 200–201.

Spiegel, M. R., *Theory and problems of probability and statistics* (New York: McGraw-Hill, 1975).

Spufford, M., *Contrasting communities: English villagers in the sixteenth and seventeenth centuries* (Cambridge: Cambridge University Press, 1974).

Spufford, M., *Small books and pleasant histories: popular fiction and its readership in seventeenth-century England* (Cambridge: Cambridge University Press, 1981).

Stevenson, L. G., The siege of Warwick Lane: together with a brief history of the Society of Collegiate Physicians (1767–1798), *Journal of the History of Medicine and Allied Sciences* **7** (1952), pp. 105–21.

Summerson, J., *Georgian London* (3rd edn, London: Barrie & Jenkins, 1978).

Sutherland, L., The City of London in eighteenth-century politics, in *Essays presented to Sir Lewis Namier*, R. Pares & A. J. P. Taylor (eds) (London: Macmillan, 1956), pp. 49–74.

Tadmor, N., "Family" and "friend" in *Pamela*: a case-study in the history of the family in eighteenth-century England, *Social History* **14** (1989), pp. 289–306.

Tate, W. E., *The parish chest: a study of the records of parochial administration in England* (Cambridge: Cambridge University Press, 1969).

Thomas, K. B., *James Douglas of the pouch* (London, Pitman 1964).
Thomas, K., Women and the Civil War sects, *Past & Present*, No. 13 (1958), pp. 42–62.
Thomas, K., The double standard, *Journal of Historical Ideas* 20 (1959), pp. 195–216.
Thomas, K., *Religion and the decline of magic: studies in popular beliefs in seventeenth-century England* (first published 1971; Harmondsworth, Penguin, 1978).
Todd, *Women writers*: J. Todd, *A dictionary of British and American women writers 1660–1800* (Totowa, NJ: Rowman & Allanheld, 1985).
Towler, J. & J. Bramall, *Midwives in history and society* (London, 1986).
Trumbach, R., The aristocratic family in England, 1690–1780. Studies in childhood and kinship (Johns Hopkins PhD thesis, 1972).
Trumbach, R., *The rise of the egalitarian family: aristocratic kinship and domestic relations in eighteenth-century England* (New York: Academic Press, 1980).
Turner, E., Bibliographie de François Rousset, *Annales de Gynécologie* 14 (1881), pp. 1–25.
Underwood, A. C., *A history of the English Baptists* (London: Baptist Union/Kingsgate Press, 1947).
Valentine, A. C., *The British establishment 1760–84: an eighteenth-century biographical dictionary* (2 volumes; Norman, Oklahoma: University of Oklahoma Press, 1970).
Versluysen, M. C., Midwives, medical men, and "poor women labouring with child": lying-in hospitals in eighteenth century London, in *Women, health and reproduction*, H. Roberts (ed.), (London: Routledge, 1981), pp. 18–49.
Vickery, A. J., *Women of the local elite in Lancashire, 1750–1825* (PhD thesis, University of London, 1991).
Waddington, I., The struggle to reform the Royal College of Physicians, 1767–1771: a sociological analysis, *Medical History* 17 (1973), pp. 107–26.
Wall, C., *The history of the Surgeons' Company, 1745–1800* (London, 1937).
Wallis, *Medics* and Phibb, *Subscriptions*: P. J. V. Wallis et al., *Eighteenth century medics (Subscriptions, Licences, Apprenticeships)* (Newcastle, 1985 & 1988), and associated subscription-lists produced by the Project for Historical Biobibliography (PHIBB).
Warne, A., *Church and society in eighteenth-century Devon* (Newton Abbot, 1969).
Watt, I., *The rise of the novel: studies in Defoe, Richardson and Fielding* (London: Chatto & Windus, 1957; reprinted Hogarth Press, 1987).
Wilson, A., The Enlightenment and infant care, *Bulletin of the Society for the Social History of Medicine*, No. 25 (1979), pp. 44–7.
Wilson, A., Childbirth in seventeenth- and eighteenth-century England (DPhil thesis, University of Sussex, 1982; copy in WIHM).
Wilson, A., William Hunter and the varieties of man-midwifery, in *William Hunter*, Bynum & Porter (eds), pp. 343–69.
Wilson, A., Illegitimacy and its implications in mid-eighteenth-century London: the evidence of the Foundling Hospital, *Continuity & Change* 4:1 (1989), pp. 103–64.
Wilson, A., The ceremony of childbirth and its interpretation, in *Women as mothers in pre-industrial England: essays in memory of Dorothy McLaren*, V. Fildes (ed.), (London: Routledge, 1990), pp. 68–107.
Wilson, A., The politics of medical improvement in early Hanoverian London, in *The medical enlightenment of the eighteenth century*, A. Cunningham & R. French (eds) (Cambridge: Cambridge University Press, 1990), pp. 4–39.
Wilson, A., The perils of early-modern procreation: childbirth with or without fear?, *British Journal for Eighteenth-Century Studies* 16:1 (1993), pp. 1–19.
Wilson, K., Urban culture and political activism in Hanoverian England: the example of vol-

untary hospitals, in *The transformation of political culture: England and Germany in the late eighteenth century,* E. Hellmuth (ed.) (Oxford, 1990), pp. 165–84.

Woodward, J., *To do the sick no harm: a study of the British voluntary hospital system to 1875* (London: Routledge & Kegan Paul, 1974).

Wrightson, K., Infanticide in earlier seventeenth-century England, *Local Population Studies*, No. 15 (1975), pp. 10–22.

Wrightson, K., Infanticide in European history, *Criminal Justice History* 3 (1982), pp. 1–20.

Wrigley, E. A. & R. S. Schofield, *The population history of England: a reconstruction* (1981).

Young, J. H., *Caesarean section: the history and development of the operation from earliest times* (London: Lewis, 1944).

Young, M. & P. Willmott, *Family and kinship in East London* (3rd edn; Harmondsworth, 1986).

Index of personal names

The names of midwives are indicated with an asterisk (*)

Addison, Joseph 86
*Agnew, Mrs, of London 68
Ahlers, Cyriacus 108
Alldist, Mrs. Elizabeth 206n.1
Allen, John MD 43n.85, 117
Altree, John, of Wolverhampton then Norfolk Street, London 172n.51
Anderson, James 118–19n.4
Anne, Queen 56
Ashplant, Timothy 192n.1
Astell, Mary 187, 189, 190
Atterbury, Francis, Bishop of Rochester 56, 70, 72, 73
Avicenna 74n.4
Ayliffe, John 118–19n.4

Ballard, George 32, 44n.107
*Ballard, [Miss], of Campden, Gloucestershire 32, 41n.48
*Ballard, [Mrs], of Campden, Gloucestershire 32
Bamber, John MD 70, 71, 73, 78nn.49–51, 83, 108, 135–41, 144n.33, 150, 161, 162, 171n.34, 200
*Barber, Elizabeth, of Acle, Norfolk 42n.50
Barnard, Sir John 157n.39
Barne, Anne 28
Barret, Robert 54, 170n.10
Barrowby, William MD 142n.10
Battie, William MD 141n.7

Baynard, Edward MD 107, 112, 164
Beale, John MD 83
Bechler, Rosemary 189
Beeston, William MD 76n.30
Behn, Aphra 187, 190
Benjamin, Marina 192n.1
Benson, George 78n.53
Bethell, Slingsby 151, 157n.39
Bichat, Marie-François Xavier 4
Birch, John MD 83, 84, 85, 90n.37, 139, 142–3n.19, 143n.22
Blackbourne, James 53
Blackbourne, John 77n.43, 78n.51
Blackmore, Sir Richard MD 77n.46
Blackstone, James 77n.44
Blackwell, Alexander 44n.107
*Blackwell, Elizabeth, of London 38, 44n.107
Blackwell, Thomas, junior 44n.107
Blackwell, Thomas, senior 44n.107
Bland, Robert MD 15, 17–18, 203
Blundell, Nicholas 27
Boehme, Jacob 189
Boerhaave, Herman MD 87, 157n.33
Boudin, Mr 53–4
*Bourgeois, Louise, of France 6, 52
Bracken, Henry MD 8, 33, 36, 75n.10, 90n.37, 110, 116–17, 163, 164, 172n.53, 182n.22
*Brancker, Hannah 41n.48

229

INDEX OF PERSONAL NAMES

Brodsky, Vivien 39n.6
Brooke, Jonathan MD 83
Broughton, Lady 51–2
Brown, John 199
Buchan, William MD 203
Buckingham family 56
Bundy, Richard 77n.43
Burnet, Gilbert 143n.22
Burney, Fanny 188, 190
Burt, James 206n.1
Burton, John MD, of York 102n.27, 125, 168
Bute, John Stuart, 3rd Earl of 158n.45
Butter, Alexander 8, 66, 96, 109, 117, 125, 139, 140
Byron, Lady 59n.2

Cadogan, William MD 166, 172n.52, 191, 203–4
Calverly, Mrs 206n.1
Calvert, Sir William 157n.39
Camper, Peter MD 140, 144n.39
Cansardine *see* Carwardine
Carter, Elizabeth 189
Carter, Matthew MD, of Dublin 117, 158n.49
Carwardine, Henry Holgate (1779–1867) 62n.47
Cavendish, Margaret, Duchess of Newcastle 187
*Cellier, Mrs Elizabeth, of London 32, 35, 154n.2
Chaber, Lois 192n.1
Chamberlen family 3, 6, 53–7, 65–72, 84, 93, 96, 99, 100, 110, 112, 117, 135, 140, 149, 192
Chamberlen, Hugh I 53, 54–7, 60n.4, 67, 68, 70, 93, 99, 111, 112, 138–9
Chamberlen, Hugh II 53, 56, 67, 68, 69, 70, 71, 73, 75n.18, 79, 83, 84, 85, 96, 107, 108, 109, 117, 135, 138–9
Chamberlen, Peter I 53
Chamberlen, Peter II 32, 53, 54, 57, 99
Chamberlen, Dr Peter MD 32, 53, 54, 56–7, 67, 99, 100
Chapman, Edmund 6, 8, 33, 36, 69–70, 71–4, 77n.47, 78n.52, 83, 84, 85, 96, 99, 100, 109, 110, 111, 112, 113–14, 115, 116, 120n.20, 125, 128, 131, 136, 139, 140, 141, 149, 152
Chapman, Mr, senior pupil of Smellie 131n.9
Cheselden, William 110
Church, Thomas 151–2
*Churchill, Mrs, of Chelsea 101n.11
Clare, Martin 78n.53
Clarges, Sir Thomas 158n.40
Clark, Mrs 49
Clark, William MD 102n.27, 142n.15
Clayton, Mr (Robert? Thomas?) 90n.37, 158n.49
Clive, Lord 158n.45
Cobden, Edward 152–3, 154
Cockburn, William MD 75n.10, 83, 107
Cogan, Thomas MD 141, 144n.39, 151, 157n.34, 197
Cole, Joshua 83, 136–7, 138, 140, 150
Collier, Jeremy 77n.43, 158n.43
Collinson, William 206n.1
Cooke, George 158n.40
Cooke, James 22, 47, 50–3, 57, 59, 96, 163
Cooper, William MD 197
Coram, Thomas 121n.51
*Cornwallis, Elizabeth, of Norwich 31
Counsell, George 78n.53, 172n.52, 208n.33
*Crewe, Phoebe, of Norwich 34, 173n.56
Crisp, Samuel 188
Croft, Dr, of the Lying-in Charity 197
*Crome, Jane, of North Elmham, Norfolk 42n.50
Croxson, Bronwyn 154n.1
Cunningham, Sandy 192n.1

Dale, Samuel, of Braintree, Essex 53
Davies, David 204
Dawkes, Thomas, of St Ives 110, 116–17, 122n.65
Deacon, Thomas 77n.43
Dease, William 143n.31
Defoe, Daniel 38
Delaney, Mrs Mary 136, 188, 203
Denman, Thomas MD 137–8, 143n.31, 150, 199, 201, 202
Dennison, Dr, of the Lying-in Charity 197
de Preville, translator of Smellie 139
Desaguliers, J.T. 77n.43
Deventer, Hendrik van 6, 11, 23n.5, 57, 66,

INDEX OF PERSONAL NAMES

79–85, 87, 95, 107, 113, 115, 117, 126, 127, 129, 130, 131, 150, 156*n*.27, 161, 162, 163, 168, 178, 179, 180, 192, 198
  followers of 79, 83–7, 95, 107, 108, 109, 113, 115, 116, 117, 118, 126, 136, 140, 141, 149, 150, 153, 161, 162, 166, 168, 172*n*.52, 177–8, 192
Dickens, Charles 2
Dick Read, Grantley *see* Read
Dionis, Pierre 6, 107
Donnison, Jean 201
Doughton, Mr 53
Doughty, Samuel 151–2
Douglas, Dr, of the Lying-in Charity 197
Douglas, James MD 68, 71, 72, 73, 83, 85, 86–7, 90*n*.36, 100, 108, 113, 116, 119*n*.11, 128, 136, 141, 149, 150
Douglas, John 8, 42*n*.62, 73, 77*n*.47, 83, 84–6, 110–14, 139, 154*n*.2, 162, 164, 166, 178
Douglas, William 83, 84, 129, 146, 148, 149, 153, 156*nn*.23–4, 208*n*.31
Downing, Nicholas 53
Dowse, Mr, surgeon 93
Drinkwater, John 69, 70, 73, 83, 108, 109
*du Coudray, Mme, of France 5
Dunn, Sir Patrick 118
D'Urban, John MD 149–50
Dusée, M. 74*n*.9, 96, 117
*Du Tertre, Marguerite, of France 6, 112
Dyke, Sir Thomas 158*n*.40

Eaton, Joseph MD 93, 101*n*.7, 142–3*n*.19
Eaton, Robert MD 93, 101*n*.7
Eden, Sir Frederick Morton 204
Egmont, John Percival, Earl of 121*n*.51
Elder, M.G. 23*n*.1
Epictetus 189
*Erney, Mrs, of Shaftesbury, Dorset 38
Exton, Brudenell MD 74, 83, 115, 120*n*.21, 149–50, 153

Fabry von Hilden, Wilhelm 52
Fara, Patricia 157*n*.38
Fiddes, Richard 143*n*.22
Fielding, Henry 187, 188
Fielding, Sarah 187
Fissell, Mary 42*n*.58
Fitzwalter, Lady 37

Fleming, Daniel 49, 51
*Fletcher, Ellen, of Liverpool 32
Flinders, Matthew, of Donington, Lincs 200
Ford, Ann (later Thicknesse) 207*n*.9
Ford, Edward, surgeon 207*n*.9
Ford, John MD (c.1736–1806) 141, 144*n*.41, 197, 201, 206*n*.2
Ford, John MD (c.1731–1807) 207*n*.9
Ford, Randolph 77*n*.43
Foreest, Pieter van 80
Fores, S.W. 4
Foucault, Michel 3
Franco, Pierre 52
Frederick, Price of Wales 156*n*.24
Freeman, Benjamin, of Woodbridge, Suffolk 53
Freke, John 69, 70, 71, 72, 75*n*.24, 76*n*.41, 78*n*.53, 83, 108, 109
French, Mr and Mrs 29

Gabbay, Flic 23*n*.1
Gabbay, John 23*n*.1
Galabin, Alfred Lewis 202
Garcia, Jo 23*n*.1
*Gates, Mrs, of Gower Street, London 136
Gay, John 56
George I, King 56, 79, 161
George II, King 152
George, Dorothy 121*n*.51, 186
Gibson, Joseph, of Edinburgh 117
Giffard, William 3, 8, 14, 15–19, 31, 33, 36, 58, 69–70, 71–3, 75*n*.18, 75*n*.19, 77*n*.42, 83, 91–101, 108, 109, 110, 111, 112, 113, 115, 116, 119*n*.9, 125, 128, 131, 136, 139, 140, 141, 162
*Gooding, Mrs, of London 93
Goold, Mrs, of Sharpham 38
Gordon, Dr., of Glasgow 123, 129
Goslead, John, surgeon 77*n*.48
Greenfield, John *see* Groeneveldt, Johannes
Grégoire the elder 142–3*n*.19
Grégoire the younger 74*n*.9, 124, 125
*Griffin, Mary, of Deal, Kent 32
Griffith, Moses MD 137, 138, 140, 144*n*.35, 146, 150, 157*n*.32
Groeneveldt, Johannes ("John Greenfield") MD 61*n*.37, 75*n*.10

INDEX OF PERSONAL NAMES

Guillemeau, Jacques 6

*H—s, Mrs, of Lambeth-Marsh 101*n*.11
Hacon, Charles, of Norwich 53
Hamilton, Sir David MD 56, 83, 87, 113
Handeside, Clifford 136–7, 138
Hanway, Jonas 199
Harley, David 31
*Harrison, Mrs, of London 93
Harvie, John MD 117–18
Haste, Philip, Jr, surgeon, of Coggeshall, Essex 120*n*.21
Hawkins, William 78*n*.51
Haywood, Eliza 188
Hearne, Thomas 31, 32, 56, 70, 73, 143*n*.22
Heineken, Herman MD 157*n*.31
Heister, Lorenz von 67, 71, 88*n*.9, 128, 131*n*.4, 163
Hess, Anne 43*n*.82
Hinton, Sir John MD 54
Hippocrates 23*n*.11
Hoden, Mrs, of Aston, Warks 49
Hodges, James 77*n*.46, 151
Hody, Edward MD 69, 73, 78*n*.53, 83, 91, 109, 149, 172*n*.52
*Holdship, Mrs, of Oxford 38
*Holland, Nanny 42*n*.58
*Holmes, Mrs, of Bridgwater, Somerset 32, 57
Holt, Ralph, man-midwife, of Liverpool 172*n*.53
*Hopkins, Mary, of Wilton, Wilts 34
Hopkins, Paul 61*n*.41
*Houlden, Mary, of Sudbury, Suffolk 38
Houstoun, James MD 86–7, 107, 117
Howard, John, of Guildford, Surrey 108
Hudson, Gill 108
Humble, Francis, surgeon and man-midwife, of Newcastle-upon-Tyne 173*n*.55
Hunter, William MD 1, 3, 5, 86, 108, 132*n*.17, 137, 140, 142*n*.18, 146, 150, 156*n*.27, 166, 167, 169, 171*n*.41, 175–81, 190, 191, 192, 199, 201, 202, 204
Huntingdon, Elizabeth Hastings, Countess of 52

Inglis, Dr, of Lanark 123

Jackson, Thomas, surgeon, of Twickenham 77*n*.48
James II, King 32, 60*n*.4
Janssen, Stephen T. 157*n*.39
Johnson, Dr 54, 68 (cf. Johnstone, Nathaniel MD *or* William MD)
Johnson, Robert Wallace 69, 140, 199, 204
Johnson, Dr Samuel 187, 189
Johnstone, Nathaniel MD *or* William MD 75*n*.14 (cf. Johnson, Dr)
Jones, Thomas, of Norwich 110, 116–17, 173*n*.56
Jones, Thomas W. (1764–1846), of Henley-in-Arden, Warks 200
Jordanova, Ludmilla 192*n*.1
Josselin, Jane 27, 34, 51
Josselin, Ralph 27, 29, 49, 51

*Kennon, Mrs, of London 171*n*.30
*Kent, Mrs Frances, of Reading, Berks 38, 44*n*.104
Kent, John, surgeon, of Wolverhampton 172*n*.51
Keppel, Augustus, Viscount, Admiral 158*n*.45
Kingston, Evelyn Pierrepont, Duke of 158*n*.45
*Kite, Mrs, of Oxford 31

La Badie, Jean de (1610–74), 79–81, 87*n*.2
Ladbroke, Sir Robert 158*n*.40
Lambert, Sir Daniel 158*n*.40
La Motte, Guillaume Mauquest de 6, 67, 69, 71, 74*n*.9, 84, 129, 130, 156*n*.22, 163, 179
Lawrence, Thomas MD 171*n*.30, 171*n*.34
Layard, Daniel Peter MD 83, 146, 148–9, 150, 153, 154, 156*n*.19, 156*n*.29
Leake, John MD 146–7, 148, 151, 157*n*.38
*Le Boursier, Mme, of France 5
Le Doux, Gilles 74*n*.9
Lennox, Charlotte 189
Levret, André 5
Lewen, Johannes van MD 117
Limborch, Dr, court physician 108
Long, Roger 77*n*.43
Lowder, William MD 143*n*.31
*Lucas, Mrs, of London 101*n*.11

INDEX OF PERSONAL NAMES

*Luddington, Mrs, of London 101n.11

Macaulay, Mrs Catherine 150
Macaulay, George MD 83, 150, 156n.30
Macdonough, Felix 16, 19, 24n.20, 146, 147, 151, 203, 208n.32
McKendrick, Neil 192n.1
Mackenzie, Colin MD, senior pupil of Smellie 131–2n.9
McLeod, Hugh 40n.32
McMath, James MD 117
Maconachy, George MD of Dublin 117
Maddock or Maddocks, Richard 144n.36, 156n.30
*Maddox, Mrs, of London 131n.9
Maittaire, Michael 77n.43, 78n.51
Makin, Bathsua 190
Manley, Mary Delariviere 187, 188
Manningham, Sir Richard MD 56, 74, 83, 85, 86, 89nn.28–9, 108, 110, 113, 114–16, 118, 119n.11, 124, 136, 138, 141, 149, 162, 163, 169n.8, 182n.22, 200
Manningham, Thomas 89n.28
Marlborough, Charles Spencer, 3rd Duke of 158n.45
*Marlton, Sarah, of Wickhambrooke, Suffolk 31
Martineau, Mr., man-midwife, of Norwich 173n.56
Mary of Modena 48
Massey, Edmund 152
Maubray, John MD 83, 107–8, 113, 118–19n.4, 154n.2, 164
Maule, Dr 142n.10
Mauriceau, François 6, 14, 20, 22, 54–5, 56, 57, 66, 69, 87, 93, 99, 111, 112, 117, 163
Mead, Richard MD 85, 127, 171n.30
*Mears, Martha, of London 201–2
Merian, Maria Sibylla 80
Middleton, Conyers 78n.51
Middleton, Starkey, junior 83, 136–7, 138, 140, 141, 142n.16, 144n.36, 150, 161, 171n.34
Middleton, Starkey, senior 142n.16, 144n.36
Milward, Edward MD 72, 77n.44, 109
Mitchell, Archibald MD 119n.7
Molyneux, Jane (later Wildbore) 59n.2

Monmouth, James Duke of 55
Montagu, Lady Mary Wortley 188, 189
*Moore, Mrs, see Simpson
Morley, Matthew MD 83, 136–7, 138, 141, 141n.8, 200
Morris, Claver MD 38
Morton, John Esq. 158n.45
Mosse, Bartholomew MD of Dublin 117–18
Mounteney, Richard 78n.53, 143n.22

Nathaniels, Elizabeth 192n.1
Nelson, James 191
Nesbit, Robert MD 83, 136–7, 138, 140, 141, 150, 166, 171n.34
Newcome, Henry 27
Newdigate, Sir Roger 158n.40, 158n.45
Newton, Sir Isaac 186
Nicholls, Frank MD 136, 137, 166–7, 171n.34, 197, 198, 199, 208n.33
Nicholls, William 78n.49
*Nihell, Elizabeth, of Haymarket, London 11, 59, 90n.37, 125, 140, 167, 198, 199, 202, 207n.4
Nihell, James MD 207n.4
Northampton, George Compton, Earl of 158n.45
Northumberland, Earl of see Smithson, Sir Hugh
Nowell, John MD 53

Ockley, Simon 78n.49, 143n.22
Orange, Anne Princess of 85
Osborne, William MD 201, 202
Oxford, Edward Harley, Earl of 78n.51
Ould, Fielding, MD of Dublin 1, 8, 14, 61n.31, 117–18, 128

Packer, Rev. Samuel 77–8n.48
Page, John, of Lutterworth, Leics 120n.21
Palfinus see Palfyn
Palfyn, Jean 66, 67, 71, 74n.9
Paré, Ambroise 6, 52, 163
Parker, Reeve 157n.38
Parsons, James MD 83, 90n.36
*Partridge, Dorothy 44n.107
Pearson, Grace 28
Pelham, Hon. Henry 151

233

INDEX OF PERSONAL NAMES

Pepys, Elizabeth 186, 187
Perfect, William 140, 171*n*.39
Peterborough, Charles Mordaunt, Earl of 61*n*.41
Peters, Dr, of Canterbury 53, 59
Petty, William 154*n*.2
Piper, Mr 29
Place, Francis 203–4
Pollock, Linda 40*n*.22, 61*n*.29
Pope, Alexander 86
Portal, Paul 6, 69
Portland, Margaret Cavendish Bentinck, Duchess of 152
Portland, Earl of 157*n*.39
Potter, Mr, senior pupil of Smellie 131*n*.9
Prior, Matthew 56, 78*n*.49
Proctor, Sir William Beauchamp 157*n*.39
Prosser, Mr, senior pupil of Smellie 131–2*n*.9
Pugh, Benjamin 75*n*.10, 76*n*.25, 84, 99, 103*n*.41, 164, 168–9, 172*n*.50

Rathlauw, Johannes Peter 75*n*.10
Read, Grantley Dick 194*n*.39
Rees, John, apothecary 77–8*n*.48
Richardson, Samuel 187, 188, 189
Roberts, Elizabeth 205
Rockingham, Charles Watson-Wentworth, 2nd Marquis of 152
*Rogerson, Ruth, of Northwich, Cheshire 32
Roonhuysen, Rogier van 67, 68, 81, 83, 135, 138, 139–40
*Rosado, Luisa, of Spain 5
Rösslin, Eucharius 5
Rousset, François 22
Rueff, Jacob 20, 21, 37
Rumbold, Valerie 192*n*.1

St André, Nathaniel 108
Samber, Robert 83, 107
Sandys, Francis MD 83, 84, 85, 88–9*n*.21, 113, 116, 142*n*.15, 146, 148–9, 150, 152–3, 156*n*.23
Savage, Wendy 2, 7*n*.2
Schaffer, Simon 192*n*.1
Schomberg, Isaac MD 136, 137, 171*n*.30
Schurman, Anna Maria van 80

Scultetus, Johannes 20, 53
Secker, Thomas 90*n*.37
*Seeley, Sarah, of Dalham, Suffolk 37
Sennert, Daniel 50, 52
Sermon, William 29
*Sexton, Mrs, of London 101*n*.11
Shapcote, John MD of Chelmsford 76*n*.30
*Simpson, Mrs (formerly Moore), of London 131*n*.9
Sims, John MD 197
Skinner, James 75*n*.18
*Slap, Mrs Anne (? of Deal, Kent) 32
Sloane, Sir Hans MD 73, 77*n*.44, 107, 114, 139, 152
Smalridge, George 143*n*.22, 158*n*.43
Smart, Christopher 166
Smellie, William 1, 2, 3, 11, 13, 14, 15, 16–19, 36, 44*n*.107, 60*n*.6, 75*n*.11, 83, 84, 85, 99, 100, 102*n*.27, 114, 123–33, 137, 139–40, 141, 145, 146, 147, 149, 150, 153, 154, 156*n*.22, 156*n*.23, 156*n*.30, 162, 163, 164, 166, 167, 168, 172*n*.53, 176, 177, 178–80, 192, 198, 200–1, 202, 203
Smith, Mr, surgeon, of Edinburgh 117
Smith, Mr, surgeon, of Newcastle-upon-Tyne 173*n*.55
Smith, Richard 192*n*.1
Smither, Mr, of Reading, surgeon 120*n*.21
Smithson, Sir Hugh (Earl of Northumberland from 1750) 145, 157*n*.39
Smollett, Tobias 124, 125, 131, 179, 198
Soranus 20, 163
Southwell, Thomas MD, of Dublin 117–18
Spufford, Margaret 30, 192*n*.1
Squire, Dr, of the Lying-in Charity 197
Stanton, Mr, of Lombard Street, London, instrument-maker 172*n*.46
Steele, Richard 86
*Stephen, Margaret, of London 201–2
Sterne, Laurence 168
Stewkely, John 27
*Stone, Sarah, of Bridgwater, Taunton and London 6, 8, 11, 14, 32, 33, 34, 36, 37, 53, 57–9, 110, 116–17, 166, 169*n*.7, 172*n*.52, 198, 208*n*.28
Strafford family 56
*Strettell, Margaret 41n.48
Stuart, Alexander MD 125, 132*n*.14

234

INDEX OF PERSONAL NAMES

Stuart, James Francis Edward 48
*Sutton, Hannah, of Knutsford, Cheshire 41n.48
Swain, Thomas, instrument-maker 78n.52
Swift, Jonathan 56
Symonds, Josiah, surgeon 84, 139

Thicknesse, Ann, see Ford
Thicknesse, Philip 125, 140, 167, 198–9
Thornton, Alice 49, 51
Todd, Janet 192n.1
Toft, Mary, of Godalming, Surrey 72, 108
Tomkyns, Thomas 129, 130
Torr, John, surgeon 150
*Tredwell, Mrs, of Oxford 42n.57
Trentham, Viscount 157n.39
Turner, Daniel 38
Turner, Matthew, man-midwife, of Liverpool 172n.53
Turner, Thomas 29

Underwood, Michael MD 209n.34

van Deventer, Hendrik see Deventer
van Foreest, Pieter see Foreest
van Lewen, Johannes see Lewen
van Roonhuysen, Rogier see Roonhuysen
Van Schurman, Anna Maria see Schurman
Verney, Sir Ralph 27
Versluysen, Margaret 3, 153–4
Viardel, Cosme 20, 183n.26
Vickery, Amanda 195n.43

Waldren, Richard 76n.26
Walker, Middleton MD 53, 56, 69, 70, 71, 73, 75n.18, 83, 108, 109, 117, 136, 138, 152, 157n.38
Walker, Chamberlen 53, 117
Walpole, Lady 113

Walpole, Sir Robert 113, 151
Ward, Judith, of Derby 49, 52
Wareing, John, man-midwife, of Liverpool 172n.53
Warren, Sir Peter 157n.39
Wathen, Mrs Elizabeth 157n.33
Wathen, Jonathan 141, 144n.40, 150, 157n.34, 158n.49, 207n.3
Wathen, Samuel MD 142n.18, 146, 150, 157n.33, 158n.49
*Weatherbone, Mrs, of London 101n.11
*Webb, Alice, of Stradishall, Suffolk 37
Weltden, Dr W. 120n.21
*West, Mary, of Blackburn, Lancs 41n.48
Wharton, George MD 72, 77n.43, 93
Wheatly, Charles 28
Whistler, Daniel MD 37
White, Charles MD, of Manchester 2, 166, 173n.54, 181, 203, 204
White, John, of Ipswich 76n.30
White, Thomas, of Manchester 173n.54
Whitelocke, Bulstrode 38, 49, 51
Whitelocke, [Mrs] 38, 51
Wildbore, Jane see Molyneux, Jane
*Wilkes, Judith, of London 48
William and Mary, King and Queen 55
*Willughby, Eleanor, of Derby, Stafford and London 41n.48, 41n.49, 59n.2
Willughby, Percival 6, 12, 14, 15, 20, 22, 29, 30, 31, 33, 36, 47, 49–53, 57, 59, 60n.6, 93, 96, 98, 100, 163, 164, 178, 183n.26
Wilson, Thomas 76n.41
Wilson, Molly 78n.51, 136
Wood or Woods, Alexander or Nally, of Oxford 69–70, 73, 76n.26
Woolhouse, Dr, of Paris 142–3n.19
Wright, Miss, of Oxford 38
Wynn, Sir Watkin Williams 158n.45
Young, Robert 75n.18

Index of places and institutions

Where appropriate (particularly for London), institutions are grouped under locality. For this purpose, and for parishes, streets, etc., *Westminster has been subsumed within London*.

Acle, Norfolk 42*n*.50
Africa 15
America 5, 29, 202
Amsterdam 68, 81, 135, 137, 140
Aston, Warks 49

Bank of England 55
Barking, Essex 144*n*.33
Bath, Somerset 180
Birmingham, Warks, 169
Blackburn Lancs 41*n*.48
Box, Wiltshire 102*n*.27
Braintree, Essex 53
Brentford, Middlesex 69, 70, 71, 109
Brentwood, Essex 69, 70, 71
Bridgwater, Somerset 32, 34, 57, 117, 200
Bristol, 34, 60*n*.50, 117, 169, 207*n*.9
Bungay, Suffolk 34
Bury, Lancs 30
Bury St Edmunds, Suffolk 34

Cambridge, Cambs. 113
  University 73, 136
Campden, Gloucestershire 32
Canterbury, Kent 53
Charitable Corporation 108
Chelmsford, Essex 76*n*.30, 164, 168–9
Cheshire 30, 164
Church of England 27, 32, 56
Church Wotton 51

City of London *see under* London
Coggeshall, Essex 120*n*.21
Colchester, Essex 142*n*.15, 144*n*.35, 157*n*.32

Dalham, Suffolk 37
Deal, Kent 32
Delft 80
Derby 6, 47, 50, 53
Devon 2
Donington, Lincs 200
Dorking, Surrey 157*n*.33
Dublin 53, 117–18, 208*n*.29
  College of Physicians 117, 208*n*.29
  Lying-in Hospital (Rotunda Hospital) 118, 145, 146
  Professorship of Midwifery 118
Dutch Republic 5, 55, 56, 66–7, 68, 79–81, 138

Earles Colne, Essex 34
East Anglia 25
Edinburgh 109, 117
Essex 33
Exeter 34, 169

France 3, 5, 6, 56, 66–7
Friendly Societies 204

Germany 5

237

INDEX OF PLACES AND INSTITUTIONS

Glasgow   123
　University   150
Godalming, Surrey   108
Guildford, Surrey   108

Halstead, Essex   68, 70, 71, 75n.18, 96, 109
Henley-in-Arden, Warks   200
Huntingdon, Hunts   156n.19

Ipswich, Suffolk   34, 76n.30
Ireland   117
Italy   5

Kendal, Cumberland   34
Knutsford, Cheshire   41n.48

Lambeth, see under London
Lanark   123, 124, 125
Lancashire   33, 164
Lancaster   110, 117
Leeuwarden   79
Leyden   73, 79, 81
Lincolnshire   33, 35
Liverpool   2, 32, 169
London   5, 6, 15–19, 28, 29, 30, 31–3, 34, 35, 36, 38, 41n.49, 47, 53, 68, 71, 79, 82–7, 94, 99, 100, 107–18, 124, 125, 127, 131, 137, 140, 141, 145–54, 168–9, 175, 177, 179, 186, 197, 200–2 (see also Westminster)
London, City of   69, 70, 71, 118, 135–6, 139, 140–1, 150, 152, 197
　Parliamentary constituency   148, 158n.40
London, diocese of   32
London (including Westminster, Southwark and Lambeth), institutions:
　City of London Lying-in Hospital (est. 1750)   146–8, 150, 151–2
　College of Physicians   32, 54, 73, 107, 136, 139, 166, 201
　Company of Barbers and Surgeons   110, 135–6, 201
　Company of Surgeons (1745–1800)   151, 157n.33, 200–1, 208n.32
　Foundling Hospital, London   38, 121n.51, 180
　General Lying-in Hospital, Westminster (est. 1752; later Queen Charlotte's)   16, 146–8, 151, 152

Guy's Hospital (est. 1725)   145, 171n.34
Guy's Hospital Lying-in Charity   24n.19
Lacy's Bagnio   108
London Hospital   145
London Medical Society   183n.31
Lying-in Charity for delivering poor married women at their own habitations (later Royal Maternity Charity), 157n.34, 197–8, 202
Lying-in Hospital, Brownlow-Street (est. 1749; British from 1746)   146–51, 153, 154
Manningham's Lying-in Infirmary (1739–?)   110, 114–16, 118, 124, 145, 146, 147, 162
Middlesex Hospital   141, 145–54, 165, 170n.26
Royal College of Surgeons (1800–)   201
Royal Maternity Charity, see Lying-in Charity for delivering poor married women at their own habitations
St Bartholomew's Hospital   69, 73, 135, 145
St George's Hospital   145
St Thomas's Hospital   145
Westminster Abbey   56
Westminster General Dispensary   15, 19
Westminster Infirmary   145
Westminster New Lying-in Hospital, Lambeth (est. 1767; later the General Lying-in Hospital)   146, 148, 151
London (including Westminster, Southwark and Lambeth), locations, parishes and streets in and near:
Aldersgate Street   147
Bartholomew Lane   157n.34
Bedford Street   78n.52
Bishopsgate   136, 197 (and see St Botolph's)
Blackfriars Bridge   146
Bow Lane   139, 143n.23
Brownlow Street, 147 (and see Lying-in Hospital)
Cheapside   197
Chelsea   94, 101n.11
Covent Garden   166
Craven Street   157n.38
Devereux Court   207n.4

238

INDEX OF PLACES AND INSTITUTIONS

Devonshire Square 157n.33
Fenchurch Street 143n.23
Gerrard Street 147
Gower Street 136
Great Suffolk Street 56
Haymarket 198
Hoxton 144n.36
Jermyn Street 147
Kennington 144n.37
Kensington 94
Lambeth 146, 151, 157n.38
Lambeth-Marsh 101n.11
Lombard Street 172n.46
Mincing Lane 139, 150
Norfolk Street 75n.19, 172n.51
Old Jewry 197
Pall Mall 147
Parliament Street, 157n.38
St Botolph's Bishopsgate 94
St James's parish, Westminster, vestry 121n.5
Southwark, 71, 94, 136, 146, 157n.38, 197
Wardour Street 147
West End, 94, 109, 118, 141
Westminster Bridge, 146
Windmill Street 147
Low Countries 108
Lutterworth, Leics 120n.21

Manchester 2, 36, 169
Middlesex (Parliamentary constituency of) 145, 148, 151, 157n.39, 158n.40
Midlands, 36, 93

National Health Service 206
Newcastle-upon-Tyne 2, 34, 169
North Elmham, Norfolk 42n.50.
Northwich, Cheshire 32
Norwich 31, 34, 41n.49, 53, 110, 117, 169, 173n.56, 173n.56
  diocese of 42n.50

Oxford 31, 38, 69–70, 71
  University 73, 166

Paris 12, 23n, 55, 86, 124, 125
  Écoles de Santé 3
  Hôtel-Dieu, *salle des accouchements* 86–7,

111, 115, 142–3n.19, 145, 147, 198
Parliament 32, 141, 147, 151
Parliamentary constituencies, *see* London, City of; Middlesex; Westminster
Peterborough, diocese of 32
Pontefract, Yorkshire 164, 168
Poor Law 204
Preshaw, Hants 27

Quarter Sessions 147

Reading, Berks 38, 120n.21
Rochester, diocese of 56

St Ives, Hunts 110, 116–17
Scotland 55, 66, 68, 73
Shaftesbury, Dorset 38
Sharpham, Somerset 38
Southampton 6
Southwark, *see* under London
Spain 5
Spalding, Lincs 89n.28
Stafford 47
Sudbury, Suffolk 38
Suffolk 33, 35, 202

Taunton, Somerset 34, 36, 57–8, 110, 117
Ticknall, Derbs 183n.26

Utrecht 68

Warwick 22, 50, 51, 53
Wells, Somerset 164
West Country 32
Westminster 71, 85, 111, 118, 136, 141
  Parliamentary constituency 148, 151, 157n.39, 158n.40
  institutions in, *see* under London
  locations in, *see* under London
Wieuward 79
Wickhambrooke, West Suffolk 31
Wilton, Wilts 34
Wolverhampton 172n.51
Women's Co-operative Guild 204–6
Woodbridge, Suffolk 53
Woodham Mortimer Hall, Essex 56, 67
York 34, 125
Yorkshire 2